Data Analysis of Medical Studies

Potter C. Chang

Data Analysis of Medical Studies

Reading and Reporting

Springer

Potter C. Chang
Department of Biostatistics, School of Public Health
University of California at Los Angeles
Los Angeles, CA, USA

ISBN 978-3-031-49983-8 ISBN 978-3-031-49984-5 (eBook)
https://doi.org/10.1007/978-3-031-49984-5

This Springer imprint is published by the registered company Springer Nature Switzerland AG
The registered company address is: Gewerbestrasse 11, 6330 Cham, Switzerland

Paper in this product is recyclable.

Preface

Frustrated by descriptions of data analysis results is a common experience among medical journal readers. This book uses published articles to show how stylish yet ambiguous and hyperbolic descriptions of data revelations can be read intelligently and how data revelations can be reported informatively. The examples show that to read intelligently, it is essential to investigate the revelations of data by scrutinizing comprehensive data descriptions. To report informatively, it is enlightening to articulate manifestations of comprehensive data descriptions. The examples also show how statistical methods have been misused.

A critical element of the examples is the realization that statistical significance is the root of the stylish yet ambiguous and hyperbolic descriptions of data revelations. The term "statistical significance" is artificial. The P-values of statistical significance tests result from testing the statistical null hypothesis that data revelations are chance occurrences. Rejecting the statistical hypothesis when the P-values are small is an abduction. Declaring data revelations statistically significant is a chic rephrasing of the assertion that they are not chance occurrences.

This book comprises 12 chapters organized in three parts. Part I consists of three chapters (Chaps. 1 to 3). Chapter 1 uses simple examples to introduce the concept of data distribution that is the foundation of statistical methods for data analysis. Chapter 2 shows the magnitude of graphical displays of data distributions. The indications and limitations of commonly used statistics are elaborated upon in Chap. 3. Part II comprises six chapters (Chaps. 4 to 9). Chapter 4 stresses that the revelations of unpaired quantitative data sets are manifested by their distributions. The distributions of statistically significant differences may overlap extensively and show pertinent similarities. Chapter 5 demonstrates that revelations of paired quantitative data sets are informatively unveiled by observation pairs instead of the observations of the data sets. The distribution of a set of before and after treatment changes may include decreases and increases even though the mean of the changes is declared statistically significant. One key message of Chap. 6 is that it is essential to present measures of risk in treatment groups when hazard ratios are used to assess the difference in risks between treatment groups. Another is that adjusted measures of risk are often oversimplifications. The fact that the revelations of paired qualitative data sets are manifested by the distribution of observation pairs, rather than the respective distributions of the data sets, is emphasized in Chap. 7. Chapter 8 shows that scatterplots that depict the observations graphically show how the observations of two quantitative variables relate. The results of regression analyses are valuable only if the regression functions are creditable characterizations of the relationships manifested by scatterplots. Chapter 9 emphasizes that associations between two qualitative variables are manifested by the percentages of observations of one variable in sub-cohorts of subjects specified by the other variable. Part III comprises three chapters (Chaps. 10 to 12). Chapter 10 uses simple examples to introduce the concepts of random samples and the sampling distributions of sample statistics. Classic tests are used in Chap. 11 to demonstrate that declaring data revelations statistically significant is a chic paraphrasing of the declaration that data revelations are not chance occurrences. The use of 95% confidence intervals to assess the replicability of data revelations is elaborated on in Chap. 12.

Composing this book has been a continuous learning process. Much was learned when examples were composed. There is much room for improvement. Comments and suggestions are highly appreciated. Errors will be acknowledged and corrected at the earliest opportunity. Suggestions including but not limited to the following are sincerely invited:

- Examples with or without demonstrations and discussions
- Comments and revisions of examples
- Clarifications of elaborations and discussions.

I am indebted to my mentors at the University of Minnesota, particularly Professors Bearman, Brown, and Boen.

Hacienda Heights, CA, USA Potter C. Chang

Abstract

Data Analysis of Medical Research is a book for the many medical journal readers frustrated by the stylish yet ambiguous and hyperbolic descriptions of data revelations. It uses published examples to show intelligent reading and informative reporting of data revelations.

The examples show that the ritual of statistical significance testing is the root of stylish yet ambiguous and hyperbolic data descriptions. The statistical null hypothesis that implies data revelations are chance occurrences is tested. The P-value, an estimate of the probability of data revelations if the statistical null hypothesis is true, is calculated by assuming a statistical model. The statistical null hypothesis is rejected, and data revelations are declared statistically significant when the P-value is small. A P-value of 0.05 or less is customarily considered sufficiently small.

The book stressed that rejecting the statistical null hypothesis is an abduction, not proof or induction. Declaring data revelations statistically significant is a chic paraphrasing of declaring data revelations are not chance occurrences. To read intelligently, it is essential to recognize the statistics portraying the data revelations and note that rejecting the statistical null hypothesis means that the statistics are not chance occurrences. It is productive to scrutinize manifestations of comprehensive data descriptions.

Descriptions of data revelations often cite P-values and 95% confidence intervals. When the P-value is smaller than 0.05, the 95% confidence interval excludes the null value of the statistic portraying the data revelation (0 if a difference and 1.0 if a ratio). The reported 95% confidence intervals are used to assess replicability. Narrow intervals suggest that the data revelations are adequately reproducible, while wide intervals suggest that they are not adequately replicable. The replicability of statistically significant data revelations is often inadequate.

Contents

Part I
Data Description

Data description is a vital element of data analysis. Data revelations are probed by examining the distributions of observations and articulated by highlighting the manifestations of the data distributions. The concept of "data distribution" is introduced in Chap. 1. Chapter 2 reviews informative graphical displays of data distributions. Indications of descriptive statistics that are often used to depict data synoptically are examined in Chap. 3.

Chapter 1
Data Distribution

Data distribution is a vital component of statistical methods for data analysis. Revelations of data are productively explored by examining the distributions of data and described by articulating manifestations of distributions. This chapter uses simple examples to introduce the concept of data distribution.

Section 1.1 reviews basic terms relating to data. Section 1.2 explains the classification of qualitative and quantitative data, which is used to organize the presentations of Part II of this book. Section 1.3 reviews simple examples of data distribution. Section 1.4 illustrates how histograms that are informative displays of data distributions may be made.

1.1 Basic Terms

This section reviews basic terms pertinent to data.

- *Observations and Data*

Symbols and numbers that indicate categories or quantitative measurements are referred to as observations or data.

- *Variable*

Traits such as gender, smoking status, heart rate, and blood pressure are referred to as variables.

- *Subjects and Participants*

Individuals who participate in a study are dubbed subjects or participants.

- *Observational Unit*

Subjects, blood samples, families, and so forth whose characteristics are observed and recorded are examples of observational units.

P. C. Chang, *Data Analysis of Medical Studies*,
https://doi.org/10.1007/978-3-031-49984-5_1

- *Data Set*

  A collection of observations is dubbed a set of data or a data set.

- *Univariate, Bivariate, and Multivariate Observations*

  An observation of one single variable is dubbed a univariate observation. Observations of two variables obtained from the same observational unit make up a bivariate observation. Observations of three or more variables obtained from the same observational unit comprise a multivariate observation.

- *Univariate, Bivariate, and Multivariate Data Sets*

  A collection of univariate observations is called a univariate data set; a collection of bivariate observations is dubbed a bivariate data set; a collection of multivariate observations is called a multivariate data set.

- *Size of Data Set*

  Usually, there is one observation per observational unit, and the number of observational units and the number of observations are equal. Either may be used as the size of such a data set. If some observational units have more than one observation, it is critical to specifically indicate whether the size of a data set is its number of observational units or observations.

- *Clusters of Observational Units*

  The observational units of observations are occasionally unclear. For instance, when glucose and cholesterol levels are determined from blood samples taken from a group of subjects before and after breakfast, the observational units could be the blood samples or the subjects. When subjects are observational units, the two blood samples of each subject (one before and one after breakfast) are subunits. When blood samples are observational units, the two blood samples of a subject constitute a cluster of observational units.

  When data are collected from a group of families and their members, either the families or their members may be considered observational units. Families are the observational units of observations such as family size, number of children per family, and family income. Family members are the observational units of observations such as gender, age, educational level, and other traits of members of the families.

  When each family is treated as an observational unit, its members are subunits. When each member is treated as an observational unit, the family constitutes a cluster of observational units.

Table 1.1 Artificial data sets

ID	Gender	Smoking status	Resting Heart rate	After-exercise Heart rate	Resting Systolic blood pressure
1	M	C	96	136	168
2	F	F	64	116	165
3	M	F	80	128	140
4	F	N	84	112	102
5	M	F	68	128	132
6	M	F	92	136	138
7	F	N	80	128	114
8	M	F	100	140	158
9	F	F	76	132	130
10	F	F	84	140	160
11	F	F	72	128	158
12	M	N	60	112	108
13	M	N	72	132	105
14	M	F	84	132	155
15	F	F	76	124	124
16	F	C	104	140	185
17	M	F	80	136	116
18	M	F	76	136	125
19	M	F	68	116	116
20	F	F	72	120	135
21	M	F	80	140	134
22	F	F	84	140	125
23	M	F	80	136	118
24	M	F	88	132	126
25	F	N	96	132	145
26	M	F	76	124	118
27	M	F	92	140	114
28	M	N	92	104	110
29	F	F	88	112	122
30	F	C	100	136	175
31	M	F	80	124	148
32	M	C	92	140	198
33	F	F	76	120	128
34	M	N	56	140	110
35	M	F	64	116	136
36	F	F	68	104	120
37	M	F	72	108	130
38	F	F	72	120	142
39	F	N	68	100	115
40	M	F	80	96	140
41	M	F	64	108	124

(continued)

Table 1.1 (continued)

			Resting	After-exercise	Resting
ID	Gender	Smoking status	Heart rate	Heart rate	Systolic blood pressure
42	M	C	88	128	170
43	M	N	60	136	112
44	M	N	80	140	104
45	F	F	88	124	126
46	M	F	84	132	135
47	M	F	84	136	122
48	F	N	76	120	110
49	M	F	96	140	112
50	F	F	92	132	155

Example 1.1.1

Table 1.1 presents five sets of artificial data ostensibly obtained from a group of 50 subjects with coronary heart disease. The first column shows numbers assigned to identify the subjects. The other columns exhibit observations. The two letters F and M displayed in the second column are observations on the variable gender. They indicate whether the subjects are female (F) or male (M). The three letters N, F, and C displayed in the third column are observations on the variable smoking status. They indicate whether subjects are rated nonsmokers (N), former smokers (F), or current smokers (C). The numbers in the fourth column are observations on the variable resting heart rate. The values in the fifth column are observations on the variable post-exercise heart rate. The sixth column exhibits observations on the variable resting systolic blood pressure.

The 50 subjects are the observational units of each of these data sets. Each unit has one observation, and the size of the data set is 50, which is the number of observational units as well as the number of observations in the data set.

When the observations of two data sets obtained from the same subject are arranged as a doublet, the doublet makes up a bivariate observation. The collection of the 50 doublets constitutes a bivariate data set; the observational units of the bivariate data set are the 50 subjects. There is one bivariate observation per unit, and the size of the bivariate data set is 50, which is the number of observational units as well as the number of bivariate observations of the data set.

For instance, the doublet consisting of the first entries of the fourth and fifth columns, 96 and 136, constitutes a bivariate observation on the variables at-rest heart rate and post-exercise heart rate. The set of 50 doublets formed by the entries of the two columns constitutes a bivariate data set. The observational units of the set of 50 bivariate observations are the 50 subjects. There is one bivariate observation per unit; the size of the data set size is 50.

Example 1.1.2

The results of a study evaluating state expenditures for tobacco control programs in fiscal year 2001 are reported in a special article of the New England Journal of Medicine (Gross and Others, 2002). The article uses a table (Table 1.2) to present

Table 1.2 Table 1 of Gross and Others (2002)

State	Expenditures for tobacco control programs per capita		2001 tobacco settlement revenue	
	2001 amount	Amount recommended by CDC[a] (dollars)	Per capita amount	Total amount[b]
Mean of 50 states	3.49	7.47	28.35	163,800,000
Pennsylvania	0.10	5.46	27.83	341,800,000
Ohio	0.13	5.52	27.52	312,400,000
Tennessee	0.24	6.00	26.61	151,400,000
Connecticut	0.30	6.50	32.42	110,400,000
Alabama	0.30	6.19	21.81	97,000,000
North Carolina	0.32	5.74	17.73	142,700,000
Louisiana	0.37	6.23	31.33	140,000,000
Missouri	0.43	6.07	25.40	142,100,000
Arkansas	0.58	7.10	19.23	51,400,000
Nevada	0.59	8.04	18.92	37,800,000
Texas	0.59	5.31	46.72	974,200,000
Oklahoma	0.59	6.58	18.63	64,300,000
Michigan	0.66	5.61	26.05	258,900,000
South Carolina	0.78	6.36	18.20	73,000,000
Kansas	0.83	6.96	19.23	51,700,000
Kentucky	0.84	6.42	25.98	105,000,000
North Dakota	1.71	12.73	35.35	22,700,000
New York	1.74	5.28	39.75	754,300,000
Idaho	1.75	9.13	17.39	22,500,000
New Mexico	1.89	7.93	20.34	37,000,000
Georgia	2.19	5.69	18.59	152,200,000
Illinois	2.26	5.46	23.25	288,700,000
Utah	2.46	7.40	12.36	27,600,000
Florida	2.49	5.35	45.76	731,300,000
Oregon	2.71	6.51	19.96	68,300,000
Virginia	2.82	5.77	17.91	126,800,000
Rhode Island	3.03	10.01	42.54	44,600,000
Washington	3.08	5.94	21.61	127,400,000
New Hampshire	3.29	9.28	35.04	43,300,000
Colorado	3.32	6.31	19.76	85,000,000
California	3.44	5.12	22.41	759,200,000
Iowa	3.52	6.78	18.42	53,900,000
New Jersey	3.80	5.60	28.50	239,800,000
Alaska	4.01	13.27	33.82	21,200,000
Maryland	4.05	5.95	26.47	140,200,000
Wisconsin	4.09	6.03	22.97	123,200,000

(continued)

Table 1.2 (continued)

State	Expenditures for tobacco control programs per capita		2001 tobacco settlement revenue	
	2001 amount	Amount recommended by CDC[a] (dollars)	Per capita amount	Total amount[b]
West Virginia	4.31	7.80	30.41	55,000,000
Delaware	4.61	11.80	29.99	23,500,000
Nebraska	4.83	8.03	21.56	36,900,000
Montana	4.85	10.65	29.04	26,200,000
Minnesota	4.92	6.11	68.50	337,000,000
South Dakota	5.15	11.77	28.62	21,600,000
Wyoming	5.62	15.39	29.97	14,800,000
Indiana	6.05	5.93	17.52	106,500,000
Arizona	7.32	6.10	17.09	87,700,000
Massachusetts	10.25	5.76	37.83	240,200,000
Hawaii	10.82	9.08	29.55	35,800,000
Vermont	12.58	13.42	40.24	24,500,000
Mississippi	12.82	6.88	74.21	211,100,000
Maine	15.47	9.01	37.10	47,300,000

[a]CDC denotes Center for Disease Control and Prevention
[b]Total amounts have been rounded to the nearest $100,000

pertinent data. The first column of the table displays identifications of the states. The top entry of each of the remaining columns is the mean of the entries in the column. It is not an observation. The following discussions allude to the second to fifth column after the entries in the first row have been excluded.

The second to the fifth columns constitute a univariate data set. The variables may be dubbed estimate, CDC recommendation, tobacco revenue settlement, and tobacco revenue settlement. The observational units of each data set are the 50 states. There is one observation per observational unit; the size of each data set is 50.

Each row exhibits four observations pertaining to a state. A doublet consisting of two entries displayed in the same row constitutes a bivariate observation. The collection of 50 such doublets constitutes a bivariate data set. The observational units of the bivariate data set are the 50 states. For instance, the second and third observations displayed in the second row, 0.10 and 5.46, respectively, constitute a bivariate observation of two variables: estimate and CDC recommendation. The 50 doublets (0.10, 5.46), (0.13, 5.52), . . ., and (15.47, 9.01) make up a bivariate data set. The observational units of the bivariate data set are the 50 states; the size of the bivariate data set is 50.

The four observations shown in the second to fifth columns of the same row constitute a multivariate observation. For instance, the observations 0.10, 5.46, 27.83, and 341,800,000 make up an observation on four variables of the observational unit Pennsylvania. They constitute a multivariate observation; the 50 multivariate observations make up a multivariate data set of size 50.

Example 1.1.3
Hillmen and Others (2004) presented the results of a study that followed 11 transfusion-dependent patients who had received a diagnosis of paroxysmal nocturnal hemoglobinuria (PNH) at least six months earlier, had a detectable GPI (deficient hematopoietic clone) and had received at least four red cell transfusions in the preceding 12 months. One feature of the article is that pertinent data of the 11 subjects 1 month before and 3 months after eculizumab treatment are displayed in Table 1 (Table 1.3).

The first column of the table exhibits the identification numbers of the subjects. The values in the remaining eight columns are quantitative observations. Each column shows the observations of a single variable and constitute a univariate quantitative data set. The observational units of the data set are the 11 subjects. There is one observation per unit; the data size of the data set is 11. The values in the second column constitute a univariate data set consisting of 11 observations of the variable before treatment hemoglobin. The size of the data set is 11, which is the number of observation units as well as the number of observations.

The observations of the same subjects on two variables constitute a bivariate observation. For instance, the doublet consisting of the 12 months before and 3 months after hemoglobin levels of patient no. 1: 10.3 and 10.0 g/dl constitute a bivariate observation. The 11 doublets (10.3, 10.0), (8.3, 8.8), ... (8.5, 10.0) constitute a set of bivariate observations. The observational units are the 11 participants. There is one bivariate observation for each unit; the size of the data set is 11.

Table 1.3 Table 1 of Hillmen and Others (2004)

Table 1 Transfusion rates, hemoglobin levels, and reticulocyte counts 12 months before and after 3 months of eculizumab treatment

	12 Mo before Eculizumab Treatment				After 3 Mo of Eculizumab Treatment			
	Transfusions		Hemoglobin	Reticulocytes	Transfusions		Hemoglobin	Reticulocytes
Patient No.	no. of units	rate[a]	g/dl	$\times 10^{-3}/mm^3$	no. of units	rate[b]	g/dl	$\times 10^{-3}/mm^3$
1	22	1.8	10.3	77.5	2	0.7	10.0	100.7
2	23	1.9	8.3	200.0	8	2.9	8.8	182.6
3	20	1.6	10.1	169.5	0	0.0	10.7	175.9
4	28	2.3	9.3	282.0	0	0.0	9.4	333.3
5	12	1.0	11.9	96.3	2	0.7	10.6	121.8
6	14	1.2	9.8	346.8	0	0.0	10.6	259.0
7	34	2.8	12.8	100.6	0	0.0	13.5	166.8
8	21	1.7	9.5	164.5	0	0.0	9.8	239.6
9	55	4.5	10.7	138.0	3	1.1	11.4	285.8
10	41	3.4	8.5	108.7	5	1.8	8.8	140.1
11	14	1.2	8.5	91.4	0	0.0	10.0	97.4
Median[c]		1.8				0.0		
Mean		2.1	10.0	161.4		0.6	10.3	191.2

[a]The rate (in units per month) was calculated as (number of units ÷ 365 days) × 30
[b]The rate (in units per month) was calculated as (number of units ÷ 84 days) × 30
[c]P = 0.003 for the change in the median rate of transfusion by the Wilcoxon signed-rank test

Example 1.1.4
DeBaun and Others (2014) present the results of a study assessing whether the incidence of infarct recurrence would be lower if children with sickle cell anemia received regular blood transfusion. Subjects were between 5 and 15 years of age, with one or more silent cerebral infarcts but no history of stroke. Of these subjects, 99 were randomly assigned to receive regular blood transfusions (transfusion group), and 97 to receive standard care (observation group). The primary endpoint was the recurrence of infarct, defined as a stroke or a new or enlarged silent cerebral infarct. Neurologic events were observed in 22 children, 6 from the transfusion group and 16 from the observation (standard care) group. The events and some baseline characteristics of the 22 children are shown in Table 2 of the article (Table 1.4).

The first column of the table exhibits the children's identification numbers. The six children from the transfusion group were designated #1 to #6; their observations are displayed in the top six rows below the label : Transfusion group. The 16 from the Observation group were designated #7 to #22; their observations are exhibited in the lower 16 rows below the label Observation group.

The third column shows whether the End-Point Classification of the event of a child is stroke, silent cerebral infarct (SCI), or transient ischemic attack (TIA). They are observations on the variable End-Point Classification. The first six entries denote the classifications of children #1 to #6; they comprise one univariate data set. The observational units are the six children from the transfusion group. There is one observation per child. The size of the data set is 6, which is the number of observational units of the data set and the number of observations in the data set.

The lower 16 entries of the third column denote the classifications of children #7 to #22. They comprise another univariate data set. The observational units of the data set are the 16 children from the transfusion group. There is one observation per child. The size of the data set is 16, which is the number of observational units of the data set as well as the number of observations in the data set.

The last column lists observations on the variable hemoglobin F. The top six entries are hemoglobin F levels of the six children from the observation group. They comprise one univariate data set. The observational units are children #1 to #6. The lower 16 entries are observations of the children of the transfusion group (#7 to #22). The observations of children #7, #8, #9, and #15 are NA indicating not available. The remaining 12 values comprise a data set. The observational units are the 12 children from the transfusion group whose hemoglobin levels were available. The size of the data set is 12, which is the number of observational units as well as the number of observations.

Whether a child is in the transfusion group or the observation group may also be used as an observation of the treatment group. The observational units are the 22 children; the size of the data sets is 22.

Table 1.4 Table 2 of DeBaun and Others (2014)

Table 2 Neurologic events and baseline characteristics, according to patient[a]

Patient No.	Time from randomization to end point	End-point classification	Neuroradiology finding[b]		TIA[c]	Age[d]	Baseline clinical characteristics		
			New infarct	Enlarged infarct			Systolic blood pressure	Steady-state hemoglobin	Hemoglobin F[e]
	mo					yr	mm Hg	g/dl	%
Transfusion group									
1	24	Stroke	+	–	–	7.9	107	6.7	4
2	35	SCI	+	+	–	8.5	85	9.8	17
3	36	SCI	+	+	–	7.5	101	10.3	19
4	36	SCI	+	+	–	9.3	107	7.9	13
5	39	SCI	+	–	–	9.1	92	7.5	2
6	36	SCI	–	+	–	8.3	107	7.2	10
Observation group									
7	6	Stroke	+	+	–	7.8	106	7.9	NA
8	19	Stroke	+	–	–	6.7	106	7.8	NA
9	30	Stroke	+	–	–	12.7	122	6.7	NA
10	36	Stroke	+	–	–	7.3	93	7.5	4
11	12	Stroke	–	+	–	6.6	107	8.0	9
12	19	Stroke	–	–	+	7.1	96	6.5	18
13	35	Stroke	–	–	–	10.3	100	6.1	0
14	16	SCI	+	–		8.0	110	7.7	8
15	27	SCI	+	–	–	6.3	103	8.4	NA
16	34	SCI	+	–	–	6.9	107	7.7	18
17	37	SCI	+	–	–	6.7	109	8.0	25
18	41	SCI		–	–	12.7	118	6.9	4
19	41	SCI	+	–	–	6.7	112	9.4	9

20	44	SCI	+	–	–	9.6	120	10.2	16
21	12	TIA	–	–	+	12.3	136	7.7	13
22	13	TIA	–	–	+	7.1	87	8.6	15

[a]The baseline characteristics were determined at the time of initial screening. NA denotes not available, SCI silent cerebral infarct, and TIA transient ischemic attack

[b]A plus sign indicates that the end point event occurred and a minus sign that the end point event did not occur

[c]The age listed is the age at randomization rather than the age at the time of initial screening

[d]Data on hemoglobin F at baseline were categorized as not available (NA) if the test was performed before the participant was 3 years of age or if the test was not performed

Example 1.1.5
Sedman and Others (1985) reported the results of a study investigating whether premature infants receiving intravenous feeding are vulnerable to aluminum toxicity. The plasma and urinary aluminum concentrations of 18 premature infants with a history of intravenous therapy are displayed in Table 1 (Table 1.5), along with gestational age, birth weight, and age when plasma and urinary were determined.

Infant Number
The first column lists the identification numbers assigned to premature infants. The numbers are not observations.

Gestational Age and Birth Weight
The second column displays gestational ages, and the third column displays birth weights. Each of these two columns exhibits one univariate data set. The observational units of each set are the 18 infants. There is one observation per unit; the size of each data set is 18, which is the number of observational units as well as the number of observations of the data set.

The entries of two columns shown in the same row are observations of two variables obtained from the same observational unit. They comprise a bivariate observation on the two variables. The 18 bivariate observations make up a bivariate data set. There is one bivariate observation per unit; the size of the data set is 18.

Urinary Excretion of Aluminum
The eighth column, the second column from the right, exhibits values of urinary excretion of aluminum determined in 13 infants, one for each. The 13 values comprise a univariate data set. The observational units are the 13 infants. The size of this data set is 13.

Plasma Aluminum Concentration
Aluminum concentrations determined from blood samples drawn from each infant on two occasions are exhibited in the sixth column under the heading: plasma aluminum.

The 36 aluminum concentrations may be regarded as observations of two data sets. The first aluminum concentration of each infant was determined when the infant was younger, and the second when the infant was older. The first concentrations of the infants may be thought of as a set of observations of the variable: first plasma aluminum concentration; the set of second concentrations of the infants may be thought of as a set of observations on the variable: second plasma aluminum concentration. The size of each set is 18; the observational units of each set are the 18 infants.

The two plasma aluminum concentrations of each infant may be considered a bivariate observation on two variables: first plasma aluminum concentration and second plasma aluminum concentration. The observational units of the bivariate observations are the 18 infants. There is one bivariate observation per unit, and the size of this bivariate data set is 18.

Table 1.5 Table 1 of Sedman and Others (1985)

Table 1 Plasma and urinary aluminum levels in 18 premature infants receiving parenteral nutrition[a]

Infant	Gestation	Birth weight	Age		Plasma aluminum	Urinary aluminum	Urinary excretion of aluminum	Urinary aluminum: Creatinine
no.	wk	g	days	Feeding	μgl liter		μgl 24 hr	
1	28	1070	1	IV	49	29		
			22	BM/F	3	35	5.0	4.3
2	28	980	1	IV	26	260		
			22	BM/F	6	28	2.9	2.2
3	32	1060	1	IV	9	170		
			18	BM/F	9	60	10.1	4.3
4	26	760	1	IV	9	35		
			22	F	26	40	5.3	6.0
5	32	1200	1	IV	3	6		
			25	F	3	8	1.8	0.5
6	30	1460	1	IV	<2	20		
			33	F	6	137	19.5	11.4
7	33	1610	1	IV	<2	15		
			21	F	<2	<2	<2.0	0.2
8	34	1440	1	IV	<2	7		
			23	F	<2	20	3.9	1.8
9	31	1980	1	IV	9	35		
			24	F	3	20		1.7
10	32	1520	42	F	4	22		
			78	F	13	20	4.7	2.2
11	32	1220	17	F	46	32		
			38	F	13	16	3.5	1.6

(continued)

Table 1.5 (continued)

Table 1 Plasma and urinary aluminum levels in 18 premature infants receiving parenteral nutrition[a]

Infant	Gestation	Birth weight	Age		Plasma aluminum	Urinary aluminum	Urinary excretion of aluminum	Urinary aluminum:
no.	wk	g	days	Feeding	μgl liter		μgl 24 hr	Creatinine
12	28	820	16	F	3	25		2.1
			37	F	6	32		2.9
13	36	2720	11	IV	39	42		3.6
			22	F	26	15	4.0	0.9
14	37	2320	22	IV	29	90		9.8
			45	IV	29	85		9.6
15	27	750	30	IV	32	30		3.4
			51	IV	23	105		13.5
16	28	990	22	IV	20	40		5.9
			46	F	4	75		3.1
17	32	1100	16	IV	172	145		14.5
			43	F	9	23	3.8	*1.9*
18	33	2608	16	IV	136	68		6.7
			32	F	6	132	27.4	11.0

[a]Aluminum was measured on two different occasions separated by an interval of three weeks. IV denotes intravenous, BM breast milk, and F formula. To convert aluminum values to micromoles per filer, divide by 27

Urinary Aluminum:Creatinine Ratio

The last column of the table exhibits 25 urinary aluminum:creatinine ratios. One is exhibited for each of 11 infants (#1 to #11), and two for each of 7 (#12 to #18). When the 25 ratios are considered one set of observations, the observational units are urinary samples; the size of the data set is 25. If one observation is determined from the ratios of each infant who had two, the resulting value of the 11 infants and the remaining seven urinary aluminum:creatinine ratios make up a new univariate data set. The observational units of the new data set are the 18 infants. There is one observation per infant; the size of the data set is 18.

Example 1.1.6

Chosidow and Others (2010) presented the results of a study assessing the efficacy and safety of oral ivermectin, compared with malathion lotion, in subjects with live head lice not eradicated by topical insecticides; 376 households were randomly assigned to receive ivermectin or malathion lotion. The primary end point was the absence of head lice on day 15. Some results are presented in the article as follows:

> . . . on day 15, 378 of the 397 patients (95.2%) in the ivermectin group were free of head lice, as compared with 352 of the 414 patients (85%) in the malathion group (absolute difference, 10.2 percentage points; 95% confidence interval [CI], 4.6 to 15.7, P < 0.001) (Table 2) . . . At the cluster level, 171 of the 185 households (92.4%) in the ivermectin group were free of head lice, as compared with 151 of 191 households (79.1%) in the malathion group (absolute difference, 13.4 percentage points; 95% CI, 6.4 to 20.0).

Percentages computed from several data sets were cited; the observational units and sizes of the data sets differ. The percentages: 95.2% and 85% (percent of participants who were free of head lice on day 15) were computed from data sets consisting of observations obtained from the 397 subjects in the ivermectin group and the 414 in the malathion group. The observational units of these data sets are the subjects. There is one observation per observational unit (subject). The number of observations in each data set equals the number of observational units.

The percentages: 92.4% and 79.1% (percent of households that were free of head lice on day 15) were computed from data sets consisting of observations pertaining to the 185 households in the ivermectin group and the 191 households in the malathion group. The observational units of these data sets are the households. There is one observation per observational unit (household). The number of observations in each data set equals the number of observational units. The sizes of the data sets are 185 and 191.

With respect to data sets consisting of observations pertaining to individuals, members of a household amount to a cluster of observational units. With respect to data sets consisting of observations pertaining to households, households are the observational units, and members of a household are subunits of the observational unit.

1.2 Data Types

Different statistical methods are more productive for different types of data. Data may be classified in many ways. The simple classification of qualitative and quantitative data is used in this book to organize its presentation. Its relationship with other often-used classifications is examined briefly.

- *Qualitative Variable and Qualitative Observations*

A qualitative variable is a trait that is observed and recorded in terms of mutually exclusive categories. There is not a generally accepted quantitative measure of the degree of difference among the categories. Traits such as sex, race, survival status, and occurrence of events are qualitative variables. Observations on such traits are qualitative. They may be denoted by alphabets, digits, or other symbols.

- *Quantitative Variable and Quantitative Observations*

A quantitative variable is a trait that is measured and recorded in numerical values representing well-defined orders and yielding realistic quantitative measures of degrees of difference. Numerical values that represent the recorded results of quantitative variables are quantitative observations. Traits such as age, heart rate, and blood pressure are quantitative variables. Their observations are quantitative.

- *Types of Qualitative Data*

Qualitative data may be nominal or ordinal; they may also be dichotomous or polytomous.

– Nominal Variable and Nominal Observations

A nominal variable is a trait that is observed and recorded in mutually exclusive categories that do not have an ordered relationship and do not yield reliable quantitative measures of degrees of difference. Alphabets, digits, or other symbols representing categories of nominal variables are nominal observations. Variables such as gender, ethnicity, and blood type are nominal. Their attributes do not have an ordered relationship.

– Ordinal Variable and Ordinal Observations

An ordinal variable is a trait that is observed and recorded in mutually exclusive categories that have an underlying ordered relationship but do not yield reliable measures of degrees of difference. Alphabets, digits, and symbols representing observations on ordinal variables are ordinal observations.

Categories of socioeconomic status, education levels, and measures of degree of pain are examples of ordinal variables. Multiple choices, such as strongly agree, agree, indifferent, disagree, and strongly disagree, are examples of ordinal data.

– Categorical Variables and Categorical Data

Qualitative variables are often referred to as categorical variables, especially if the variables are nominal. A set of qualitative observations is often referred to as a set of categorical observations or a categorical data set.

– Dichotomous Variable and Dichotomous Observations

A qualitative variable that has only two possible categories is a dichotomous variable. Qualitative observations that belong to only two categories are dichotomous observations.

The two categories of a dichotomous variable may be referred to as the YES and the NO categories for convenience. For instance, the female and male categories may be referred to as the YES and the NO categories of the variable female. Similarly, having or not having a disease may be regarded as the YES and the NO features of a dichotomous variable, say disease. Survived and not survived are the YES and the NO features a dichotomous variable, say survival.

– Polytomous Variable and Polytomous Observations

A qualitative variable that has three or more possible categories is a polytomous variable. Qualitative observations that belong to three or more are polytomous observations.

– Categories of qualitative variables denoted by digits

Categories of qualitative variables are sometimes denoted by digits. The digits may reflect orders of the categories if the variables are ordinal. When there are many possible values, the values may sometimes be treated as quantitative observations.

- *Continuous and Discrete Variables*

Variables are labeled discrete and continuous in mathematical statistics. This classification is important to discussions of mathematical properties of statistical methods. Continuous and discrete variables are quantitative. What constitutes continuous and discrete variables is illustrated here by examples.

When observations of a variable are recorded as counts, the variable is regarded as a discrete variable. The number of children, number of cigarettes smoked per day, number of heartbeats per minute, number of blood cells per unit volume, and number of bacteria per unit are examples of discrete variables. They are quantitative.

When observations of a variable can be measured more precisely and recorded in finer units, the variable is considered a continuous variable. Age, weight, height, blood pressure, cholesterol level, and aluminum level are examples.

- *Binary and Bernoulli Variable*

A binary variable is one that has only two possible values 0 and 1. It is an important discrete variable and is also known as a Bernoulli variable in statistics. It is basically a quantitative variable. A set of observations of a binary variable is called a binary data set.

Binary observations are often the result of assigning the values 0 and 1 to dichotomous observations. Generally, the value 1 is assigned to YES observations, and the value 0 is assigned to NO observations. This brings about much convenience. The sum of a set of binary observations is the number of YES observations in the data set; the mean of a set of binary observations is the proportion of YES observations. Nevertheless, the values 0 and 1 do not necessarily represent an ordered relationship, and their difference is not necessarily a realistic measure of the degree of difference.

Example 1.2.1
Some of the observations displayed in Table 1.1 are qualitative, and some are quantitative. The observations exhibited in the second column belong to either of two categories F and M. They are observations of a dichotomous qualitative variable. There is no ordered relationship between the two categories; the variable is nominal. If the value 1 is assigned to F and 0 to M, the resulting values constitute a binary data set.

The observations exhibited in the third column belong to one of three categories. They are observations of a polytomous qualitative variable. It may be argued that the risk of coronary heart disease may be highest among current smokers, second highest among former smokers, and lowest among never smoked subjects. The three categories have an ordered relationship; the variable smoking status may be regarded as an ordinal variable. The letters N, F, and C denote nominal observations. The three categories may be denoted by digits in many ways, such as 1, 2, and 3 or 1, 10, and 100. The digits are correct reflections of the order of the three categories. However, differences among the digits are not reliable measures of the degree of difference.

Entries of the fourth and fifth columns are heart rates. Their magnitudes are reliable indications of the ordered relationship among the heart rates; differences among the entries are reliable measures of degrees of difference. For instance, it is generally agreed that 60 bpm is slower than 70 bpm, and 90 bpm is faster than 70 bpm. The degree of difference between 60 bpm and 70 bpm is 10 bpm; the degree of difference between 70 bpm and 90 bpm is 20 bpm. 120 bpm is considered twice as fast as 60 bpm. The heart rates are quantitative observations; they are observations of a discrete variable.

Entries of the sixth column are systolic blood pressures. Their magnitudes are reliable indications of an ordered relationship; differences among the entries are reliable measures of their degrees of difference. For instance, it is generally agreed that 110 mmHg is higher than 100 mmHg but lower than 140 mmHg. The degree of difference between 100 mmHg and 110 mmHg is 10 mmHg; the degree of difference between 100 mmHg and 140 mmHg is 40 mmHg.

Heart rate is a discrete variable; blood pressure is a continuous variable.

Example 1.2.2
The four sets of observations displayed in Table 1 of Gross and Others (2002) (Table 1.2) are quantitative. The observations shown in each column are numerical

values that have an ordered relationship and yield reliable measures of the degree of difference.

Example 1.2.3
All eight data sets displayed in Table 1 of Hillmen and Others (2004) (Table 1.3) are quantitative.

Example 1.2.4
Several types of data are displayed in Table 2 of DeBaun and Others (2014) (Table 1.4). The second column of the table displays observations of a quantitative variable: time from randomization to end point. The observations are numerical values that have an ordered relationship and yield reliable measures of the degree of difference. They constitute a quantitative data set. The data sets presented in the seventh to tenth columns age, systolic blood pressure, steady-state hemoglobin, and hemoglobin F are quantitative observations.

The third column lists observations of a polytomous qualitative (categorical) variable: end-point classification. The observations belong to one of three categories stroke, silent cerebral infarct (SCI), and transient ischemic attack (TIA).

If stroke was considered a more severe event than SCI, and SCI a more severe event than TIA, the three classifications would be ordinal.

The fourth to the sixth columns use + and – signs to denote observations of three dichotomous variables new infarct, enlarged infarct, and transient ischemic attack (TIA), respectively. The signs + and – indicate YES and NO, respectively. If the value 1 is assigned to each + and the value 0 is assigned to each, the resulting data sets are binary.

The first column shows the identification numbers of the subjects, which are usually not considered observations. However, the column also indicates whether a subject was in the transfusion or the observation group. Such indications may be used as observations of a dichotomous nominal variable, say treatment group.

Example 1.2.5
Acker and Others (2018) presented the results of a study that randomly assigned patients with severe ischemic mitral regurgitation to undergo either mitral valve repair or chordal-sparing replacement. The primary outcome was the left ventricular end-systolic volume index (LVESVI) 12 months after randomization which is a quantitative variable.

One outcome was the New York Heart Association (NYHA) classification. It is a qualitative and ordinal measure ranging from I to IV, with higher classes indicating higher severity. The New York Heart Association (NYHA) classes of a group of patients make up a set of ordinal qualitative observations.

Possible scores of the Minnesota Living with Heart Failure questionnaire range from 0 to 105. The scores are ordinal observations, with higher scores indicating worse conditions. They may be treated as quantitative observations, although their differences may not be reliable reflections of the degrees of diffidence in the severity of conditions.

Example 1.2.6
Albers and Others (2018) presented the results of a study that randomly assigned patients with proximal middle cerebral artery occlusion, an initial infarct size of less than 70 ml, and a ratio of the volume of ischemic tissue on perfusion imaging to infarct volume of 1.8 or more to receive endovascular therapy plus standard medical therapy (endovascular therapy group) or standard medical therapy alone (medical therapy group). The article stated: *The primary efficacy outcome was the ordinary score on the modified Rankin Scale (range, 0 [no symptom] to 6 [death]) on day 90*; .... The scores are ordinal. A higher score indicates a more severe disability; 0 indicates no symptom, 1 indicates no clinically significant disability, 2 indicates slight disability, 3 indicates moderate disability, 4 indicates moderately severe disability, 5 indicates severe disability, and 6 indicates death. Differences among the scores are not reliable measures of the degree of difference in severity.

Example 1.2.7
Walker and Others (2014) presented the results of a study that randomly assigned 1310 adult smokers who were motivated to quit to receive cytisine or nicotine replacement therapy. The baseline characteristics of the subjects are depicted in Table 1. Two of the characteristics are the number of cigarettes smoked per day and cigarette dependence. The number of cigarettes smoked per day is a quantitative variable that is discrete. A footnote of the table states: *Cigarette dependence was measured with the Fagerstrom Test of Cigarette Dependence. On a scale of 1 to 10, a score above 5 indicates high cigarette dependence, and a score of 5 or below indicates low cigarette dependence.* Cigarette dependence is an ordinal qualitative variable; cigarette dependence scores are ordinal observations.

1.3 Data Distribution

The first task of data analysis is to explore data revelations. Observations are organized to show how they are distributed among categories or distinct values. Data revelations are manifested by the distributions.

Definition: Data Distribution

The distribution of a set of observations comprises percentages of the observations belonging to the categories among the observations or equaling the distinct values among the observations.

1.3.1 Distribution of Qualitative Data

To explore the revelations of a set of qualitative observations, the observations are reviewed, and the categories among the observations are identified. Percentages of observations belonging to the categories are determined and used to display how the observations are distributed among the categories. Revelations of the data set are manifestly exposed.

Definition: Distribution of Qualitative Data

The distribution of a set of qualitative observations comprises percentages of the observations belonging to the categories among the observations.

Example 1.3.1.1

To explore the revelation of the observations of the variable gender displayed in Table 1.1, the observations were reviewed. It was immediately evident that the observations are dichotomous and belong to either of two categories, F or M. It was determined that the percentages of F and M are 40% and 60%, respectively. The two percentages comprise the distribution of the set of dichotomous observations and manifest of the revelation of the 50 observations cogently.

To explore the revelations of the observations of the variable: smoking status displayed in Table 1.1, the observations were reviewed first. It was determined that the observations are polytomous and belong to three categories N, F, or C. The percentages of never smoked, formerly smoked, and currently smoking subjects are 20%, 70%, and 10%, respectively. The percentages reveal how the 50 observations are distributed among the three categories and comprise the distribution of the 50 observations. They present a cogent manifestation of the revelations of the observations.

Example 1.3.1.2 DeBaun (371, 8)

The fourth column of Table 2 of DeBaun and Others (2014) (Table 1.4) uses "+" and "−" signs to denote whether neuroradiology findings are new infarcts. To explore of the revelation of the 16 dichotomous observations of the observation group, it was determined that the percentages of "+" and "−" are 69% and 31%, respectively. The two percentages divulge how the observations are distributed between the two categories and constitute the distribution of the set of 16 dichotomous observations. They present a cogent description of the revelation of the 16 dichotomous observations.

The third column of the table reveals that the observations of the variable: classifications of end points belong to one of three categories. Among the observations of the 16 children from the observation group, 44% are stroke, 44% are SCI, and 12% are TIA.

The three percentages divulge how the observations distribute among the three categories and constitute the distribution of the set of 16 polytomous observations. They present a cogent description of the revelation of the 16 polytomous observations.

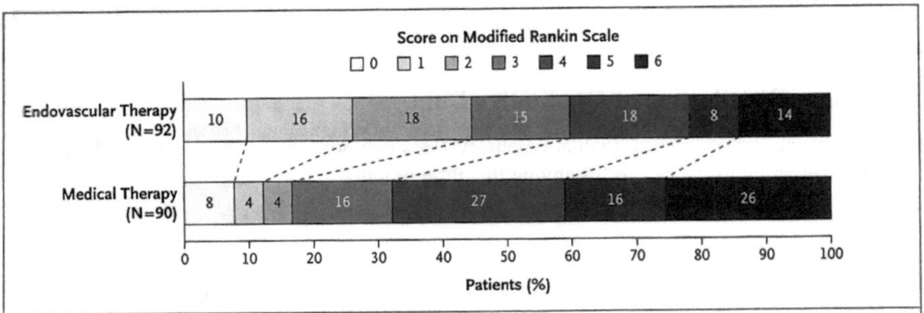

Figure 2. **Scores on the Modified Rankin Scale at 90 Days.**
Patients in the endovascular-therapy group received endovascular therapy plus standard medical therapy. Patients in the medical-therapy group received standard medical therapy alone. Scores on the modified Rankin scale range from 0 to 6, with 0 indicating no symptoms, 1 no clinically significant disability, 2 slight disability, 3 moderate disability, 4 moderately severe disability, 5 severe disability, and 6 death. There was a significant difference favoring the endovascular-therapy group over the medical-therapy group in the overall distribution of scores (unadjusted common odds ratio, 2.77; 95% CI, 1.63 to 4.70; P<0.001).

Fig. 1.1 Figure 2 of Albers and Others (2018)

Example 1.3.1.3
Figure 2 of Albers and Others (2018) (Fig. 1.1) uses the widths of sections of a horizontal bar to denote the percentages of patients whose scores on the modified Rankin scale equal each of seven possible values. The top bar shows 10%, 16%, 18%, 15%, 18%, 8%, and 14% the percentages of subjects in the endovascular therapy group whose scores were 0, 1, 2, 3, 4, 5, and 6, respectively. These percentages portray how the scores of the 92 subjects are distributed among seven values and constitute the distribution of the 92 scores. The bottom bar shows 8%, 4%, 4%, 16%, 27%, 16%, and 26% of the subjects in the medical therapy group whose scores were 0, 1, 2, 3, 4, 5, and 6, respectively. These percentages depict how the scores of the 90 subjects distribute among the seven values and constitute the distribution of the 90 scores.

1.3.2 Distribution of Quantitative Data

To explore the revelations of a set of quantitative observations, the observations are examined to identify distinct values and determine percentages of observations equaling the values. The percentages show how the observations distribute among distinct values and comprise the distribution of the observations.

Definition: Distribution of Quantitative Data

The distribution of a set of quantitative observations is comprised of percentages of observations equaling the distinct values among the observations.

When the number of distinct values among a set of observations is large, the percentages of observations equaling distinct values may not manifest the revelations of the data clearly. In this case, percentages of observations in thoughtfully specified intervals may present an expressive description of the distribution of the observations and manifest the revelations of the data lucidly.

Example 1.3.2.1

To explore revelations of the resting heart rates listed in Table 1.1, the heart rates were inspected to identify distinct values and compute percentages of heart rates equaling the values. The percentages comprise the distribution of the 50 resting heart rates. They are exhibited in Table 1.6 and displayed graphically in Fig. 1.2.

Table 1.6 Percentages of resting heart rates equaling distinct values

Heart rate	56	60	64	68	72	76	80	84	88	92	96	100	104
Number	1	2	3	4	5	6	8	6	5	4	3	2	1
Percent	2%	4%	6%	8%	10%	12%	16%	12%	10%	8%	6%	4%	2%

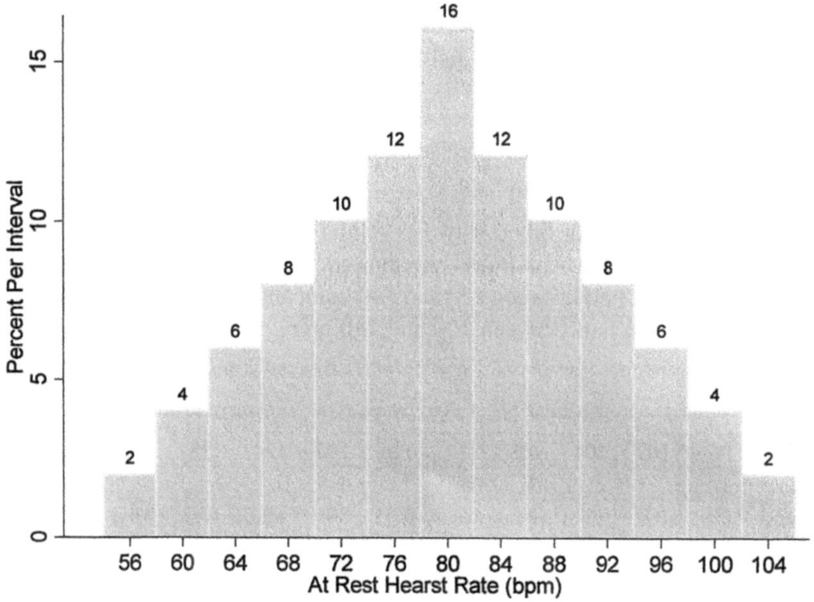

Fig. 1.2 Percentages of resting heart rates equaling distinct values

The table is a frequency table; it shows percentages and numbers of heart rates equaling distinct values. Figure 1.2 shows a histogram. It uses heights of bars of identical widths to signify percentages of heart rates equaling distinct values. Labels are marked along a vertical line, the vertical axis (y-axis), to specify magnitudes of percentages signified by heights of bars; labels are marked along a horizontal line, the horizontal axis (x-axis), to specify magnitudes of heart rates signified by distances from the vertical line.

Table 1.6 and Fig. 1.2 present precise delineations of the distribution of the set of heart rates and unveil the following:

- The 50 heart rates are distributed between 56 and 104 bpm.
- The distribution of the heart rates is symmetric, with a cluster of heart rates concentrated in the vicinity of 80 bpm and equal percentages of rates distributed in its left half below 80 bpm and its right half above 80 bpm.

Example 1.3.2.2
To explore revelations of the after-exercise heart rates listed in Table 1.1, distinct values were identified, and percentages of rates equaling the values were computed. The percentages show how the heart rates are distributed among 12 distinct values and constitute the distribution of the set of 50 heart rates.

The percentages are exhibited in Table 1.7 and displayed graphically in Fig. 1.3. The table is a frequency table; it shows numbers and percentages of heart rates equaling distinct values. Figure 1.3 shows a histogram. It uses heights of bars of identical widths to signify percentages of heart rates equaling distinct values. Labels are marked along a vertical line, the vertical axis (y-axis), to specify magnitudes of percentages signified by heights of bars; labels are marked along a horizontal line, the horizontal axis (x-axis), to specify magnitudes of heart rates signified by distances from the vertical line.

Table 1.7 and Fig. 1.3 present precise delineations of the distribution of the set of heart rates and unveil the following:

- The heart rates are distributed between 96 and 140 bpm.
- The distribution of the heart rates is asymmetric. The bulk of the heart rates (76%) cluster in its right half between 120 and 140 bpm, and the remaining 24% disperse sparsely in its left half between 120 and 140 bpm.

Table 1.7 Numbers and percentage post-exercise heart rates equaling distinct values

Values	96	100	104	108	112	116	120	124	128	132	136	140
Number	1	1	2	2	3	3	4	4	5	7	8	10
Percent	2%	2%	4%	4%	6%	6%	8%	8%	10%	14%	16%	20%

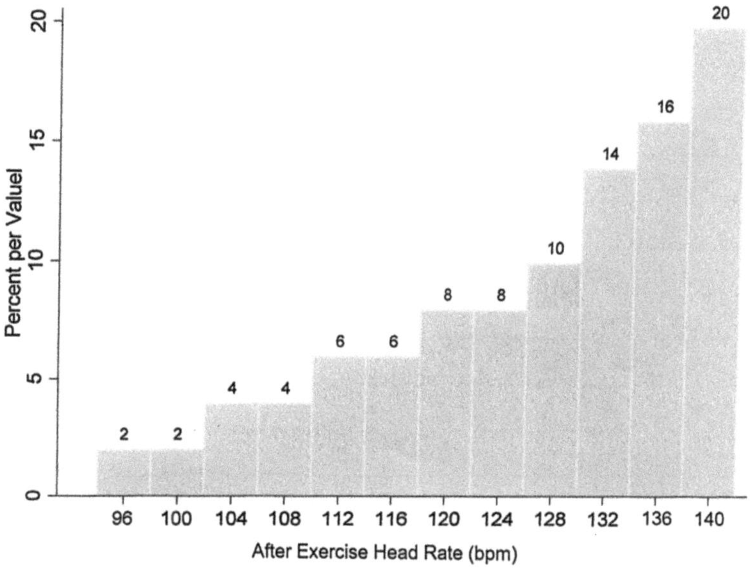

Fig. 1.3 Percentages of after-exercise heart rates equaling distinct values

Example 1.3.2.3

To explore revelations of the systolic blood pressures listed in Table 1.1, distinct values were identified, and numbers and percentages of pressures equaling the values were determined. The percentages are shown in Table 1.8. They unveil how the pressures are distributed among 34 values and constitute the distribution of the set of 50 systolic blood pressures.

The percentages of pressures equaling the 34 distinct values show that the pressures vary widely from as low as 102 mmHg to 198 mmHg. However, they do not expressively present the properties of the distribution. It is not clear whether the distribution is symmetric and whether there is a cluster of pressures concentrated in its middle.

To exhibit properties of the distribution of the blood pressures manifestly, numbers and percentages of pressures in 10 intervals are displayed in Table 1.9. The intervals are mutually exclusive and encompass the values of the 50 pressures. They are unmistakably specified so that it is clear to which interval every blood pressure belongs. The widths of the intervals are identically 10 mmHg. The lower boundary of the first interval is slightly lower than the lowest pressure (102 mmHg); the upper boundary of the last interval is slightly higher than the highest pressure (198 mmHg). Each interval includes pressures larger than or equal to its lower boundary but smaller than its upper boundary.

Figure 1.4 exhibits a graphical display of the percentages of pressures shown in Table 1.9. The widths of its bars are identical; the heights of its bars signify sizes of

Table 1.8 Systolic blood pressures equaling distinct values

Pressure	102	104	105	108	110	112	114	115	116	118	120	122	124	125	126	128	130	132	134	135	136	138	140
Number	1	1	1	1	3	2	2	1	2	2	1	2	2	2	2	1	2	1	1	2	1	1	2
Percent	2%	2%	2%	2%	6%	4%	4%	2%	4%	4%	2%	4%	4%	4%	4%	1%	6%	2%	2%	4%	2%	2%	4%

Pressure	142	145	148	150	155	158	160	165	168	170	175	185	198
Number	1	1	1	1	2	1	1	1	1	1	1	1	1
Percent	2%	2%	2%	2%	4%	2%	2%	2%	2%	2%	2%	2%	2%

Table 1.9 Percentages and numbers of systolic blood pressures in ten left-closed intervals

Interval	# in interval (frequency)	% in interval (relative frequency)
≥100 to <110	4	8%
≥110 to <120	12	24%
≥120 to <130	10	20%
≥130 to <140	8	16%
≥140 to <150	5	10%
≥150 to <160	4	8%
≥160 to <170	3	6%
≥170 to <180	2	4%
≥180 to <190	1	2%
≥190 to <200	1	2%
Sum	50	100%

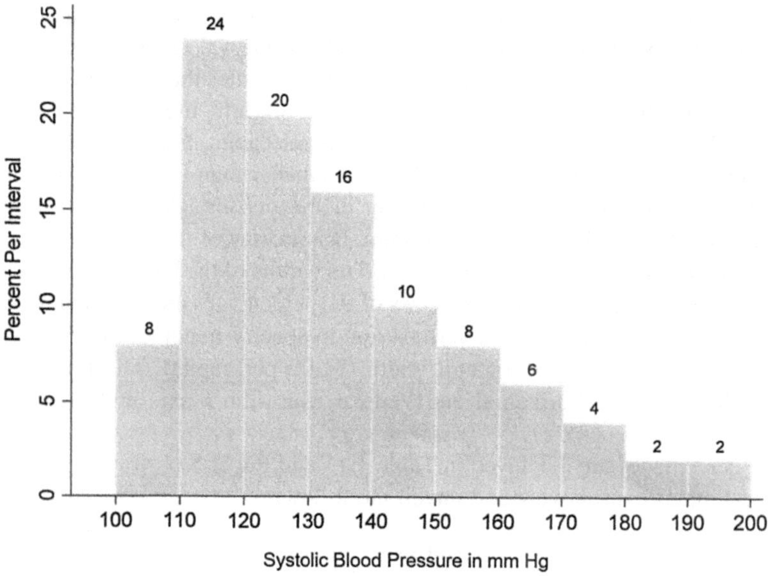

Fig. 1.4 Percentages of systolic blood pressures in ten left-closed intervals

percentages of pressures in intervals. The graph is a histogram and shows expressively how the pressures are distributed.

Table 1.9 and Fig. 1.4 submit the following regarding the distribution of the blood pressures.

- The distribution of the systolic blood pressures varies in a wide range between approximately 100 mmHg and 200 mmHg.

- The distribution is asymmetric. The bulk of the pressures (68%) cluster in its lower half between 100 mmHg and 150 mmHg, and the remaining 28% disperse sparsely in its higher right half between 150 mmHg and 200 mmHg.

Example 1.3.2.4
To explore revelations of the estimates of 2001 state expenditures for tobacco control programs displayed in Table 1 of Gross and Others (2002) (Table 1.2), the estimates were inspected to ascertain distinct values and determine numbers and percentages of estimates equaling the values. The percentages are shown in Table 1.10. They constitute the distribution of the 50 estimates and unveil that the estimates are distributed widely between 10 cents per capita and 15.47 dollars per capita. They, however, do not convey the revelations of the data clearly.

To depict the distribution of the estimates that shows revelations of the estimates manifestly, the numbers and percentages of estimates in 16 intervals were determined and are displayed in Table 1.11. The intervals are mutually exclusive and are unmistakably specified so that it is clear to which interval every estimate belongs. The lower boundary of the first interval is slightly smaller than the lowest estimate, and the upper boundary of the last interval is slightly higher than the highest estimate. The widths of the intervals are \$1.00 per capita. Each includes estimates larger than or equal to its lower boundary and smaller than its upper boundary.

Figure 1.5 exhibits a graphical display of the percentages of estimates in the 11 intervals of Table 1.11. It is a histogram. Boundaries of the intervals are marked along a horizontal line, the horizontal axis. The widths of the bars are commensurate with the widths of the intervals. The sizes of the percentages are signified by areas of bars. Labels are marked along a vertical line to specify magnitudes of percentages signified by heights of bars of unit width (\$1.00 per capita). The horizontal and vertical lines are the horizontal and vertical axes (the x-axis and y-axis) of the histogram.

The percentages are displayed in Table 1.11 and Fig. 1.5 portray the distribution of the estimates expressively and unveil the following:

- The distribution varies widely from close to zero to close to \$16.00 per capita.
- The distribution is asymmetric. While 82% of the estimates cluster in the lower portion of the distribution between 0 and \$5.00 per capita, 18% disperse sparsely in the higher portion of the distribution between \$5.00 and \$16.00 per capita.
- The percentage of the estimates below \$1.00 per capita is remarkably high (32%).

Example 1.3.2.5
Anavekar and Others (2004) summarized the results of a study evaluating the effects of captopril and valsartan. A total of 14,527 patients with acute myocardial infarction complicated by clinical or radiological signs of heart failure, left ventricular dysfunction, or both were included in the study. Figure 1 of the article (Fig. 1.6) exhibits a graphical display of the distribution of baseline estimates of glomerular filtration rate (GFR) of the 14,527 subjects. The display is a histogram. It uses heights of bars of identical width to depict numbers of baseline GFR estimates in 30 intervals. The

Table 1.10 Estimates of 2001 state expenditure for tobacco control programs equaling distinct values

Estimates	0.10	0.13	0.24	0.30	0.32	0.37	0.43	0.58	0.59	0.66	0.78	0.83	0.84	1.71	1.74	1.75
# of estimates	1	1	1	2	1	1	1	1	3	1	1	1	1	1	1	1
% of estimates	2%	2%	2%	4%	2%	2%	2%	2%	6%	2%	2%	2%	2%	2%	2%	2%

Estimates	1.89	2.19	2.26	2.46	2.49	2.71	2.82	3.03	3.08	3.29	3.32	3.44	3.52	3.80	4.01	4.05
# of estimates	1	1	1	1	1	1	1	1	1	1	1	1	1	1	1	1
% of estimates	2%	2%	2%	2%	2%	2%	2%	2%	2%	2%	2%	2%	2%	2%	2%	2%

Estimates	4.09	4.31	4.61	4.83	4.85	4.92	5.15	5.62	6.05	7.32	10.25	10.82	12.58	12.82	15.47	
# of estimate	1	1	1	1	1	1	1	1	1	1	1	1	1	1	1	
% of estimates	2%	2%	2%	2%	2%	2%	2%	2%	2%	2%	2%	2%	2%	2%	2%	

Table 1.11 Percentages and numbers of estimates of 2001 state expenditure for tobacco control programs in intervals

Right-open interval	Frequency # in interval	Relative frequency % in interval
≥0.00 to <1.00	16	32%
≥1.00 to <2.00	4	8%
≥2.00 to <3.00	6	12%
≥3.00 to <4.00	7	14%
≥4.00 to <5.00	8	16%
≥5.00 to <6.00	2	2%
≥6.00 to <7.00	1	4%
≥7.00 to <8.00	1	4%
≥8.00 to <9.00	0	0%
≥9.00 to <10.00	0	0%
≥10.00 to <11.00	2	4%
≥11.00 to <12.00	0	0%
≥12.00 to <13.00	2	4%
≥13.00 to <14.00	0	0%
≥14.00 to <15.00	0	0%
≥15.00 to <16.00	1	2%
SUM	50	100%

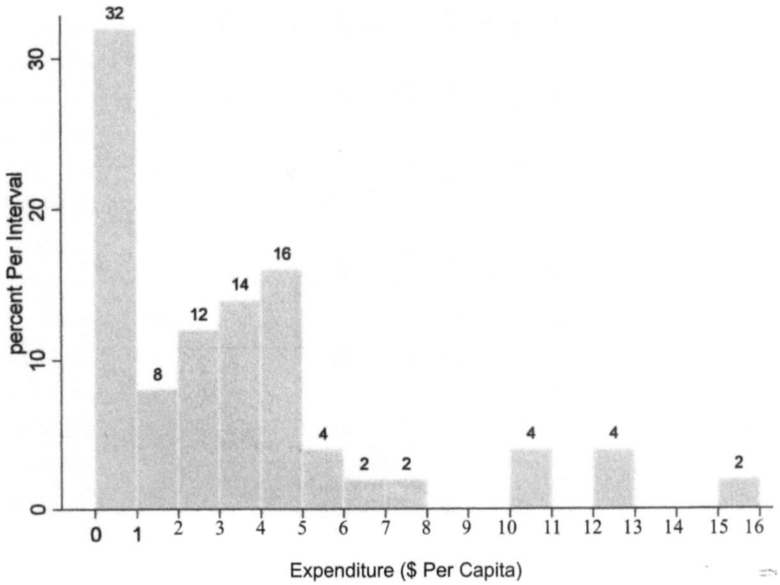

Fig. 1.5 Percentages of estimates of 2001 state expenditure on tobacco control programs in 11 intervals

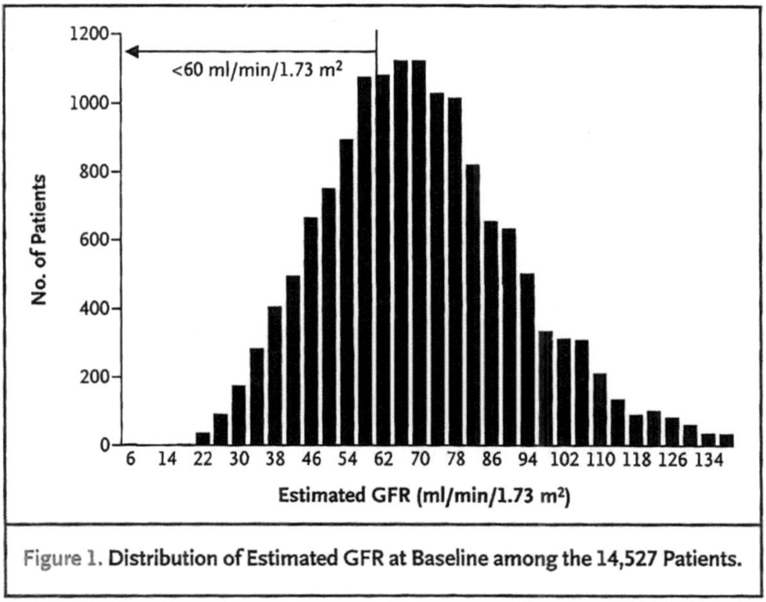

Fig. 1.6 Figure 1 of Anavekar and Others (2004)

widths of the intervals are identically 4 ml/min/1.73 m^2. The midpoints of every other interval are marked along a horizontal line, the horizontal axis of the histogram. The histogram reveals that the distribution of the GFR estimates is basically symmetric and varies between 20 and 140 ml/min/1.73 m^2, with a bulk in its middle.

Example 1.3.2.6

Weintraub and Others (2014) presented the results of a study comparing the long-term survival of patients receiving percutaneous coronary intervention (PCI) with that of patients receiving coronary artery bypass grafting (CABG). Propensity scores for CABG—estimates of the probability of being selected for CABG—were determined. Figure 1 of the article (Fig. 1.7) uses histograms to display the distributions of scores of 86,244 patients who received CABG and those 103,549 who received PCI.

The figure uses heights of vertical bars to depict the number of participants whose scores were in intervals varying from 0.00 to 1.00. The widths of the intervals are identically 0.02. The midpoints of the intervals are marked along a horizontal line; numbers signified by heights of bars are indicated by labels marked along a vertical line.

The green bars constitute a histogram that is a graphical display of the distribution of the scores of the subjects who received PCI. It shows that the distribution is asymmetric with fewer scores dispersed in its right half above 50 and more scores clustered in its left half below 50. The brown bars constitute a histogram that is a graphical display of the distribution of the scores of the subjects who received

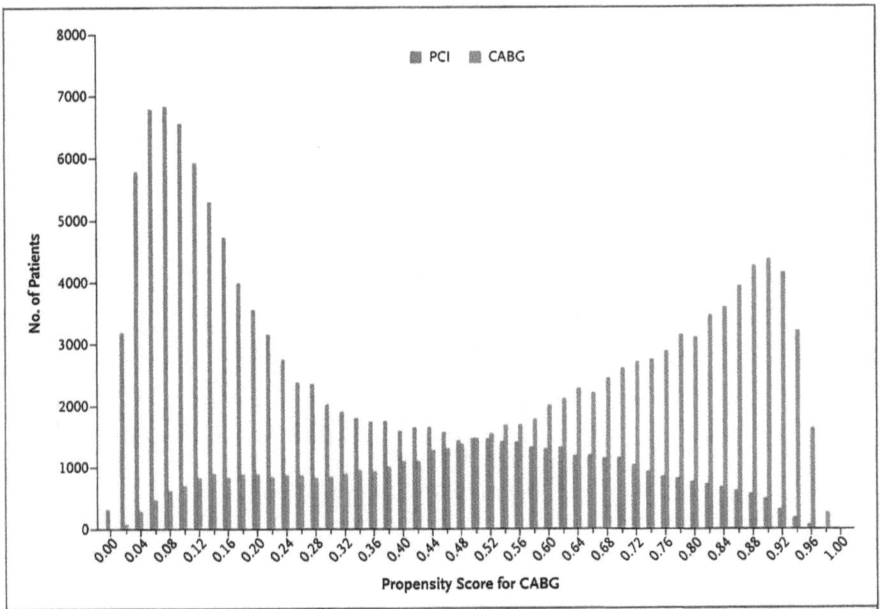

Figure 1. **Propensity Scores for Coronary Artery Bypass Grafting (CABG) in the Percutaneous Coronary Intervention (PCI) and CABG Populations.**
The propensity score for CABG is the probability given baseline variables that any patient in either group would be selected for CABG.

Fig. 1.7 Figure 1 of Weintraub and Others (2014)

CABG. It shows that the distribution is asymmetric with fewer scores dispersed in its left half below 50 and more scores clustered in its left half above 50.

- *Data Distributions and Distributions of Random Variables*

Data distributions are data counterparts of the distributions of random variables. The properties of a random variable are precisely specified by a function known as its probability function (discrete random variable) or density function (continuous random variable). Precise delineations of data distributions depicting percentages of observations equaling distinct values are data counterparts of probability functions of discrete random variables; expressive descriptions of data distributions depicting percentages of observations in intervals are data counterparts of density functions of continuous random variables.

1.4 Making Frequency Table and Histogram

The first two phases of the *eDeD* approach to data analysis are probing productively and describing informatively revelations of data. Revelations of data are productively probed by scrutinizing frequency tables or histograms that are cogent descriptions of data distributions and informatively related by articulating manifestations of data distributions. When the number of distinct values among a set of observations is not small relative to the number of observations, a frequency table and histogram displaying percentages of observations equaling distinct values may not manifest the revelations of data clearly. Frequency table and histogram displaying percentages of observations in thoughtfully specified intervals unveil revelations of data manifestly. How intervals are specified so that frequency tables and histograms are vivid manifestations of data revelations is demonstrated in this section.

- *Essential Properties of Distributions of Quantitative Observations*

Location, variation, and skewness are three essential properties of distributions of quantitative observations. Revelations of observations are upshots of these properties. When the distribution of a set of quantitative observations is depicted by a frequency table or histogram displaying percentages or numbers of observations in intervals, it is vital to specify the intervals thoughtfully so that the three essential properties of the distribution are distinctly manifested.

– *Location*

The location of the distribution of a set of observations is marked by the values of the smallest and largest observations that spell out the range of the observations. When the distribution of a set of quantitative observations is depicted by a frequency table displaying percentages of observations in intervals, the lower boundary of the lowest interval and the upper boundary of the highest interval is an improvised range of the distribution and a contrived label of the location of the distribution.

The location of the distribution of a set of observations may be marked by a value that is smaller than or equal to and larger than or equal to 50% of the observations. It is the median of the observations and an operative label of the location of the center of the distribution.

If the distribution of a set of quantitative observations features a single cluster of observations in its middle, the location of the cluster of observations is dubbed the central location of the distribution. The median of such a set of observations is a useful designation of its central location.

– *Variation*

Individuals are in different conditions and respond to treatments in varying ways. Individual differences play a critical role in medical research.

The degree of difference among a set of observations is manifested by the distribution of the observations. It is called the variation, dispersion, or variability of the distribution. The width of the range of the distribution is a crude measure of the variation of the distribution. There are several more inclusive measures of variation; their indications are examined in Chap. 3.

– *Skewness*

Distributions of quantitative data are often asymmetric and demonstrate a notably lower percentage of observations dispersed in one half and a higher percentage of observations clustered in the other half of its range. In statistics, an asymmetric data distribution is dubbed a skewed distribution. It is skewed to right, right skewed, or positively skewed when the percentage of larger observations in the right half of its range is noticeably smaller than the percentage of smaller observations in the left half of its range. It is skewed to left, left skewed, or negatively skewed when the percentage of smaller observations in its left half is noticeably smaller than the percentage of larger observations in its right half.

• *Table Displaying Percentages of Observations in Intervals*

When the distribution of a set of observations is depicted by a table displaying percentages or numbers of observations in intervals, it is critical to note the following:

– *Range*

The lower boundary of the lowest interval and the upper boundary of the highest interval of a frequency table comprise the range of the intervals. The lower boundary of the first interval may be the same or slightly smaller than the smallest distinct value of the observations; the upper boundary of the last interval may be the same or slightly larger than the largest distinct value of the observations.

– *Boundaries of Intervals*

It is vital to specify boundaries of intervals explicitly so that it is clear to which interval every observation belongs. It is shrewd to use convenient values.

Intervals may be left-closed (right-opened), left opened (right-closed), or closed. A left-closed (right-opened) interval includes all observations larger than or equal to its lower boundary but smaller than its upper boundary, a left-opened (right-closed) interval includes all observations larger than its lower boundary but smaller than or equal to its upper boundary, and a closed interval includes all observations larger than or equal to its lower boundary but smaller than or equal to its upper boundary. The intervals of Table 1.9 and Table 1.11 are left-closed (right-opened).

Boundaries of intervals may be specified by using signs such as $\leq$, $\geq$, $<$, and $>$. They may also be specified by units finer than the unit in which observations are recorded. For instance, when blood pressures are recorded in mmHg, a right-closed interval may be written as 100.1 to 110.0 mmHg, a right-opened interval may be written as 100.0 to 109.9 mmHg, and a closed interval may be written as 100.0 to 110.0 mmHg.

– *Widths and Number of Intervals*

Intervals of identical widths are usually used. The width of intervals is chosen so that properties of data distributions are expressively manifested and revelations of data are clearly disclosed. Usually, 10 to 20 intervals are adequate. If it is necessary to use intervals of unequal widths, limit the number of widths as much as feasible.

– *Percentages or Numbers of Observations*

Frequency table may display percentages or numbers of observations in intervals or both. The sum of the percentages is 100% or close to it; the sum of the numbers equals the number of observations in the data set exactly. The percentages are dubbed relative frequencies and the numbers frequencies. It is important to display percentages of observations in intervals if there are more than one data set, and the numbers of observations in the data sets differ.

– *Number of Possible Values in Intervals:*

If observations are recorded in coarse discrete values, it is critical to make sure that the numbers of possible values included in the intervals are commensurate with the widths of the intervals. When the widths of intervals are identical, it is critical that the intervals include identical numbers of possible values. (See Example 1.4.3.)

• *Histograms Displaying Frequencies of Intervals*

Histograms are graphical displays of frequency tables. They use areas of bars to denote percentages or numbers of observations. It is important to consider the following when a histogram is made:

– *Areas and Heights of Bars*

Bars are drawn so that their areas are accurate indications of magnitudes of percentages or numbers of observations in intervals. The widths of the bars are commensurate with the widths of the intervals. When the widths of the bars are identical, the heights of the bars are indicators of the magnitudes of percentages or numbers. If the widths of bars are unequal, it is essential to ensure that magnitudes of percentages or numbers are accurately reflected by the areas of bars.

– *Percentages or Numbers of Observations in Intervals*

It is judicious to use areas of bars to signify percentages instead of numbers of observations. This is particularly important when there are two or more data sets, and the numbers of observations in the data sets differ noticeably. In this case, distinctions among the distributions of the data sets are distracted by differences in the sizes of bars displaying numbers of observations in intervals.

– *Using a Computer to Make Frequency Tables and Histograms*

Computer algorithms for statistical data analysis are widely available. Their use requires only that data be stored in appropriate files. Default options of procedures making frequency tables and histograms displaying numbers and percentages of observations equaling distinct values require only the name of the variable by which the set of observations is labeled. Frequency tables and histograms displaying numbers and percentages of observations in intervals produced by default options are often unsatisfactory if observations are quantitative and there are many distinct values. Expressive descriptions of data distributions may be obtained by using appropriate options.

The intervals may be left closed or left opened. Percentages and numbers in some intervals may differ slightly when the intervals are left closed and left opened.

Example 1.4.1
The histogram of Fig. 1.4 depicts the distribution of the 50 systolic pressures listed in Table 1.1 expressively and manifests the revelations of the set of pressures cogently. It was printed by a computer algorithm using 100 as the lower boundary of the first interval and 10 as the constant width.

The histograms of Figs. 1.8 and 1.9 are also description of the 50 systolic blood pressures. They do not unveil the revelations of the 50 systolic blood pressure as cogently as the histogram of Fig. 1.4. Figure 1.8 was printed by a computer algorithm specifying 100 as the lower boundary of the first interval and 5 as the constant width. Figure 1.9 was printed by specifying 100 as the lower boundary of the first interval and 20 as the widths of the intervals. Both are not as informative as the histogram of Fig. 1.4. Clearly, 10 mmHg is an optimal width of the intervals when the distribution of the 50 systolic blood pressures is depicted.

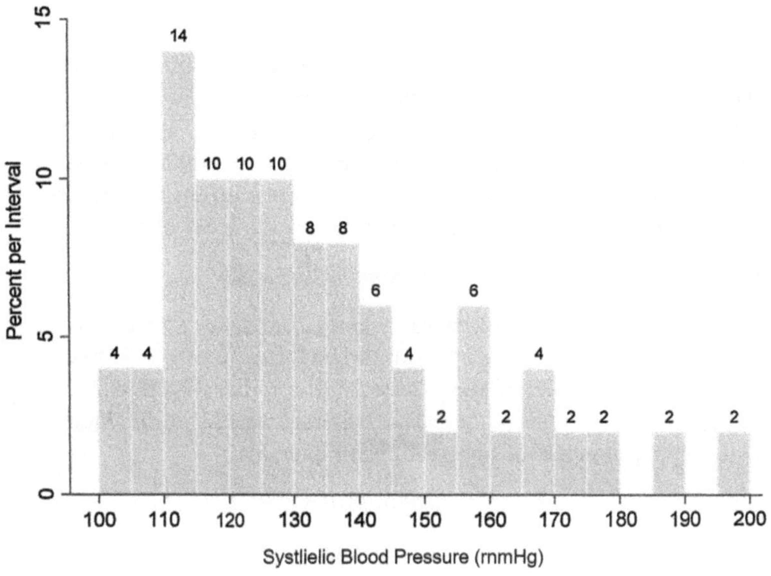

Fig. 1.8 Percentages of systolic blood pressures in 20 intervals of 5 mmHg

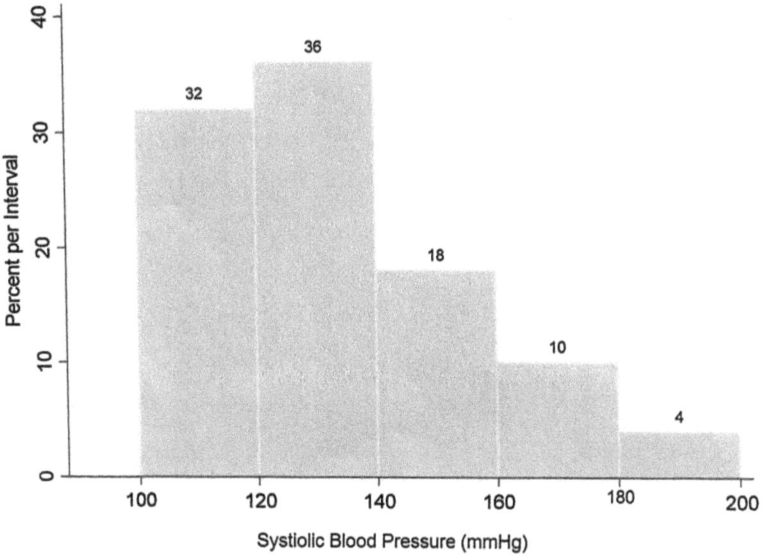

Fig. 1.9 Percentages of resting systolic blood pressures in 5 intervals of width 20 mmHg

Example 1.4.2 Gross (347, 14)

The histogram of Fig. 1.5 displays percentages of estimates of the state expenditures for tobacco control programs in the fiscal year of 2001 in right-opened intervals ranging from 0 to 16 dollars per capita. The widths of the intervals are identically $1.00 per capita.

Figure 1.10 presents a histogram depicting percentages of estimates in intervals of width $2.00 per capita. It shows more regularity and demonstrates a smoother pattern than the histogram of Fig. 1.5. However, it does not convey the important message that the estimates of as much as 32% of states are below $1.00 per capita. This important message is explicitly indicated by the histogram of Fig. 1.5.

Example 1.4.3

The histogram shown in Fig. 1.11 was made to demonstrate the importance of making sure that the numbers of possible values included in intervals are commensurate with the widths of the intervals. The histogram uses intervals of identical widths (5 bpm) varying from 55 to 105 bpm to depict the distribution of the resting heart rates shown in Table 1.1.

This histogram has several merits. Its range: {55 to 105 bpm} is just slightly wider than the range of the observations and is specified by convenient values, and the widths of its intervals (5 bpm) are identical and opportune; boundaries of the intervals are expressed in apt values. However, the histogram differs from the precise delineation of the set of heart rates shown by Fig. 1.2. The difference is artificial because some intervals include unequal numbers of possible values.

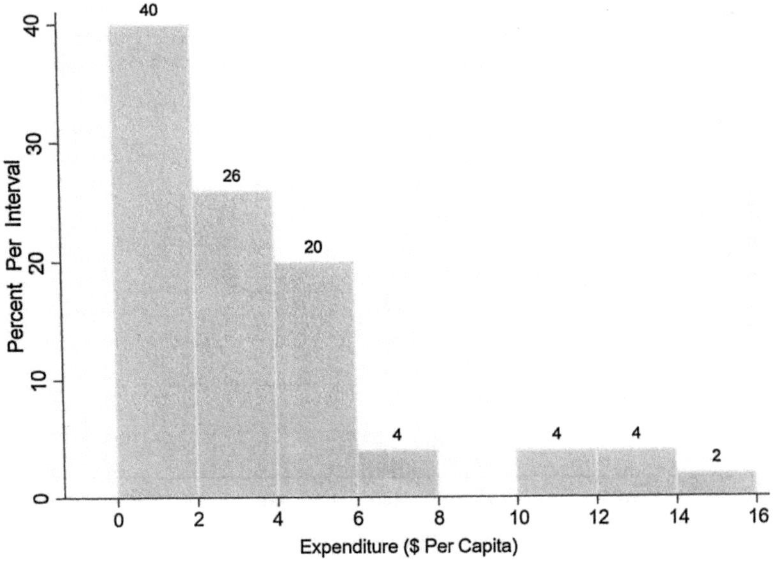

Fig. 1.10 Percentages of estimates in intervals of $2.00 per capita

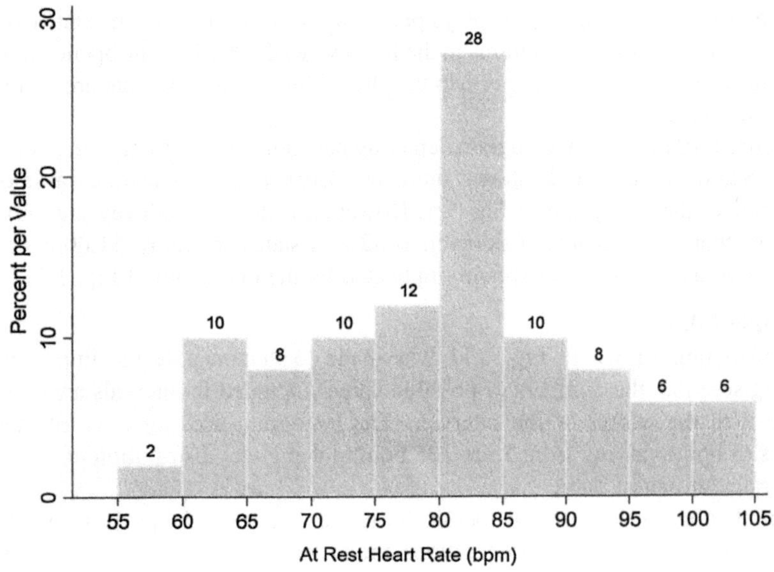

Fig. 1.11 Percentages of resting heart rates in ten intervals

The set of heart rates was determined as the number of beats per 15 seconds but recorded as beats per minute. All heart rates are multiples of 4. Intervals such as (≥ 55 to <60) and (≥ 65 to <70) include only one possible value each (56 and 68, respectively); intervals such as (≥ 60 to <65) and (≥ 80 to <85) include two possible values each (60, 64 and 80, 84, respectively). The histogram demonstrates misleading irregularities. It is not an accurate description of the distribution of the 50 heart rates.

Remark There are many other graphical displays of data distribution other than histograms. They are shown in Chap. 2.

Review Questions

1. How does the classification of qualitative and quantitative variables relate to the classification of discrete and continuous variables?
2. How can a data set consisting of a large number of observations be organized so that revelations of the observations are cogently manifested?
3. What constitutes a data distribution?
4. How is the phenomenon that individuals differ markedly reflected by the distributions of data of medical research?
5. What are the three essential properties of data distributions?
6. When the bars of a histogram denote percentages or numbers of observations in intervals, why is it critical to make sure that the widths of the bars are commensurate with the widths of the intervals?
7. Why is it important to use histograms to show percentages instead of numbers of observations?
8. What are the criteria for choosing widths of class intervals when histograms are made to expressively depict the distributions of quantitative data sets?

Exercise

1.E.1. Urine output was monitored routinely in a critical care unit. Those of 50 patients in hypovolemic shock are shown in Table 1.12. Of these patients, 25 survived and were transferred to intensive care units, and the remaining 25 died.

(a) Inspect the two sets of urine outputs and elaborate their revelations.
(b) Use frequency tables to show how the two sets of urine outputs distribute.
(c) Use histograms to display the distributions of the two data sets.
(d) Elaborate suggestions of the distributions.

1.E.2. Table 1.13 shows ratings of degree of pain of 20 participants of a study before and after administration of a pain reliever. The ratings were measured on a scale ranging from 0 (no pain) to 10 (most severe pain).

(a) Inspect the two sets of ratings and elaborate what each set reveals.
(b) Use a frequency table to show how each set of ratings distribute.
(c) Display the distributions graphically.
(d) Elaborate suggestions of the distributions, particularly whether they unveiled how the ratings of the subjects changed.

Table 1.12 Urine outputs (ml/h) of 50 patients with hypovolemic shock

Survivors	10	15	20	25	30	35	40	15	20	25	30	35	40	20	25	30	35	40	25	30	35	40	30	35	40
Nonsurvivors	10	15	20	25	30	35	40	10	15	20	25	30	35	10	15	20	25	30	10	15	20	25	10	15	20

Table 1.13 Before-and-after treatment rating of pain

Subject ID	1	2	3	4	5	6	7	8	9	10	11	12	13	14	15	16	17	18	19	20	21	22	23	24	25
Before	9	8	7	6	5	4	3	9	8	7	6	5	4	9	8	7	6	5	9	8	7	6	9	8	7
After	7	8	9	6	7	8	9	5	6	7	8	9	4	5	6	7	8	9	3	4	5	6	7	8	9

(e) Determine the difference between the before and after ratings of each subject and elaborate suggestions of the differences.
(f) Use a frequency table to show how before-and-after differences distribute.
(g) Display the distribution of the before-and-after difference graphically.
(h) Elaborate suggestions of the distribution of the before-and-after differences.

1.E.3. One entry of Table 1 of Gross and Others (2002) (Table 1.2) is the amount recommended by the CDC for expenditure on tobacco control programs. For each state, express its estimate of expenditure for tobacco-control programs as a fraction of CDC recommendation.

(a) Scrutinize the fractions and elaborate what they reveal.
(b) Use a table to show how the fractions are distributed.
(c) Display the distribution graphically.
(d) Elaborate suggestions of the distribution.

1.E.4. The 2001 tobacco settlement revenues per capita are also shown in Table 1 of Gross and Others (2002) (Table 1.2). For each state, express its estimate of expenditure for tobacco-control programs as a fraction of tobacco settlement revenue.

(a) Scrutinize the fractions and elaborate what they reveal.
(b) Use a frequency table to show how the fractions are distributed.
(c) Display the distribution graphically.
(d) Elaborate suggestions of the distribution.

1.E.5. Use a histogram displaying percentages of heart rates in intervals of width: 5 bpm to depict the post-exercise heart rates shown in Table 1.1. Discuss the relative advantage of this histogram and the one shown in Fig. 1.3.

References

Acker, M. A., et al. (2018). Mitral-valve repair vs. replacement for severe ischemic-artery stenosis. *The New England Journal of Medicine, 370*(1), 23–32.

Albers, G. W., et al. (2018). Thrombectomy for stroke at 6 to 16 hours with selection by perfusion imaging. *The New England Journal of Medicine, 378*, 708–718.

Anavekar, N. S., et al. (2004). Relation between renal dysfunction and cardiovascular outcomes after myocardial infarction. *The New England Journal of Medicine, 351*, 1285–1295.

Chosidow, O., et al. (2010). Oral ivermectin versus malathion lotion for difficult-to-treat head lice. *The New England Journal of Medicine, 362*, 896–905.

DeBaun, M. R., et al. (2014). Controlled trial of transfusions for silent cerebral infarcts in sickle cell anemia. *The New England Journal of Medicine, 371*, 699–710.

Gross, C. P., et al. (2002). State expenditure for tobacco-control programs and the tobacco settlement. *The New England Journal of Medicine, 347*(14), 1080–1086.

Hillmen, P., et al. (2004). Effect of Eculizumab on hemolysis and transfusion requirements in patients with paroxysmal nocturnal hemoglobinuria. *The New England Journal of Medicine, 350*(6), 552–559.

Sedman, A. B., et al. (1985). Evidence of aluminum loading in infants receiving intravenous therapy. *The New England Journal of Medicine, 312*(21), 1337–1343.

Walker, N., et al. (2014). Cytisine versus nicotine for smoking cessation. *The New England Journal of Medicine, 371*(25), 2353–2362.

Weintraub, W. S., et al. (2014). Comparative effectiveness of revascularization strategies. *The New England Journal of Medicine, 366*(16), 1467–1476.

Chapter 2
Graphical Displays of Data Distribution

Revelations of data are informatively manifested by graphical displays of data distributions. To read intelligently narratives of revelations of data, it is productive to review graphical displays of data distributions. To informatively report revelations of data, it is productive to articulate indications of graphical displays of data distributions. There are many types of graphical displays of data distribution. Examples of some often used ones are reviewed in this chapter. The use of box plots is reviewed in Chap. 3.

2.1 Pie Chart

Distributions of qualitative data sets are sometimes depicted by graphs that use sizes of sections of pies to denote percentages. Such graphs are known as pie charts. Not all pie charts are descriptions of data distributions. Sections of pie charts may be parades of values of means, rates, or some other quantities.

Example 2.1.1
The results of a study that screened 11,168 adolescent athletes in the England Football Association are summarized by Malhotra and Others (2015). All-cause mortality was related in the article as follows:

> Of the 92 professional clubs, 86 (93%) responded to the questionnaire regarding all-cause mortality. During a mean follow-up period of 10.6 ± 8.3 years, there were 23 deaths. The causes of death included road traffic accidents (7 deaths [30%]), cancer (5 [22%]), and suicide (1, [14%]). Cardiac disorders accounted for 8 deaths (355), all of which were sudden and occurred during exercise (Fig. 2).

The causes of the 23 deaths constitute a set of qualitative data in five categories. The percentages of the five causes comprise the distribution of the set of polytomous data. Figure 2 (Fig. 2.1) depicts the percentage graphically. Magnitudes of

P. C. Chang, *Data Analysis of Medical Studies*,
https://doi.org/10.1007/978-3-031-49984-5_2

Fig. 2.1 Figure 2 of Malhotra and Others (2015)

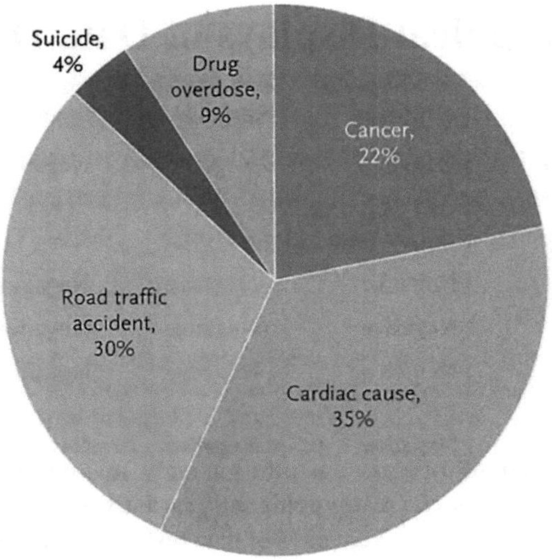

Figure 2. **Causes of Death among the 23 Screened Adolescent Soccer Players Who Died.**

percentages are signified by the sizes of sections of a pie. It is a pie chart and depicts the distribution of a qualitative data set.

Example 2.1.2

D'Acremont and Others (2014) presented the results of a study exploring the spectrum of causes of fever in African children. One result was described as follows:

> Overall, the conditions of 133 of the 1005 patients (13.2%) fulfilled the criteria for severe disease. A total of 160 illnesses were diagnosed in these patients, as shown in Fig. 3.

Figure 3 of the article (Fig. 2.2) uses the sizes of sections of a pie to denote the percentages of diagnoses. Malaria is most common (23%), followed by non-radiologically confirmed pneumonia (16%) and upper respiratory tract infection (15%). The sum of the percentages is 100.2%; its minute difference from 100% is the result of rounding off. The percentages comprise the distribution of the 160 qualitative observations; the pie presents a precise delineation of the distribution of the set of qualitative data.

Example 2.1.3

Gross and Others (2002) reported that values of 2001 tobacco settlement funds of 45 states were available. Allocation of these funds by the 45 states in aggregate was related as follows:

> State governments in aggregate distributed roughly $6.5 billion in settlement funds in 2001. Approximately 6 percent of these funds were devoted to tobacco-control programs (Fig. 1).

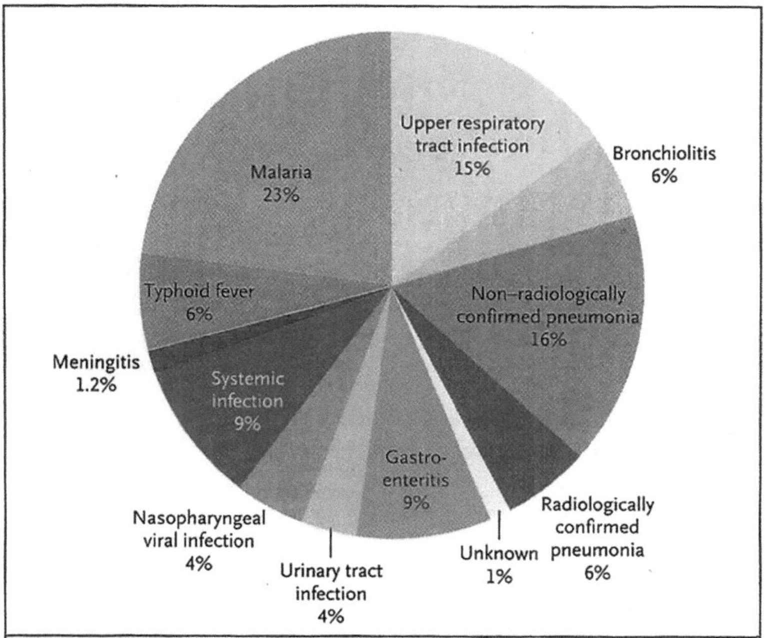

Figure 3. Distribution of All 160 Diagnoses among 133 Febrile Children with Severe Illness.

Numbers are percentages of all diagnoses. The distribution of features of severe illness was as follows: 42 cases of jaundice, 37 of respiratory distress, 27 of impaired consciousness, 19 of seizures, 14 of severe anemia (hemoglobin level, <5 g per deciliter), 9 of severe dehydration, 7 of marasmus, 5 of cardiovascular failure, 4 of plasmodium hyperparasitemia, 2 of renal failure, and 2 of meningismus. Percentages may not sum to 100 because of rounding.

Fig. 2.2 Figure 3 of D'Acremont and Others (2014)

> In aggregate, health care and medical expenditures made up approximately 41 percent of the total state settlement allocations; long-term care and medical research received 3 percent and 4 percent, respectively. Tobacco-growing communities received about 5 percent, and over one third of the funds were distributed to other non-health related programs, such as education, child and adolescent services, budget reserves, and miscellaneous programs.

Figure 1 (Fig. 2.3) uses the sizes of sections of a pie chart to denote the 6 percentages, which are percentages of an aggregate of \$6.5 billion and not percentages of observations of a qualitative data set belonging to categories. The pie chart is not a description of a data distribution.

Fig. 2.3 Figure 1 of Gross and Others (2002)

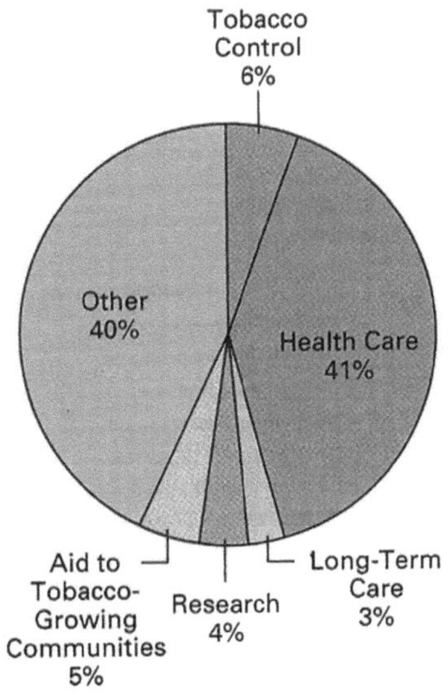

Figure 1. Allocation of Tobacco-Settlement Funds for Fiscal Year 2001.

The settlement funds allocated by the 45 states for which allocation data were available totaled roughly $6.5 billion. The "Other" category includes education (3.8 percent of the total settlement funds allocated), child and adolescent services (3.7 percent), budget reserve (13.7 percent), and miscellaneous (18.7 percent). Percentages do not total 100 because of rounding.

2.2 Bar Chart

Graphs that use rectangular bars to denote quantities are known as bar charts. When the bars of a bar chart denote percentages or numbers of observations belonging to categories, equaling distinct values, or falling in intervals, the bar chart presents a comprehensive description of the data distribution. If the bars of a bar chart denote quantities such as the means, rates, or ratios, the bar chart is not a description of the data distribution.

Example 2.2.1

Molina and Others (2014) presented the results of a study evaluating the efficacy and safety of posaconazole compared with benznidazole in adults with chronic *Trypanosoma cruzi* infection. Twenty-six eligible patients were randomly assigned to each of three treatment groups: the benznidazole group (150 mg twice daily), high-dose posaconazole group (400 mg twice daily), and low-dose posaconazole group (100 mg twice daily). A real-time polymerase chain reaction (rtPCR) assay for *Trypanosoma cruzi* DNA was performed at 8, 12, 16, 24, and 40 weeks after the end of the treatment period. The primary end point of the study was consistently negative results for the detection of *T. cruzi* DNA by rtPCR assays over the entire follow-up

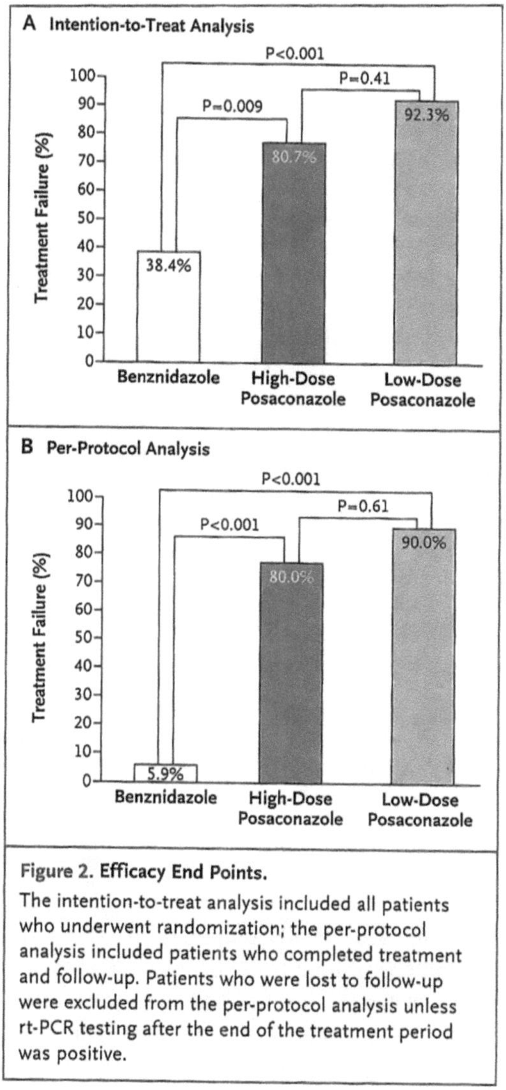

Fig. 2.4 Figure 2 of Molina and Others (2014)

period. Fig. 2 of the article (Fig. 2.4) uses the heights of bars to denote percentages of subjects who did not test positive on rtPCR over the entire follow-up period. Each percentage is a synoptic description of a dichotomous data set.

Example 2.2.2

Change in New York Heart Association (NYHA) class is one outcome of the study reported by Acker and Others (2018) (Example 1.2.5). The article stated: "Figure 2 *shows NYHA classification and mortality over time.*" Figure 2 (Fig. 2.5) uses the sections of vertical bars to denote percentages of observations belonging to each of

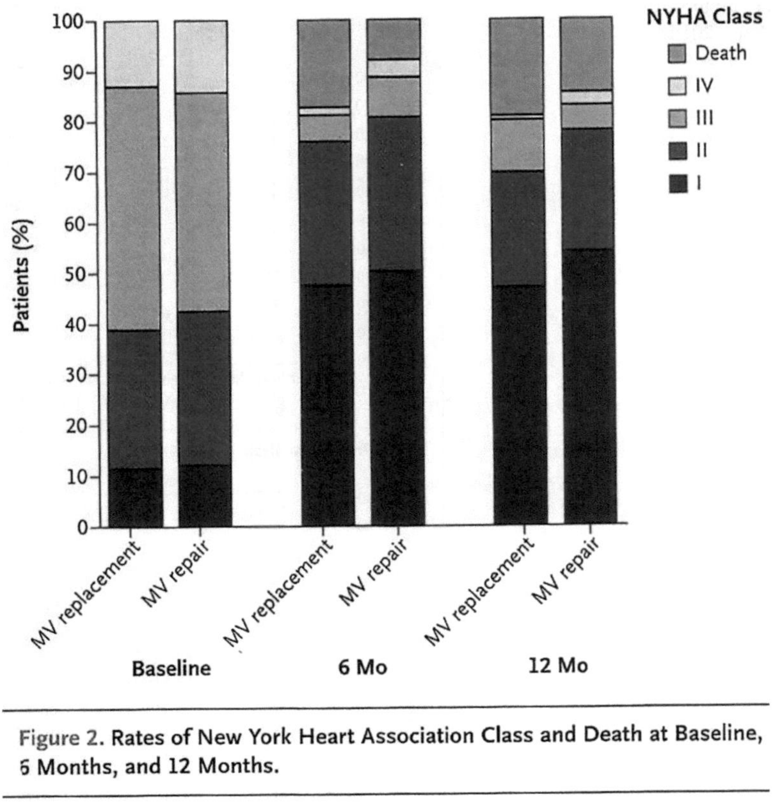

Fig. 2.5 Figure 2 of Acker and Others (2018)

five categories: NYHA class I, II, III, and IV, and died. The percentages are descriptions of qualitative data sets. Each bar depicts the distribution of one.

For instance, the first bar suggests that in the MV (mitral-valve) replacement group, the percentages of participants whose baseline NYHA classes were IV, III, II, and I were approximately 12%, 49%, 19%, and 10%, respectively. These percentages unveil how the observations of the 125 subjects of the MV replacement group were distributed among the four categories and constitute the distribution of the 125 qualitative observations. The fifth bar shows that in the MV replacement group, the percentage of subjects who died was approximately 20%, and the percentages of surviving participants whose NYHA classes were IV, III, II, and I were approximately 1%, 9%, 25%, and 45%, respectively. These percentages unveil how the observations of the 125 subjects of the MV replacement group were distributed among the five categories and constitute the distribution of the 125 qualitative observations.

Example 2.2.3
Figure 2 of Albers and Others (2018) (Fig. 1.1) uses widths of sections of horizontal bars to denote percentages of patients whose scores on the modified Rankin scale were 0, 1, 2, 3, 4, 5, or 6. Each bar depicts the distribution of one set of observations and shows how the scores of a group of patients distribute among the seven possible values.

2.3 Stem-and-Leaf Displays

A quick and easy way to bring to light revelations of a set of quantitative observations is to use a stem-and-leaf display (Tukey, 1977) to depict the distribution of the observations if the number of observations is not large. The display exhibits the numbers of observations equaling distinct values as well as values of observations. Different colors or shades may be used to indicate observations of subgroups of subjects.

One flaw of stem-and-leaf displays is that they display numbers instead of percentages of observations. The sizes of stem-and-leaf displays may differ noticeably when the numbers of observations in the data sets differ. Differences among the distributions of the data sets are distracted by differences in the sizes of stem-and-leaf displays. One advantage is that values of observations are shown, and a second advantage is that different symbols may be used to denote subgroups of subjects in different conditions.

Example 2.3.1
Figure 2.6 shows a stem-and-leaf display that portrays the distribution of the 50 systolic blood pressures shown in Table 1.1 eloquently. This figure uses integers exhibited on the left of a vertical line to label stems. Each digit on the right of the line is a leaf and represents one blood pressure. Each row of digits makes up a stem denoting an assortment of blood pressures.

For instance, 10 is the label of the first stem; the single digits 2, 4, 6, and 8 are leaves on the stem and denote four pressures 102, 104, 106, and 108 mmHg,

```
Stem        Leaves
  10 | 2 4 6 8
  11 | 0 0 0 2 2 4 4 5 6 6 8 8
  12 | 0 2 2 4 4 5 5 6 6 8
  13 | 0 0 2 4 5 5 6 8
  14 | 0 0 2 5 8
  15 | 0 5 5 8
  16 | 0 5 8
  17 | 0 5
  18 | 5
  19 | 8
```

Red: Current smoker, Blue: Never smoked, and Black: Former smoker

Fig. 2.6 A stem-and-leaf display depicting 50 systolic blood pressures respectively. 17 is the label of the eighth stem; the two digits 0 and 5 are its leaves and represent two pressures 170 and 175 mmHg, respectively. The label of the last stem is 19. This stem has just one leaf 8, representing a blood pressure of 198 mmHg.

The stem-and-leaf display presents basically the same information as the histogram of Fig. 1.4b. It shows the blood pressures distributed asymmetrically between 102 and 198 mmHg and that the majority clustered below 170 mmHg. One flaw is that it shows numbers instead of percentages of pressures; one merit is that the values of observations are explicitly shown.

One feature of Fig. 2.6 is that it uses different colors to indicate smoking status. The systolic blood pressures of never-smoked subjects were 124 mmHg or lower, and the pressures of current smokers were 168 mmHg or higher. Such information is not unveiled by the histogram of Fig. 1.4.

- *Making Stem-and-Leaf Displays*

Stem-and-leaf displays are easily made when the number of observations is not prohibitively large. One way is to sort observations of a data set into logical and convenient assortments. When observations of the same assortment are written in a row, each row is a stem; the observations in the assortment are leaves on the stem. When observations of the same assortment are written in a column, each column is a stem, and the observations in the assortment are leaves on the stem. Such a stem-and-leaf display is a histogram and a perceptive description of the distribution of the observations. It is more informative than a histogram displaying numbers of observations in that values of observations are shown.

Stem-and-leaf displays may be refined by using different shades or colors to denote observations of subgroups of subjects. Figure 2.6 is one example. It was made by the following process.

1. Table 1.1 was reviewed to assess the magnitudes of the blood pressures. As the pressures vary from 102 to 198 mmHg, it was decided that stems representing blood pressures in increments of 10 mmHg, such as 100, 110, and 120 mmHg, might yield an eloquent description of the distribution of the 50 blood pressures. 10, 11, . . ., 20 were used to label the stems, and single digits were used to label the leaves.
2. A vertical line was drawn near the left margin of a piece of paper. 10, 11, . . ., and 20 were written on the left side of the vertical line as the stem labels.
3. The first observation was 168. To denote this blood pressure by a leaf, the digit 0 was written on the right side of the vertical line as a leaf on the stem with the label 16.
4. To denote the second blood pressure 165, the digit 5 was written on the right side of the vertical line as a leaf on the stem labeled 16.
5. A rough stem-and-leaf display was completed by using leaves on appropriate stems to denote the 50 blood pressures.
6. The leaves on each stem were arranged in ascending order.

7. Leaves representing the pressures of never-smoked subjects were changed to blue color; leaves representing the pressures of current smokers were changed to red color.

Example 2.3.2

To explore revelations of the estimates of 2001 state expenditure on tobacco control programs compiled by Gross and Others (2002) (Table 1.2), a simple variation of stem-and-leaf display (Fig. 2.7) was made to display the distribution of the estimates by the following process:

1. The estimates were glanced over. It was decided that stems displaying estimates in increments of $1.00 per capita work well.
2. A vertical line was drawn near the left margin of a piece of paper.
3. The estimates 0.10, 0.13,. . ., and 0.84 were written in the first row as leaves on the first stem.
4. The estimates of 1.71, 1.74, 1.75, and 1.89 were written in the second row as leaves on the second stem.
5. The process continued until the digit 15.47 was written in the bottom row as a leaf on the last stem.
6. Leaves denoting estimates for six tobacco states were changed to red.

The stem-and-leaf unveils the same information as the histogram of Fig. 1.5. It shows that the estimates of many states are below $1.00 per capita, and those of most are below $5.00 per capita. One merit is that it shows exact values of estimates; one flaw is that it shows numbers and not percentages of estimates. It has the additional merit that it shows that the estimates of all six tobacco-producing states are below $3.00 per capita, and those of four are below $1.00 per capita.

| 0.10 0.13 0.24 0.30 0.30 0.32 0.37 0.43 0.58 0.59 0.59 0.59 0.66 0.78 0.83 0.84
| 1.71 1.74 1.75 1.89
| 2.19 2.36 2.46 2.49 2.71 2.82
| 3.03 3.08 3.29 3.32 3.44 3.52 3.80
| 4.01 4.05 4.09 4.31 4.61 4.83 4.85 4.92
| 5.15 5.62
| 6.05
| 7.32
|
|
| 10.25 10.82
|
| 12.58 12.82
|
|
| 15.47

†: Tobacco producing states in red

Fig. 2.7 Estimates of 2001 State Expenditure on tobacco control programs in Canadian Dollars per capita†

Fig. 2.8 First plasma aluminum levels of premature infants (μg/liter)

```
2         9
2  3      9
2  3  4   9  20  26  29  32  39  46  49  136  172
-----------------------------------------------------------------
Red:   One day of age and intravenous feeding.
Blue:  Older than 10 days of age and intravenous feeding.
Green: Formula feeding and more than 10 days of age.
```

Example 2.3.3

Example 1.1.5 suggests that the first plasma aluminum concentrations of the premature infants exhibited in Table 1 of Sedman and Others (1985) (Table 1.5) may be considered a set of earlier concentrations. The set of earlier concentrations was inspected. It is not immediately clear what they unveil. The stem-and-leave display shown in Fig. 2.8 was made and reviewed. It yields valuable detailed information, including the following:

- The earlier plasma aluminum concentrations of the 18 premature infants vary widely from below 2 to as high as 172 μg/liter.
- The earlier plasma aluminum concentrations of the premature infants who still required intravenous feeding when they were older than 10 days of age were 20 μg/liter or larger. Two were exceptionally large (136 and 172 μg/liter).

2.4 Dot Diagram

Distributions of quantitative data sets are often depicted by dot diagrams when the number of observations is not large. A dot diagram uses dots to denote observations. Magnitudes of observations are signified by the positions of dots. When magnitudes of observations are signified by the heights of dots; observations of the same magnitudes are denoted by dots of the same height. When magnitudes of observations are signified by the positions marked along a horizontal line, observations of the same magnitudes are denoted by columns of dots at the same position along the horizontal line.

Dot diagrams have the same shortcomings as stem-and-leaf displays in that they show numbers, not percentages, of observations. Differences among the distributions of the data sets are distracted by differences in the numbers of dots when the numbers of observations in the data sets differ noticeably. They also have the advantage that different symbols may be used to denote subgroups of subjects in different conditions.

Example 2.4.1

A study was performed to ascertain whether patients with heart failure and a normal ejection fraction have abnormalities in active relaxation and an increase in passive stiffness. Forty-seven patients who had a history of heart failure and a normal left ventricular ejection fraction (>50%) were identified. Ten patients without cardiovascular disease served as controls. The results of the study are presented by Zile and

Fig. 2.9 Figure 3 of Zile and Gaasch (2004)

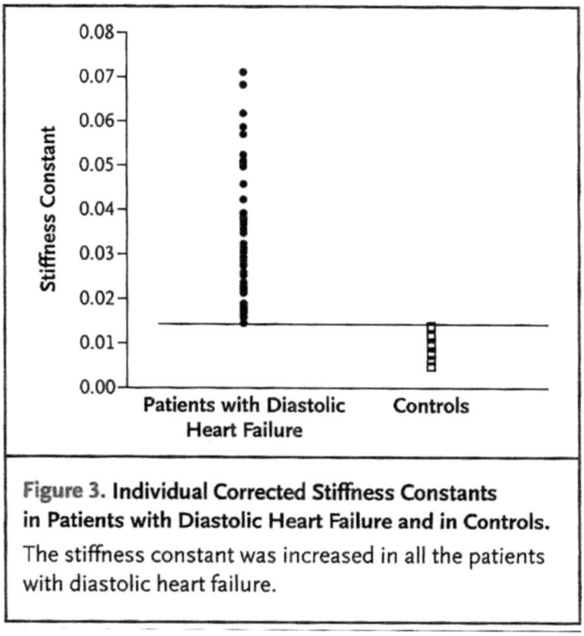

Gaasch (2004). The article stated: "*As shown in Figure 3, the chamber-stiffness constant was higher in the patients with diastolic heart failure than in the controls.*"

Figure 3 of the article (Fig. 2.9) uses assortments of dots to depict chamber stiffness constants. The heights of the dots signify the magnitudes of the chamber stiffness constants according to the labels marked along a vertical line, the vertical axis of the graph. Each assortment of dots is a dot diagram and depicts the distribution of the chamber stiffness constants of a group of subjects.

The dot diagram on the right shows that the chamber stiffness constants of the controls were all below 0.015 and lower than those of the patients with diastolic heart failure. The constants of the patients with diastolic heart failure are widely and asymmetrically distributed. While the majority of constants clustered in the lower region between 0.015 and 0.04, the remaining constants were scattered in the higher region between 0.04 and 0.070.

Example 2.4.2
Perrine and Others (1985) presented the results of a study evaluating globin biosynthesis during the natural evolution of the fetal globin switch under conditions of hyperinsulinemia. Ratios of β-globin synthesis to total non-α-globin in 10 infants of diabetic mothers and 11 infants of normal mothers at 36–39 weeks of gestation are depicted by two assortments of dots in Fig. 1 (Fig. 2.10). The heights of the dots signify the magnitudes of the ratios in accordance with the labels marked along a vertical line. Each assortment of dots is a dot diagram and depicts the distribution of the ratios of one group of infants.

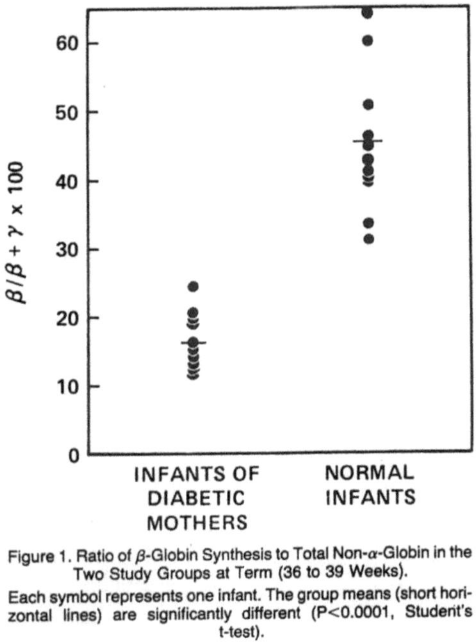

Fig. 2.10 Figure 1 of Perrine and Others (1985)

The dot diagrams show that the ratios of the infants of diabetic mothers are distributed in a low range between 10 and 25 and are lower than those of all infants of normal mothers, which are distributed in a higher and wider range between 30 and 65.

Example 2.4.3

Petersen and Others (2010) reported the results of a study that recruited 95 healthy Asian Indian men, a group known to have a high prevalence of nonalcoholic fatty liver disease. Two single-nucleotide polymorphisms (SNPs) in the gene encoding apolipoprotein C3 (APOC3) that are known to be associated with hypertriglyceridemia were genotyped. Liver triglyceride content and APOC3 genotypes were also assessed in a group of 163 healthy non-Asian Indian men. The liver triglyceride contents in the APOC3 variant allele carriers and the wild-type homozygotes are depicted in Fig. 1 of the article (Fig 2.11) by arrays of dots. The heights of the dots represent the magnitudes of the contents. Each array of dots depicts the distribution of a set of liver triglyceride contents.

The dot diagram on the left of panel A shows that the liver triglyceride contents of the wild-type homozygotes are distributed in a low and narrow range between approximately 0 and 5 percentage points. The distribution is skewed to the right, with most of the contents clustered below 2 percentage points. The dot diagram on the right reveals that the liver triglyceride contents of APOC3 variant allele carriers are distributed in a markedly wider range between 0 and 50%. The contents of many are larger than 5 percentage points.

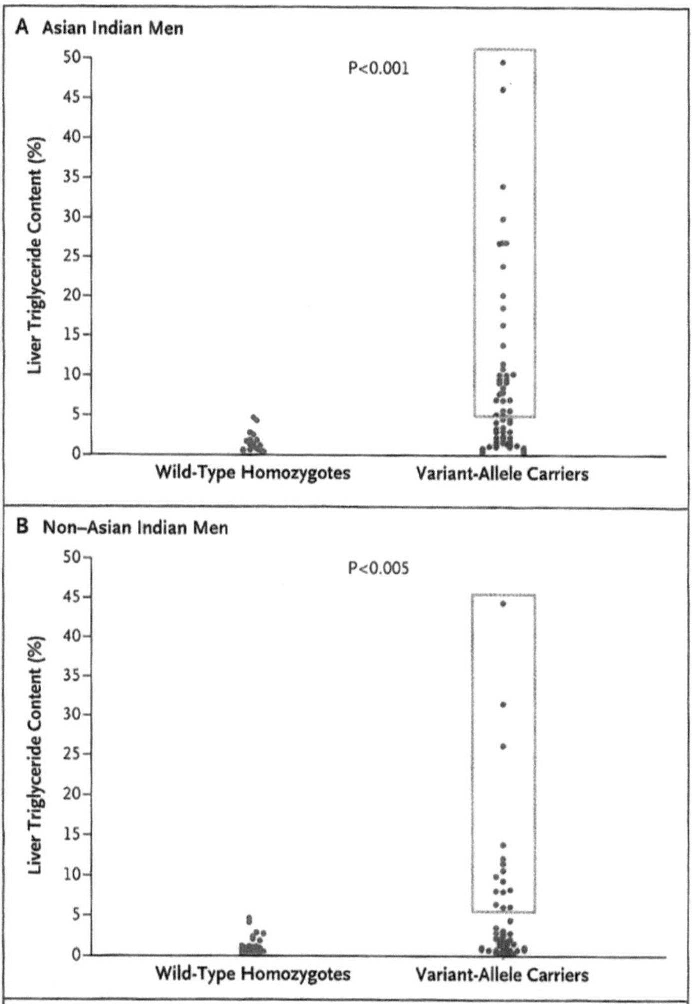

Figure 1. Scattergrams of Liver Triglyceride Content in Asian Indian and Non–Asian Indian Men.

Carriers of *APOC3* variant alleles (C-482T, T-455C, or both) were compared with *APOC3* wild-type homozygotes (C-482 and T-455) in terms of liver triglyceride content. Results are shown for two groups of Asian Indian men (Panel A) and for two groups of non–Asian Indian men (Panel B). The boxes delineate subjects who had nonalcoholic fatty liver disease (hepatic lipid content >5.5%), all of whom were carriers of the variant allele.

Fig. 2.11 Figure 1 of Petersen and Others (2010)

One feature of the figure is that it uses a box to enclose the liver triglyceride contents of subjects who had nonalcoholic fatty liver disease (hepatic lipid content >5.5%). The box reveals that the liver triglyceride contents of APOC3 variant allele carriers who had nonalcoholic fatty liver disease were larger than 5 percentage points and that those of wild-type homozygotes who did not have nonalcoholic fatty disease were smaller than 5 percentage points. A salient revelation is that the hepatic triglyceride contents of the APOC3 variant allele carriers without nonalcoholic fatty liver disease were lower than those of the APOC3 variant allele carriers with nonalcoholic fatty liver disease and comparable with those of wild-type homozygotes.

Example 2.4.4

The results of a study assessing the prevalence of alcoholic myopathy and cardio-myopathy are presented by Urbano-Marquez and Others (1989). The study determined the muscular strength of a group of 50 asymptomatic alcoholic men and a group of 50 controls—male physicians and medical students who reported drinking less than 20 g of alcohol a day. Measurements of muscle strength of the two groups of men are depicted by dot diagrams in Fig. 2 of the article (Fig. 2.12).

The dot diagrams reveal that muscular strength measurements of alcoholic men are distributed in a wide range from as low as 10 to as high as 30 kg. The measurements of the controls, on the other hand, were distributed in a narrower and higher range between 23 and 34 kg. The muscular strength measurements of the stronger alcoholic men are comparable with those of the weaker nonalcoholic controls.

One feature of the dot diagrams is that muscular strength measurements of the same magnitude are represented by a row of dots of the same height. The number of subjects having the same measurements of muscular strength is clearly indicated, and the distributions of the two sets of measurements are picturesquely portrayed.

Another feature is that different symbols are used to denote two types of subjects. Subjects with histologically normal muscle are denoted by solid dots, and subjects with histological myopathy are denoted by open circles. All controls had histologically normal muscle, and 46% (23) of the alcoholic men had histologic myopathy. Additionally, the muscular strength measurements of most (21 of 23) alcoholic men with histologic myopathy were below 20 kg and lower than those of the controls.

Example 2.4.5

Monath and Others (2011) presented the results of a study investigating the safety and immunogenicity of a yellow fever vaccine. Healthy subjects between 18 and 40 years of age were randomly assigned to receive vaccines containing 0.48 μg or 4.8 μg of antigen or placebo. Blood samples were obtained on days 0, 21, 31, and 42 to determine the neutralizing antibody titer, which was measured by the $PRNT_{50}$ titer, the highest serum dilution inhibiting 50% or more of the plaques.

Figure 1 of the article (Fig. 2.13) uses the heights of dots to denote neutralizing antibody titers of subjects in the low- and high-dose groups. Labels are marked along a vertical line—the vertical axis—to indicate magnitudes of titers signified by the heights of dots. The labels are spaced in such a way that each label is twofold the

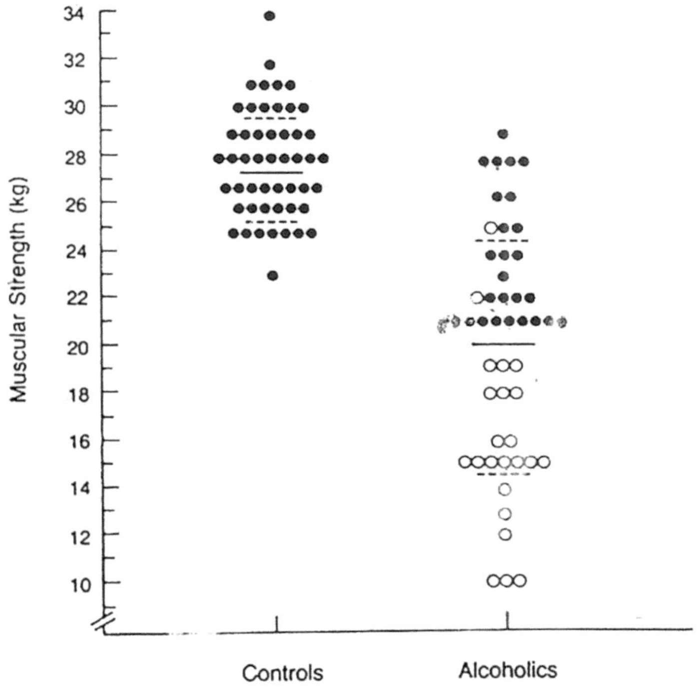

Figure 2. Measurements of Muscular Strength in 50 Alcoholic Patients and 50 Controls.

Strength was measured in the nondominant deltoid muscle (see Methods). The difference in the means is significant (P<0.001). Means are shown by solid lines, and standard deviations by dashed lines; patients with histologically normal muscle are shown by solid circles, and patients with histologic myopathy by open circles.

Fig. 2.12 Figure 2 of Urbano-Marquez and Others (1989)

label below it. Days are shown on a horizontal line. Each array of dots depicts the distribution of a set of $PRNT_{50}$ titers.

The figure yields much valuable information including the following:

- The baseline neutralizing antibody titers of all subjects were five in both groups.
- On day 21, 13% (3 of 24) of neutralizing antibody titers in the low-dose group and 32% (7 of 22) of those in the high-dose group were 20 or larger.
- On day 31, 63% (15 of 24) of neutralizing antibody titers in the low-dose group and 100% (22 of 22) of those in the high-dose group were 20 or larger.
- On day 42, 46% (11 of 24) of neutralizing antibody titers in the low-dose group and 100% (22 of 22) of those in the high-dose group were 20 or larger.

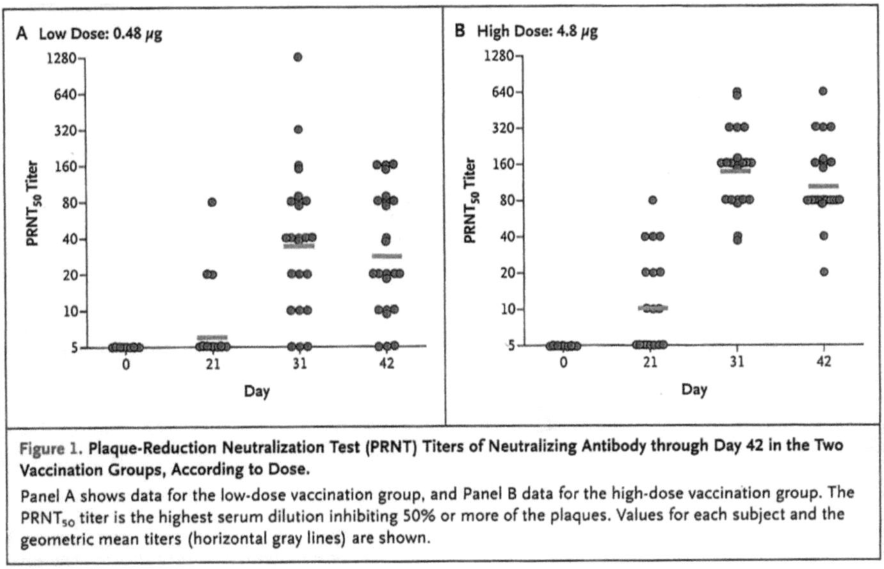

Fig. 2.13 Figure 1 of Monath and Other (2011)

2.5 Amalgamated Histograms

Histograms are important graphical displays of data distribution. The distributions of two or more sets of observations on the same variable are frequently exhibited by histograms in one figure. Such figures have the advantage that they assume less space than separate histograms, multiple dot diagrams, and multiple stem-and-leaf displays. There are several variations.

Example 2.5.1
The results of an evaluation of the effect of estrogen plus progestin on the quality of life are summarized by Hays and Others (2003). Data were obtained from the 16,608 postmenopausal women of the Women's Health Initiative (WHI) trial. These women were randomly assigned to receive estrogen plus progestin (8506 women) or placebo (8102 women). The quality of life was assessed with the use of the RAND 36-item Health Survey at baseline and at one year. The distributions of changes from baseline to year 1 in three quality-of-life measures are depicted in Fig. 2 of the article. The figure shows four panels. Panels A and B are shown in Fig. 2.14.

Each panel uses bars with two sections to present two overlapping histograms. The base section of each bar is purple; the top section of a bar may be blue or red. The height of a bar with a blue top section signifies the percentages of women in the control group whose changes were in the interval. The height of the purple base section of the bar signifies the percentages of women in the estrogen plus progestin group whose changes were in the interval. The height of a bar with a red top section

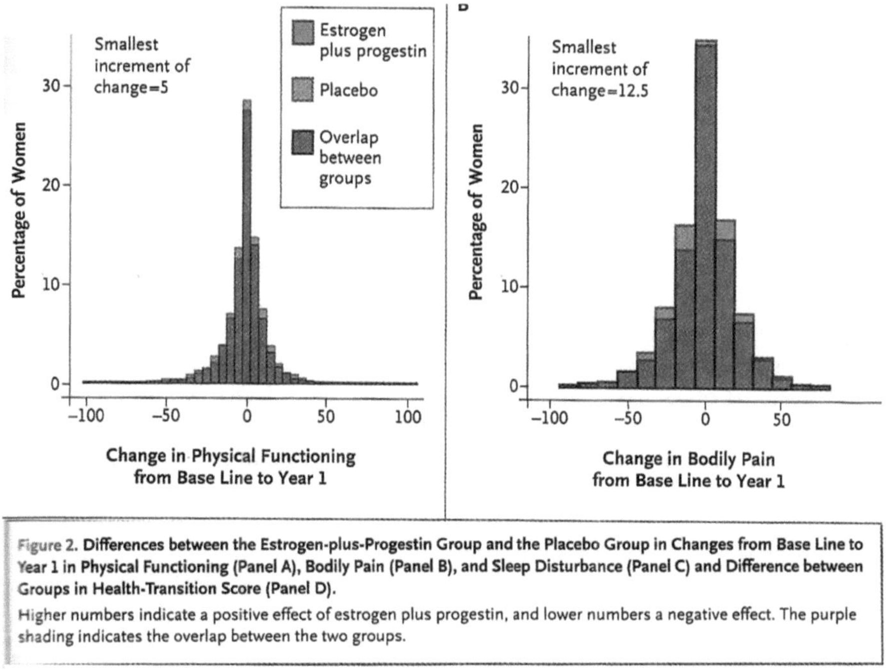

Fig. 2.14 Panels A and B of Fig. 2 of Hays and Others (2003)

signifies the percentages of women in the estrogen plus progestin group whose changes were in the interval. The height of the purple base section of the bar signifies the percentages of women in the placebo group whose changes were in the interval.

In other words, the bars with blue top sections and the purple base sections of bars with red top sections depict the distribution of the changes in the control group, and the purple base sections of the bars with red top sections and the bars with red top sections depict the distribution of the changes in the estrogen plus progestin group.

Panel A reveals the following regarding the changes in physical functioning in the two groups of women:

- The distributions of the changes in the two groups are similar. They vary widely from declines of as much as 50 points to increases of as much as 50 and overlap completely.
- The top sections of the bars on the left of zero are all blue and suggest that the placebo group has slightly higher percentages of declines.
- The top sections of the bars on the right of zero are all red and suggest that the estrogen plus progestin group has slightly higher percentages of increases.

For convenience, this type of amalgamated histogram is dubbed overlaid histogram in this book.

Example 2.5.2

The results of a study assessing whether infants at risk for congenital malformations could be identified prenatally by measurements of enzyme activity are presented by Buehler and Others (1990). The measurement of epoxide hydrolase activity in 16 patients with fetal hydantoin syndrome and 100 randomly selected pregnant women is depicted graphically in Fig. 1 of the article (Fig. 2.15).

The figure uses histograms to depict the distributions of measurement of epoxide hydrolase activity of the two groups of subjects. Gray bars show that the distribution of the 100 randomly selected pregnant women varied widely between 7.5% and 122.5% of the standard. The dark bars show that the distribution of the 16 patients varied in a narrow range between 7.5% and 37.5% of the standard.

The epoxide hydrolase activity of 16 patients with fetal hydantoin syndrome was lower than that of approximately 70% of the randomly selected women.

One feature of the figure is that the dark bars are depicted in front of the gray bars. The distribution of the patients overlaps the lower portion of the distribution of the pregnant women. The epoxide hydrolase activity of the 16 patients with fetal hydantoin syndrome was lower than that of a large percentage of pregnant women.

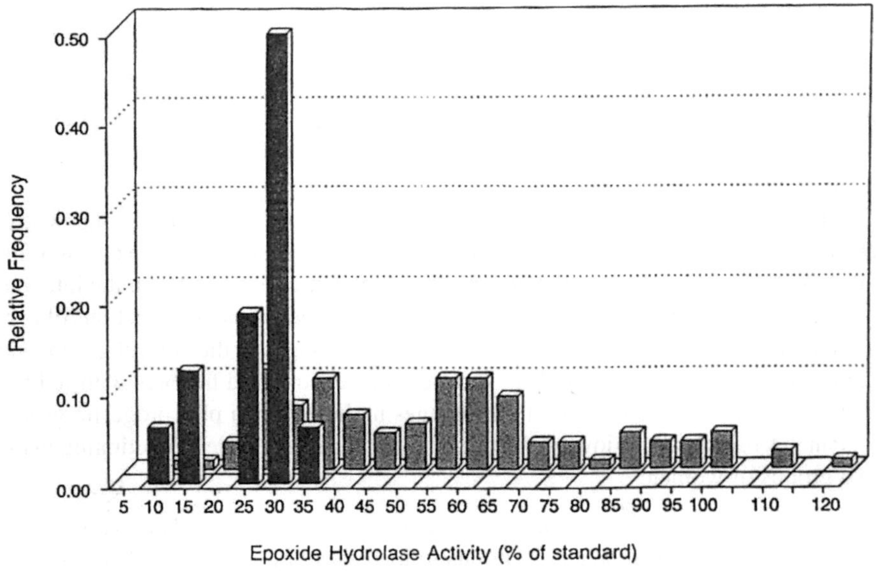

Figure 1. Distribution of Epoxide Hydrolase Activity in 100 Random Samples of Amniocytes (Gray Bars) and in Fibroblasts (12 Samples) or Amniocytes (4 Samples) from Infants Determined Retrospectively or Prospectively to Have the Fetal Hydantoin Syndrome (Solid Bars).

The enzyme activity in the samples from patients with the fetal hydantoin syndrome was less than 35 percent of the standard, whereas it ranged from 8 to 120 percent of the standard in the random samples of amniocytes.

Fig. 2.15 Figure 1 of Buehler and Others (1990)

This type of amalgamated histogram is called a double-layer histogram in this book. It has a minor shortcoming; the precise percentage denoted by the bars of the histogram on the back is uncertain. In this case, epoxide hydrolase activity measurements of randomly selected pregnant women were all below 37.5% of the standard and were comparable with those of approximately 30% of the subjects with fatal hydantoin syndrome.

Example 2.5.3 Russell (371, 4)

Russell and Others (2014) presented the results of two studies evaluating the safety and effectiveness of a wearable "bionic" pancreas that uses data from a continuous glucose monitor to control the delivery of insulin and glucagon. One study used 20 adults and the other 32 adolescents with type 1 diabetes mellitus as subjects. Subjects in both studies received therapy with the bionic pancreas for 5 days and therapy with their own insulin pumps for 5 days in random orders. During each monitoring period, glucose levels were determined every 2 hours. The mean of the glucose levels of each subject determined during the monitoring period was computed and used as a summary measure of the glucose levels of the subject during the period.

The mean glucose levels on days 2 through 5 of the two monitoring periods are depicted in Fig. 4 of the article. Panels A and B of the figure are shown in Fig. 2.16. Panel A uses the heights of bars to denote the numbers of adults whose mean glucose levels were in the interval. A blue bar denotes the number of mean glucose levels in the interval during the bionic pancreas period; an adjoining red bar denotes the number of mean glucose levels in the same interval during the control period. The blue bars make up a histogram and depict how the mean glucose levels during the

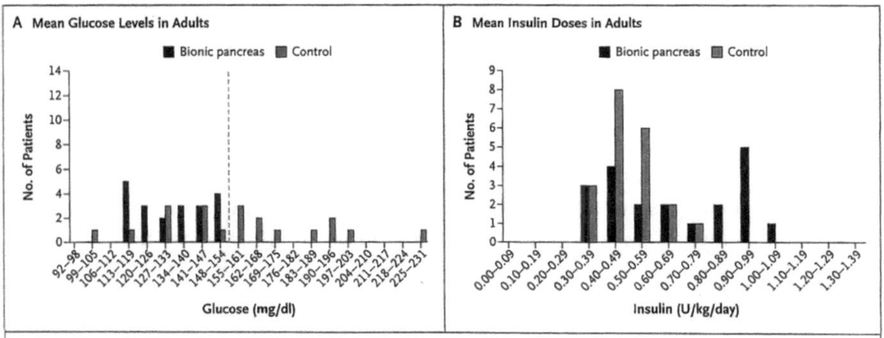

Figure 4. **Histogram Distributions of Mean Glucose Levels and Insulin Doses among Adults and Adolescents.**

Panel A shows a histogram distribution of the mean glucose levels on continuous monitoring in adults during the bionic-pancreas period and the control period. The distribution shows the number of patients with mean glucose levels divided into intervals of 7 mg per deciliter on days 2 through 5. The dashed red line indicates a mean glucose level of 154 mg per deciliter, which corresponds to a glycated hemoglobin level of 7%. Panel B shows a similar histogram distribution of total daily doses of insulin in the adults, divided into intervals of 0.1 U per kilogram of body weight per day. Panels C and D show similar histogram distributions for the adolescents, with a cutoff point for the mean glucose level of 168 mg of glucose per deciliter, which corresponds to a glycated hemoglobin level of 7.5%. To convert the values for glucose to millimoles per liter, multiply by 0.05551.

Fig. 2.16 Panels A and B of Fig. 4 of Russell and Others (2014)

bionic pancreas period are distributed; the red bars make a histogram and depict how the mean glucose levels during the control period are distributed.

The red bars suggest that the distribution of the mean glucose levels of the adults during the control period varies in a wide range from approximately 99 mg/dl to approximately 231 mg/dl. The blue bars suggest that the distribution of the mean glucose levels of the adults during the bionic pancreas period varies in a lower and narrower range from approximately 113 to approximately 154 mg/dl and overlaps the lower portion of the distribution during the control period. The mean glucose levels during the bionic pancreas period were lower than the mean glucose levels during the control period.

For convenience, this type of amalgamated histogram may be dubbed an intermingled histogram. A special feature of Fig. 4A is that a red vertical line is shown to mark the therapeutic goal recommended for adults by the American Diabetic Association (154 mg/dl). The figure reveals that the mean glucose levels of all adults attained the therapeutic goal during the bionic pancreas period and that those of 11 (55%) did not attain the therapeutic goal during the control period.

2.6 Frequency Polygon

Distributions of quantitative observations are often depicted by frequency polygons or frequency curves that are adaptations of histograms. A frequency polygon uses line segments, and a frequency curve uses a curve to connect the tops of the bars of a histogram. They bring to light the location, variation, and skewness of data distributions picturesquely. One merit is that the distributions of several data sets are displayed in one figure.

In mathematical statistics, properties of distributions of discrete random variables are specified by functions known as probability functions, and properties of continuous random variables are specified by functions known as density functions. Frequency polygons and frequency curves denoting percentages of observations equaling distinct values are data counterparts of graphical displays of probability functions of discrete random variables. Frequency polygons and frequency curves denoting percentages of observations in class intervals are data counterparts of graphical displays of density functions of continuous random variables.

Example 2.6.1
Kimm and Others (2002) summarized the results of the National Heart, Lung, and Blood Institute Growth and Health Study. This study followed 1213 black and 1166 white 9- to 10-year-old girls for 10 years. Energy expenditure needed by leisure activities beyond activities of daily living was assessed by the Habitual Activity Questionnaire (HAQ). Scores of HAQ, expressed as MET-times per week, were determined to estimate weekly metabolic equivalence of recorded activities.

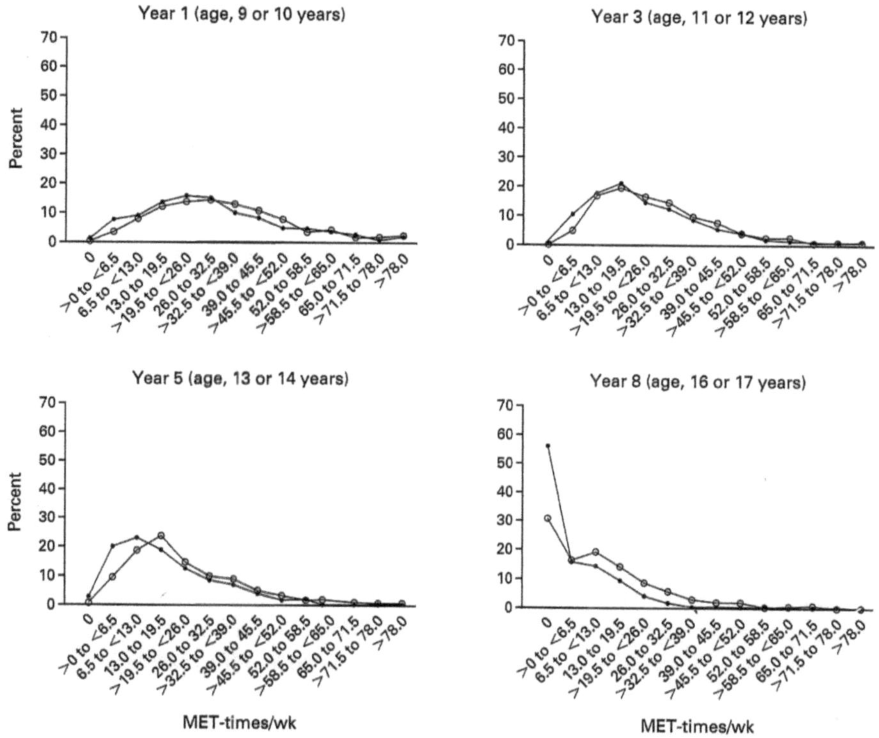

Figure 1. Frequency Distribution of Habitual Activity Questionnaire Scores According to Year of Study and Race. Scores are expressed in MET-times per week. Solid circles represent black girls, and open circles white girls.

Fig. 2.17 Figure 1 of Kimm and Others (2002)

The following is a narrative of the HAQ scores of the black and white girls:

> HAQ scores were skewed toward the lower end of the distribution at base line for both groups and shifted more to the left with time (Fig. 1). Racial differences became more notable at older ages, particularly at the lower end of the distributions.

This narrative is corroborated by Fig. 1 of the article (Fig. 2.17). It uses frequency polygons to depict the distributions of HAQ scores. The heights of dots or circles on the polygons signify the percentages of HAQ scores in intervals marked on a horizontal line, the horizontal axis. Labels on a vertical line, the vertical axis, indicate the magnitudes of percentages signified by the heights of the dots or circles. A polygon formed by line segments connecting dots depicts the distribution of HAQ scores of black girls; a polygon formed by line segments connecting open circles depicts the distributions of HAQ scores of white girls. They clarify the above narrative.

- *HAQ scores were skewed toward the lower end of the distribution at base line for both groups and shifted more to the left with time.*

This refers to the manifestations of the frequency polygons that the percentage of the area enclosed under the lower half of the polygon depicting the distribution of year-1 HAQ scores is larger than the area enclosed under the higher half of the polygon and that this distinction was amplified when the subjects were older. In statistical jargon, the distributions of the scores are skewed to the right (right skewed or positively skewed), and the degrees of right skewness are amplified when the girls are older.

- *Racial differences became more notable at older ages, particularly at the lower end of the distributions.*

This alludes to the manifestation of frequency polygons that the percentages of low scores among black and white girls, e.g., <19.5, were close when the girls were 11–12 years of age and younger but differed notably when the girls were 13 or 14 years of age and older.

Example 2.6.2
An article by the SUPPORT Study Group of the Eunice Kennedy Shriver NICH Neonatal Research Network (2010) reported the results of a study that compared the effects of target ranges of oxygen saturation of 85–89% and 91–95% on preterm infants. Subjects of the study included 1316 infants who were born between 24 weeks 0 days and 27 weeks 6 days of gestation. The primary outcome was a composite of severe retinopathy of prematurity, death before discharge from the hospital, or both. The median of the actual levels of oxygen saturation of each infant was determined and used as a summary measure of the actual levels of oxygen saturation of the infant. Figure 3 (Fig. 2.18) uses frequency polygons to depict the distributions of the median levels of oxygen saturation of the two groups of infants.

The frequency polygons suggest that the distributions of actual levels of oxygen saturation of the two groups of infants differed subtly. They vary in similar ranges and overlap considerably. In the high target group, the actual levels of oxygen saturation of most infants attained the target range (91–95%), and those of a rather small percentage of the infants were larger than the target range. In the lower target range group, on the other hand, the actual levels of oxygen saturation of most infants were larger than the target range (85–89%), and those of approximately 10% or more of the infants were even larger than the higher target range.

Example 2.6.3
Stramer and Others (2004) presented the results of a study that analyzed all antibody nonreactive donations that were positive for HIV-1 and HCV RNA on nucleic acid amplification testing of pools of 16–24 donations by the main blood collection programs in the United States during the first three years of nucleic acid screening (1999 through 2002). Figure 1 of the article (Fig. 2.19) uses frequency curves to depict distributions of logarithms (base 10) of alanine aminotransferase levels. The heights of points on the curves denote percentages of levels in class intervals. Labels are marked along a vertical line, the vertical axis, to indicate values of percentages signified by the heights of points on the curves. Logarithms (base 10) of alanine aminotransferase levels are marked along a horizontal line the horizontal axis.

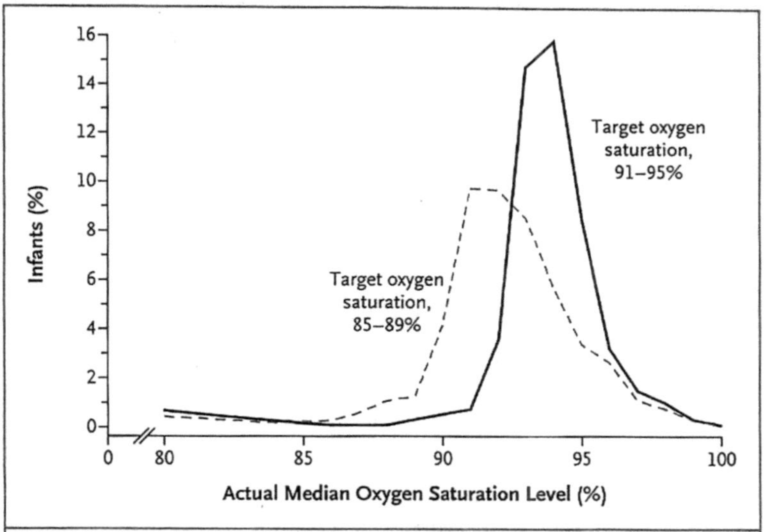

Figure 3. Actual Median Oxygen Saturation with Oxygen Supplementation in the Two Treatment Groups.
The medians of the distributions were significantly different on the basis of a rank-sum test (P<0.001). The 80% level of oxygen saturation shown includes all values at or below 80%.

Fig. 2.18 Figure 3 of SUPPORT Study Group of the Eunice Kennedy Shriver NICHD Neonatal Research Network

The frequency curves divulge much valuable information, including the following:

1. The two green curves are comparable; they are both relatively symmetric and vary from approximately 0.5–2.5 on the log scale (3.3–330 IU/l). They suggest that the distributions of aminotransferase levels of the two groups of donors with nonreactive nucleic acid test, nonactive and positive HCV antibody acid test, are comparable.
2. The two brown curves are skewed to the right and vary between 1.0 and above 3.0 approximately on the log scale. They suggest that the distributions of aminotransferase levels of the two groups of donors with positive nucleic acid test, positive and nonreactive HCV antibody test, are highly skewed to the right and vary widely from below 10.0 to above 1000.0 IU/l. The aminotransferase levels of most donors are below 120 IU/liter.
3. The distributions of aminotransferase levels of the two groups of donors with nonreactive nucleic acid tests (green curves) disperse in narrower ranges and overlap the lower halves of the distributions of aminotransferase levels of the two groups of donors with positive nucleic acid tests (brown curves). The two groups

Fig. 2.19 Figure 1 of Stramer and Others (2004)

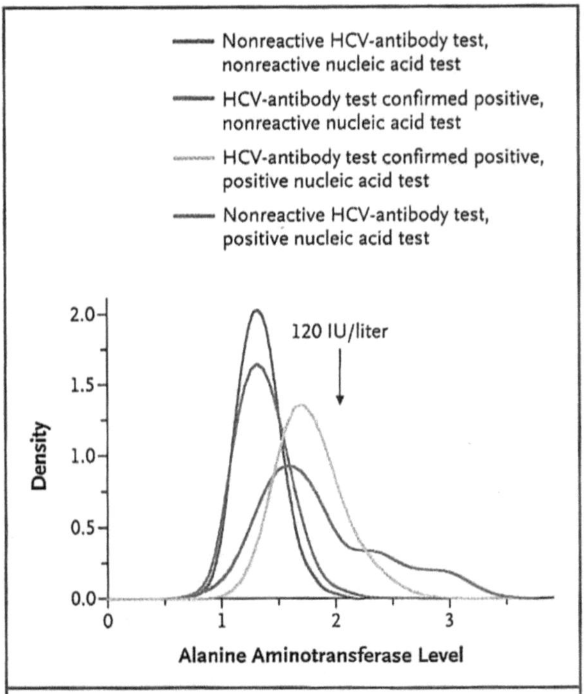

Figure 1. **Distribution of Alanine Aminotransferase Levels According to HCV Status.**

The alanine aminotransferase values, which are given on a base 10 logarithmic scale, in each of the four groups were used to estimate probability densities.

of positive nucleic acid test donors, HCV antibody test positive or nonreactive, had higher percentages of large enzyme levels (120 IU/liter or larger) than the two groups of nonreactive nucleic acid test donors.

2.7 Cumulative Distribution Curves

Cumulative and reverse cumulative distribution curves are graphical displays of data distributions that are particularly useful when percentages of large or small observations are of interest. They are also called ogives.

Cumulative distribution curves and reverse cumulative curves may be right closed (left open) or right open (left closed).

- A right-closed cumulative distribution curve displays right-closed cumulative percentages—percentages of observations in a data set that are smaller than or as small as selected values.
- A right-open cumulative distribution curve displays right-open cumulative percentages—percentages of observations in a data set that are smaller than selected values.
- A left-closed reverse distribution curve displays left-closed reverse cumulative percentages—percentages of observations in a data set that are larger than or as large as selected values.
- A left-open reverse cumulative distribution curve displays left-open reverse cumulative percentages—percentages of observations in a data set that are larger than selected values.

For a given value, the sum of the right-closed cumulative percentage and the left-open reverse cumulative percentage is 100%. The sum of the right-open cumulative percentage and the left-close reverse cumulative percentage is 100%.

Remark Right-closed cumulative distribution curves are data analogies of graphical displays of cumulative distribution functions of random variables that characterize the probability of random variables smaller than or equal to the given values.

- *Statistical Properties of Data Distributions Suggested by Cumulative Distribution Curves*

Cumulative and reverse cumulative distribution curves are most useful for the purpose of depicting percentages of large or small observations. They also unveil the essential properties of data distributions. Appraising essential properties of data distributions by reviewing cumulative and reverse cumulative distribution curves is relatively technical. It is briefly elaborated in the following:

Range The two points on the horizontal axis where a cumulative distribution curve ascends from 0% to 100% or a reverse cumulative distribution descends from 100% to 0% comprise the range of the curve. It is a crude assessment of the range of the distribution.

Center The value where a cumulative distribution curve ascends to 50% or a reverse cumulative distribution curve descends to 50% is the median of the data distribution and an indication of the location of the center of the data distribution.

Skewness The skewness of a data distribution is indicated by the following:

- Symmetry is suggested when the left and right halves of a cumulative or a reverse cumulative distribution curve are mirror images of each other and suggest that the percentages of observations in the left half and right half of the range of the distribution are close.
- Right skewness is suggested when the right half of a cumulative distribution curve ascends at a noticeably slower rate than its left half or the right half of a reverse cumulative distribution curve descends at a noticeably slower rate than its

left half. In other words, right skewness is suggested if a cumulative distribution curve or a reverse cumulative distribution curve submits that the percentage of larger observations in the right half of the range of the data distribution is noticeably lower than the percentage of smaller observations in the left half of the range of the distribution.

- Left skewness is suggested when the left half of a cumulative distribution curve ascends at a noticeably slower rate compared with its right half or the left half of a reverse cumulative distribution curve descends at a noticeably slower rate compared with its right half. In other words, left skewness is suggested if a cumulative distribution curve or reverse cumulative distribution curve submits that the percentage of smaller observations in the left half of the range of the data distribution is noticeably lower than the percentage of larger observations in the right half of the range of the distribution.

Example 2.7.1

Lange and Others (2004) presented the results of a study evaluating the effect of folate therapy on the risk of angiographic restenosis after coronary stent placement. The study randomly assigned patients who had undergone successful coronary stenting to receive folate therapy or a placebo. Coronary angiograms were obtained at baseline, immediately after stenting, and at follow-up (six months after stenting). The primary angiographic end point was the minimal luminal diameter within the target lesion at follow-up.

Figure 1 of the article (Fig. 2.20) uses cumulative distribution curves to depict distributions of minimal luminal diameters at baseline, immediately after stenting, and at follow-up. The curves may be closed or open cumulative distribution curves. This example assumes that they are right-closed cumulative distribution curves and heights of points on the curves signify the right-closed cumulative percentages—percentages of minimal luminal diameters smaller than or as small as values marked along the horizontal line. The cumulative distribution curves yield valuable information, including the following:

Before stenting (baseline)

The two curves on the left depict the distributions of the baseline minimal luminal diameters of the two treatment groups. They virtually coincide and suggest that the distributions are nearly identical. More specifically:

- The two curves rise from approximately 5% to 100% between 0 and 1.5 mm. This suggests that the baseline minimal luminal diameters of the two groups vary between approximately 0 and 1.5 mm.
- The curves reach 50% at approximately 0.5 mm. The minimal luminal diameters of approximately 50% of the subjects are less than 0.5 mm; those of the remaining 50% disperse between 0.5 and 1.5 mm.
- The curves are asymmetric; they rise at a fast rate before reaching 90% at 1.0 mm and at a much slower rate after reaching 90%. They are skewed to the right. In

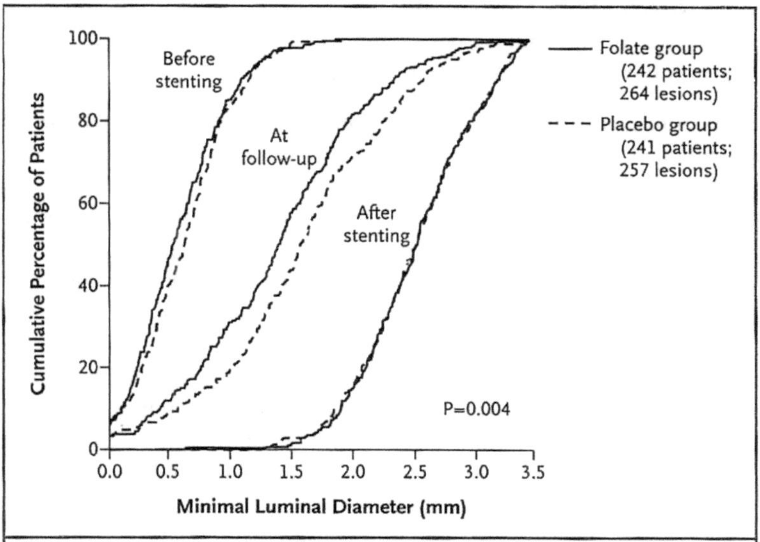

Figure 1. Cumulative Distribution of the Minimal Luminal Diameter before and Immediately after Stent Implantation and at Follow-up Angiography in the Folate Group and the Placebo Group.
A significant shift to the left is seen at follow-up in the folate group, indicating that the minimal luminal diameter was smaller in this group than in the placebo group.

Fig. 2.20 Figure 1 of Lange and Others (2004)

both groups, approximately 90% of the diameters are distributed between 0 and 1.0 mm, and those of the remaining 10% are scattered sporadically between 1.0 and 1.5 mm.

Immediately after stenting

The two curves on the right depict the distributions of the minimal luminal diameters determined immediately after stenting. They coincide completely. The two distributions are virtually identical. More specifically:

- The two curves rise from 0% to 100% between approximately 1.25 and 3.5 mm and suggest that the after-stenting diameters of the two groups of participants vary between approximately 1.25 and 3.5 mm.
- The curves reach 50% at approximately 2.5 mm; the centers of the distributions are in the vicinity of 2.5 mm.
- The distributions are slightly skewed to the left. They rise at a slower rate to approximately 10% between 1.25 and 2.0 mm and then at a faster rate to 100% between 2.0 and 3.5 mm.

Follow-up (six months after stenting)
The two curves in the middle depict the distributions of the minimal luminal diameters at follow-up (6 months after stenting).

- The distributions of the diameters of the two groups of patients are relatively symmetric and vary widely in comparable wide ranges from close to 0 to close to 3.5 mm.
- The solid curve is shifted to the left of the dotted curve. It reaches 50% at approximately 1.25 mm, and the dotted curve reaches 50% at approximately 1.5 mm. The center of the distribution of the diameters of the folate group is in the vicinity of 1.25 mm, and the center of the distribution of the diameters of the placebo group is in the vicinity of 1.5 mm.
- The folate group had a larger percentage of smaller lesions than the folate group. For instance, the percentage of diameters smaller than 1.0 mm was nearly 30% in the folate group and approximately 20% in the control group; the percentage of diameters shorter than 1.5 was nearly 50% in the folate group and approximately 40% in the control group.

Example 2.7.2
In addition to the dot plots of Fig. 1 (Fig. 2.13), Monath and Others (2011) also used reverse cumulative distribution curves to depict $PRNT_{50}$ titers on day 42. Figure 2 (Fig. 2.21) shows three descending curves and refers to the curves as cumulative reverse distributions. Although it is not explicitly indicated, the wording of the article suggests that they are left-closed reverse cumulative distribution curves. The heights of points on the curves signify the percentages of neutralizing antibody titers as larger as or larger than the values shown on the horizontal axis.

The left-closed reverse cumulative distribution curves reveal that the high-dose group had higher percentages of large neutralizing antibody titers. For instance:

- The percentage of day 42 neutralizing antibody titers larger than 10 was 100% in the high-dose group, approximately 70% in the low-dose group, and 0% in the control group.
- The percentage of day 42 neutralizing antibody titers larger than 20 was approximately 95% in the high-dose group, approximately 45% in the low-dose group, and 0% in the placebo group.

Review Questions
1. What are the relative advantages of stem-and-leaf display, dot diagram, and histogram?
2. How can stem-and-leaf display and dot diagram be made to describe differences among subsets of subjects in addition to distributions of data?
3. What are the relative advantages of the different kinds of amalgamated histograms?
4. Is it important to state clearly whether cumulative distribution curves are right closed or right open or reverse cumulative distribution curves are left open or left closed?

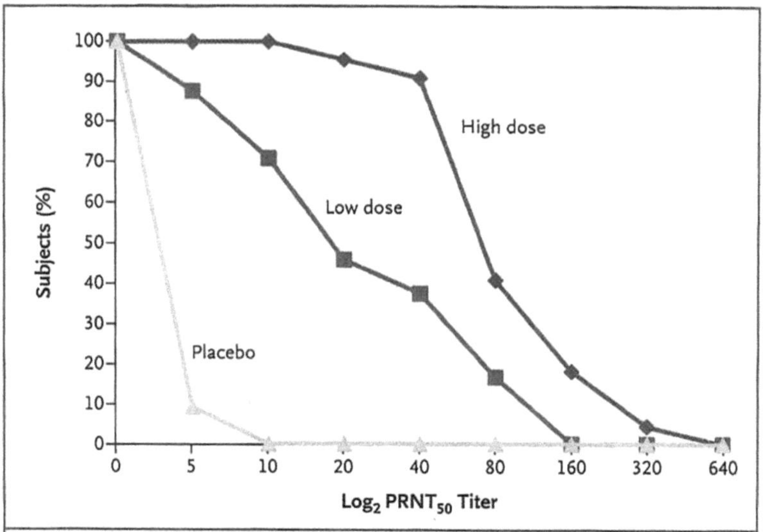

Figure 2. Cumulative Reverse Distribution of Plaque-Reduction Neutralization Test (PRNT) Titers of Neutralizing Antibody at Day 42, According to Study Group.

The $PRNT_{50}$ titer is the highest serum dilution inhibiting 50% or more of the plaques.

Fig. 2.21 Figure 2 of Monath and Others (2011)

Exercise

2.E.1. Use a pie chart and a bar chart to depict the sexes of the 50 subjects whose data are shown in Table 1.1. Discuss the relative advantages of using these graphs and a table to depict the set of observations.

2.E.2. Review the urine outputs displayed in Table 1.12.

(a) Use stem-and-leaf displays, dot diagrams, and histograms to depict the distributions of the two sets of urine outputs.

(b) Discuss the relative advantages of stem-and-leaf display, dot diagram, and histogram for the purpose of depicting the revelations of the two sets of urine outputs.

2.E.3. Appraise the before and after treatment pain indices displayed in Table 1.13.

(a) Use histograms, stem-and-leaf displays, and dot diagrams to depict the distributions of the two sets of indices.

(b) Discuss the relative advantages of stem-and-leaf displays and dot diagrams for the purpose of depicting the distributions of the two sets of indices.

(c) Elaborate revelations of the two distributions with respect to the effect of the treatment.
(d) Use a histogram, stem-and-leaf display, and dot diagram to depict the distribution of the differences between the before and after pain indices of the subjects.
(e) Elaborate revelation of the distribution of the differences that is not unveiled by the distributions of the before and after indices.

2.E.4. Fractions of CDC recommendations that were spent for tobacco control programs were computed for Problem 1.E.4.

(a) Use a stem-and-leaf display, dot diagram, frequency polygon, and cumulative distribution curve to depict the distribution of the fractions. Identify the six tobacco-producing states whenever feasible.
(b) Discuss the relative advantages of these graphical displays of the distribution of the fractions for the purpose of exploring the revelations of the fractions.

2.E.5. Fractions of tobacco settlement revenue that were spent for tobacco control programs were computed Problem 1.E.5.

(a) Use a stem-and-leaf display, dot diagram, frequency polygon, and cumulative distribution curve to depict the distribution of the fractions. Identify the six tobacco-producing states whenever feasible.
(b) Discuss the relative advantages of these graphical displays of the distribution of the fractions for the purpose of exploring the revelations of the fractions.

2.E.6. Review Fig. 1B of Petersen and Others (2010) (Fig. 2.11) and elaborate what it unveils.
2.E.7. Review Fig. 2B of Hays and Others (2003) (Fig. 2.14) and elaborate what it unveils.
2.E.8. Review Fig. 4B of Russell and Others (2014) (Fig. 2.16).

(a) Elaborate what this graph unveils.
(b) Discuss how useful this graph is for the purpose of depicting changes in individual subjects.

References

Acker, M. A., et al. (2018). Mitral-valve repair vs. replacement for severe ischemic-artery stenosis. *The New England Journal of Medicine, 370*(1), 23–32.

Albers, G. W., et al. (2018). Thrombectomy for stroke at 6 to 16 hours with selection by perfusion imaging. *The New England Journal of Medicine, 378*, 708–718.

Buehler, B. A., et al. (1990). Prenatal prediction of risk of the fetal hydantoin syndrome. *The New England Journal of Medicine, 322*(22), 1567–1572.

D'Acremont, V., et al. (2014). Beyond malaria—Causes of fever in outpatient Tanzanian children. *The New England Journal of Medicine, 370*(9), 809–817.

Gross, C. P., et al. (2002). State expenditure for tobacco-control programs and the tobacco settlement. *The New England Journal of Medicine, 347*(14), 1080–1086.

Hays, J., et al. (2003). Effects of estrogen plus progestin on health-related quality of life. *The New England Journal of Medicine, 348*(19), 1839–1854.

Kimm, Y. S. S., et al. (2002). Decline in physical activity in black girls. *The New England Journal of Medicine, 347*(10), 709–715.

Lange, H., et al. (2004). Folate therapy and in-stent restenosis after coronary stenting. *The New England Journal of Medicine, 350*(26), 2673–2681.

Malhotra, A., et al. (2015). Outcomes of cardiac screening in adolescent soccer players. *The New England Journal of Medicine, 379*(6), 524–534.

Molina, I., et al. (2014). Randomized trial of posaconazole and benznidazole for chronic chagas' disease. *The New England Journal of Medicine, 370*(20), 1899–1908.

Monath, T. P., et al. (2011). An inactivated cell-culture vaccine against yellow fever. *The New England Journal of Medicine, 364*(14), 1326–1333.

Perrine, S. P., et al. (1985). Delay in the fetal globin switch in infants of diabetic mothers. *The New England Journal of Medicine, 312*, 334–338.

Petersen, K. F., et al. (2010). Apolipoprotein C3 gene variants in nonalcoholic fatty liver disease. *The New England Journal of Medicine, 362*(12), 1082–1089.

Russell, S. J., et al. (2014). Inpatient glycemic control with a bionic pancreas in type 1 diabetes. *The New England Journal of Medicine, 371*(4), 313–325.

Sedman, A. B., et al. (1985). Evidence of aluminum loading in infants receiving intravenous therapy. *The New England Journal of Medicine, 312*(21), 1337–1343.

Stramer, S. L., et al. (2004). Detection of HIV-1 and HCV infection among antibody-negative blood donors by nucleic acid-amplification testing. *The New England Journal of Medicine, 351*(6), 760–768.

SUPPORT study Group of the Eunice Kennedy Shriver NICHD neonatal research network. (2010). Target ranges of oxygen saturation in extremely preterm infants. *The New England Journal of Medicine, 362*(21), 1959–1969.

Tukey, J. W. (1977). *Exploratory Data Analysis*. Eddison-Wesley Publishing Company.

Urbano-Marquez, A., et al. (1989). The effect of alcoholism on skeletal and cardiac muscle. *The New England Journal of Medicine, 320*(7), 409–415.

van Bone, L., et al. (2014). Proteome-wide analysis and EXCL4 as a biomarker in systemic sclerosis. *The New England Journal of Medicine, 370*(5), 433–443.

Zile, M. R., & Gaasch, W. H. (2004). Diastolic heat failure-abnormalities in active relaxation and passive stiffness. *The New England Journal of Medicine, 350*(19), 1953–1959.

Chapter 3
Descriptive Statistics

Revelations of data are routinely described synoptically by values of descriptive statistics that are measures of properties of data distributions. To read such descriptions intelligently, it is essential to be able to appreciate the indications of the statistics. To report informatively, it is vital to stress the manifestations of the distributions of the observations.

This chapter examines indications of often-used descriptive statistics. As much as values of descriptive statistics can be easily computed by computers, computation procedures are not stressed.

3.1 Percentage and Proportion

Percentage and proportion are expressions of the same quantity. The percentages of a set of qualitative observations belonging to categories constitute the distributions of the set of observations. They expose informatively revelations of qualitative data.

Percentages and proportions may be computed from numbers of observations or numbers of observational units. Usually, there is one observation per observational unit. The percentage (proportion) of observations of a data set meeting a criterion is also the percentage (proportion) of observational units of the data set meeting the criterion. Occasionally, some observational units have more than one observation. In this case, when revelations of data are articulated by percentages or proportions, it is critical to make it clear whether they are percentages (proportions) of observations or percentages (proportions) of observational units.

A proportion of observations of a data set meeting a criterion is simply:

$$\begin{aligned}&\text{Proportion of observations of a data set meeting a criterion}\\&\quad=\frac{\text{Number of observations of the data set meeting the criterion}}{\text{Number of observations in the data set}}.\end{aligned}\tag{3.1.1}$$

P. C. Chang, *Data Analysis of Medical Studies*,
https://doi.org/10.1007/978-3-031-49984-5_3

A proportion of observational units of a data set meeting a criterion equals:

$$\text{Proportion of observational units of a data set meeting a criterion} = \frac{\text{Number of observational units of the data set meeting the criterion}}{\text{Number of observational units in the data set}}. \quad (3.1.2)$$

A percentage of observations of a data set meeting a criterion is simply the proportion of observations of the data set meeting the criterion expressed as a percentage.

$$\text{Percentage of observations of a data set meeting a criterion} = (\text{Proportion of observations of the data set meeting the criterion}) \times 100\% \quad (3.1.3)$$

A percentage of observational units of a data set meeting a criterion is simply the proportion of observational units of a data set meeting the criterion expressed as a percentage.

$$\text{Percentage of observational units of a data set meeting a criterion} = (\text{Proportion of observational units of the data set meeting the criterion}) \times 100\% \quad (3.1.4)$$

In this book, unless specifically indicated, there is one observation per observational unit. Percentages and proportions are percentages and proportions of observations as well as percentages and proportions of observational units. On the rare occasions that some observational units have more than one observation, it is specifically indicated whether a percentage or proportion is a percentage or proportion of observations or a percentage or proportion of observational units.

- *Percentages of YES Observations of Dichotomous Data Sets*

The two categories of a dichotomous data set are often designated YES and NO categories for convenience. The percentages of YES and NO observations of a data set comprise the distribution of the data set and cogently unveil the revelations of the data set. The sum of the percentages (proportion) of YES and NO observations of a dichotomous data set is 100% (1.0). When the value of the percentage (proportion) of YES observations is known, the percentage (proportion) of NO observations is also known. Revelation of a dichotomous data set is depicted synoptically by the percentage (proportion) of YES observations. It suffices to use the percentage (proportion) of YES observations to relate the revelation of a dichotomous data set.

Example 3.1.1

DeBaun and Others (2014) (Example 1.1.4) reported that *exit MRIs were completed for 185 of the 196 subjects (94%).* Whether a subject completed exit MRI is a dichotomous observation. The 196 subjects are the observational units of a set of 196 dichotomous observations. The proportion of subjects completed exit MRIs was computed as:

$$\begin{aligned}&\text{Proportion of subjects completed exit MRI}\\&=\frac{\text{Number of subjects who completed exit MRI}}{\text{Number of subjects}}=\frac{185}{196}=0.94.\end{aligned}$$

The percentage of subjects completed exit MRIs was computed as:

$$\begin{aligned}&\text{Percentage of subjects completed exit MRI}\\&\quad=(\text{Proportion of subjects completed exit MRI})\times 100\%=94\%.\end{aligned}$$

The percentage of subjects completed exit MRI: 94% yields that the percentage of subjects did not complete exit MRI equals 100% – 94% = 6%. The two percentages comprise the distribution of the set of 196 dichotomous observations. They manifest the revelation of the set of dichotomous observations eloquently.

There is one observation per subject. The percentage 94% is a percentage of observational units (subjects) as well as a percentage of observations.

Example 3.1.2

Table 1 of Sedman and Others (1985) (Table 1.5) presents several sets of observations obtained from 18 premature infants. Some sets include one observation per infant, two observations per infant, and one or two observations per infant. Percentages computed from these data sets may be percentages of observations or percentages of observational units.

Thirty-six plasma aluminum levels are displayed, two per infant. Percentages may be computed from these 36 plasma aluminum levels in several ways. For instance, 15 of the 36 plasma aluminum levels were higher than 10μg/liter.

$$\begin{aligned}&\text{Percentage of plasma aluminum levels above10 μg/liter in the set of 36}\\&=\frac{\text{Number of plasma aluminum levels above 10 μg/liter}}{\text{Number of plasma aluminum levels}}\\&=\frac{15}{36}15\times 100\%=42\%.\end{aligned}$$

The plasma aluminum levels of four of the infants are both above 10 μg/liter.

$$\text{Percentage of infants whose two plasma aluminum levels are both above } 10\ \mu g/\text{liter}$$
$$= \frac{\text{Number of infants whose two plasma aluminum levels are both above } 10\ \mu g/\text{liter}}{\text{Number of infants}}$$
$$= \frac{4}{18} 15 \times 100\% = 22\%.$$

The two percentages (42% and 22%) and their indications differ. One (42%) was computed from the set of 36 plasma aluminum levels. It is a percentage of observations. The other (22%) was computed from plasma aluminum levels of the 18 infants. It is a percentage of observational units.

Example 3.1.3
Chosidow and Others (2010) (Example 1.1.6) uses percentages to depict and compare the effects of oral ivermectin and malathion lotion on subjects with live head lice. Some are percentages of subjects, and some are percentages of households.

For instance, 95.2% and 85% are percentages of subjects in the two treatment groups who were free of head lice on day 15 of the study. The percentage 95.2% was computed from the set of data consisting of observations of 397 subjects in the ivermectin group, and 85% was computed from the set of data consisting of observations of 414 subjects in the malathion group. The subjects are the observational units of these data sets. There is one observation per subject; the percentages are percentages of observational units (subjects) as well as percentages of observations.

The percentages 92.4% and 79.1% are percent of households who were free of head lice on day 15 of the study. They were computed from the sets of data consisting of observations of households. Households are the observational units of these data sets. There is one observation per unit, and 92.4% and 79.1% are the percentages of observational units and the percentages of observations, respectively.

- *Polytomous Data Sets*

When observations of a data set belong to three or more categories, the observations are polytomous, and the data set is a polytomous data set. Revelations of a polytomous data set are manifested by percentages of observations belonging to the categories, which constitute the distribution of the observations and fully unveil the revelations of the observations.

Example 3.1.4
Table 2 of DeBaun and Others (2014) (Table 1.4) shows the neurologic events of 16 of the 97 subjects in the observation group. These are 16 of a set of 97 polytomous observations. The observations belong to four categories: stroke, SCI (silent cerebral inaction), and TIA (transient ischemic attack), and no neurologic event. The numbers of subjects whose neurologic events are stroke, SCI, and TIA cases are 7, 7, and 2, respectively. They yield that the percentages of subjects whose neurologic are events stroke, SCI, and TIA, and no neurologic event were are 7%, 7%, 2%, and

84%, respectively. The four percentages comprise the distribution of the set of 97 polytomous observations and fully unveil the revelations of the set of observations.

Example 3.1.5
Zheng and Others (2018) presented the results of a study that randomly assigned 36 subjects who had unilateral arm paralysis for more than 5 years to undergo C7 nerve transfer plus rehabilitation or rehabilitation alone. One outcome was the change in the score on the Modified Ashworth Scale from baseline to month 12. The scale is an assessment of spasticity in the paralyzed arm ranging from 0 to 5, with a higher value indicating more severe spasticity. Table 1 uses 0 (1), 1 (4), 2 (13), 3 (0), and 4 (0) to depict the baseline scores for elbow rotation of 18 subjects in the surgery group. Here, 0, 1, 2, 3, and 4 are scores, and the numbers in parentheses are the numbers of scores. They indicate that the numbers of subjects in the surgery group whose baseline scores were 0, 1, 2, 3, and 4 are 1, 4, 13, 0, and 0, respectively. The numbers yield that the percentages of subjects in the surgery group whose baseline scores were 0, 1, 2, 3, and 4 were 5.5%, 22.2%, 72.2%, 0%, and 0%, respectively.

The baseline scores on the Modified Ashworth Scale of the 18 subjects in the surgery group constitute a set of 18 polytomous observations. The five percentages comprise the distribution of the set of 18 polytomous observations and fully unveil the revelation of the observations.

- *Quantitative Data Sets*

Revelations of quantitative data sets are productively exposed by reviewing their distributions. The three essential properties of data distribution, location, variation, and skewness, are all important considerations. Indications of the three properties of data distribution may be brought to light compositely by one or a few percentages of germane observations.

Example 3.1.6
Figure 1.5 shows that the distribution of the estimates of 2001 state expenditures on tobacco control programs compiled by Gross and Others (2002) (Example 1.3.2.4) varies widely from $0.10 to $15.47 per capita and is highly skewed to the right. The revelation of the estimates is tellingly brought to light by the percentage of estimates as low as $1.0 per capita or lower (32%) or the percentage of estimates as low as $5.0 per capita or lower (82%). The percentages are integrated indications of the low center, the wide variation, and the high right skewness of the distribution.

Example 3.1.7
Figure 2 of Albers and Others (2018) (Fig. 1.1) shows that the distributions of scores on the modified Rankin scale in the endovascular therapy group and the medical therapy group varied widely and encompassed the range of the scale {0 to 6}. Revelations of the scores are not immediately clear. The article reports:

> The percentage of patients who were functional independent, defined as a score on the modified Ranking scale of 0 to 2, at 90 days was 45% in the endovascular therapy group, as compared with 17% in the medical-therapy group (risk ratio, 2.67; 95% CI, 1.60 to 4.48, P<0.001).

The percentages (45% and 17%) are informative synoptic descriptions of the scores. They bring to light revelations of the scores eloquently; their difference highlights the subtle distinction between the distributions of the scores of the two groups informatively. (See Example 6.1.5 for suggestions of the risk ratio 2.67, 95% CI, 1.60 to 4.48, and P<0.001.

3.2 Mean and Standard Deviation

Revelations of quantitative observations are often portrayed by means and standard deviations. The mean of a set of quantitative observations is a useful label of the location of the center of the distribution of the observations. It is in the middle of a data distribution when the distribution is relatively symmetric. The standard deviation is an integrated measure of variation—the degree of difference among the observations. It is technical, and its indication is intangible. Except for the notion that a larger standard deviation suggests a higher degree of difference among observations, it is unclear what degrees of difference is indicated by value of a standard deviation.

The wide use of the mean and standard deviation has much to do with the fundamentally important Gaussian distributions, which are often referred to as normal or Normal distributions. Gaussian distribution is often a required conditions of statistical hypothesis tests and confidence interval construction methods; it is also a key element of large sample theories. The properties of a Gaussian distribution are completely specified by its density function and two quantities known as its mean and standard deviation. The mean of a Gaussian distribution specifies the location of its center and the standard deviation is a measure of its variation. They are dubbed location and shape parameters.

The mean and standard deviation of a set of quantitative observations may be used to make some useful conjectures about the distribution of the observations if it is known that the distribution of the observations features a prominent cluster of observations in its middle and is relatively symmetric. However, data distributions are frequently unmistakably asymmetric.

3.2.1 Mean

The mean of a set of quantitative observations is often used to label the center of the distribution of the observations. If the distribution of setoff observations is relatively symmetric, the mean of the observations is an operative label of the location of the center of the distribution. When the distribution is conspicuously asymmetric, the mean is not in the middle of the distribution; it is a label of the location of the center of the distribution in a technical way.

Definition: Mean

The mean of a set of quantitative observations is the resulting value when the sum of the observations is divided by the number of observations.

The difference between the mean of a set of observations and one of the observations is called a deviation. The mean of a set of quantitative observations has the important property that the sum of its deviations from the observations is zero.

When the mean of a set of observations is written as *MEAN* and one of the observation is written as *OBSERVATION,* the deviation of the mean from the observation is *DEVIATION* = *MEAN* – *OBSERVATION.* One important property of the mean is:

The sum of the deviations of the mean of a set of observations from the observations is zero.

The deviation of the mean of a set of observations from one of the observations may be considered a measure of the distance between the mean and the observation. When a set of observations are arranged along a line in ascending order and spaced in accordance with their magnitudes, the mean of the observations has the following important property:

The aggregated distance between the mean of a set of observations and the observations smaller than it equals the aggregated distance between the mean and the observations larger than it.

Example 3.2.1.1

Figure 3.1 displays the distributions of four sets of pain indices. The indices vary from 0 to 10, with a higher value indicating a more severe pain. The ranges of the four sets of indices are identically {0 to 9}. This suggests that the locations of the distribution of the four sets of indices are identical, but the centers of the distributions of some sets differ.

Data set 3.1	Data set 3.2	Data set 3.3	Data set 3.4
4 5		0 1	8 9
3 4 5 6		0 1 2 3	6 7 8 9
2 3 4 5 6 7	0 1 2 3 4 5 6 7 8 9	0 1 2 3 4 5	4 5 6 7 8 9
1 2 3 4 5 6 7 8	0 1 2 3 4 5 6 7 8 9	0 1 2 3 4 5 6 7	2 3 4 5 6 7 8 9
0 1 2 3 4 5 6 7 8 9	0 1 2 3 4 5 6 7 8 9	0 1 2 3 4 5 6 7 8 9	0 1 2 3 4 5 6 7 8 9
----------------------	------------------------	------------------------	------------------------------
Pain indices	Pain indices	Pain indices	Pain indices

Fig. 3.1 Distributions of four sets of fake pain indices

Set 3.1
The mean of the pain indices of Set 3.1 equals:

$$\begin{aligned}\text{MEAN} &= (0+1+2+3+4+5+6+7+8+9+0+1+\cdots+4+5)/30 \\ &= 135/30 = 4.5.\end{aligned}$$

The distribution of this set of pain indices features a cluster of indices in its middle and is symmetric. The mean of the indices 4.5 is an operative label of the center of the distribution. The deviations of the mean from the smaller indices are:

$$4.5\text{–}0.0 = 4.5, 4.5\text{–}1.0 = 3.5, 4.5\text{–}2.0 = 2.5, 4.5\text{–}3.0 = 1.5, 4.5\text{–}4.0 = 4.5, \ldots, \text{etc.}$$

The deviations of the mean from the larger indices are:

$$\begin{aligned}&4.5\text{–}5.0 = -0.5, 4.5\text{–}6.0 = -1.5, 4.5\text{–}7.0 = -2.5, 4.5\text{–}8.0 = -3.5, 4.5\text{–}9.0 \\ &\quad = -4.5, \ldots, \text{etc.}\end{aligned}$$

The sum of the positive deviation equals 27.5, the sum of the negative deviation equals – 27.5, and the sum of all deviations is 0. If the mean of the set of indices, 4.5, is used to mark the center of their distribution, it has the property that the aggregated distance between it and the smaller indices on its left equals the aggregated distance between it and the larger indices on its right.

Sets 3.2
The distribution of this set of pain indices is symmetric. It is apparent that 4.5 is an operative label of the center of the distribution. The sum of the set of indices is 135; the mean of the indices is 4.5. The deviations of the mean from the smaller indices are:

$$4.5\text{–}0.0 = 4.5, 4.5\text{–}1.0 = 3.5, 4.5\text{–}2.0 = 2.5, 4.5\text{–}3.0 = 1.5, 4.5\text{–}4.0 = 4.5, \ldots, \text{etc.}$$

The deviations of the mean from the larger indices are:

$$\begin{aligned}&4.5\text{–}5.0 = -0.5, 4.5\text{–}6.0 = -1.5, 4.5\text{–}7.0 = -2.5, 4.5\text{–}8.0 = -3.5, 4.5\text{–}9.0 = \\ &-4.5, \ldots, \text{etc.}\end{aligned}$$

The sum of the positive deviations equals 37.5, the sum of the negative deviations equals – 37.5, and the sum of all deviations is 0. If the mean of the set of indices, 4.5, is used to mark the center of their distribution, it has the property that the aggregated distance between it and the smaller indices on its left equals the aggregated distance between it and the larger indices on its right.

Set 3.3
The distribution of Set 3.3 is skewed to the right, with fewer larger indices dispersing in its higher right half and more smaller indices clustering in its lower left half.

The sum of the 30 pain indices is 95, yielding a mean of 3.17. There are 18 indices smaller than the mean and 12 larger than the mean. The mean 3.17 is not in the middle of the distribution of the pain indices. The deviations of the mean from the 18 smaller indices are:

$$3.17–0.0 = 3.17, 3.17–1.0 = 2.17, 3.17–2.0 = 1.17, 3.17–3.0 = 0.17, \ldots, \text{etc.}$$

The deviations of the mean from the 12 larger indices are:

$$3.17–4.0 = -0.83, 3.17–5.0 = -1.83, 3.17–6.0 = -2.83, 3.17–7.0 = -3.83, \ldots, \text{etc.}$$

The sum of the negative deviations is –32.0, and the sum of the positive deviations is 32.0. The sum of the deviations of the mean from all indices is zero. When the mean of the set of indices 3.17 is used to mark the center of their distribution, it has the property that the aggregated distance between it and the smaller indices on its left equals the aggregated distance between it and the larger indices on its right.

Set 3.4

The distribution of set 3.4 is skewed to the left; fewer smaller indices disperse in its lower left half, and more.

Larger indices cluster in the higher right half.

The sum of the 30 pain indices is 175; thus, the mean of the indices is 5.83. There are 12 indices smaller than 5.83 and 18 larger. The mean 5.83 is not in the middle of the distribution of the pain indices.

The deviations of the mean from the 12 smaller indices are:

$$5.83–0.0 = 5.83, 5.83–1.0 = 4.83, 5.83–2.0 = 3.83, 5.83–4.0 = 1.83, 5.83–5.0 = 0.83, \ldots, \text{etc.}$$

The deviations of the mean from the 18 larger indices are:

$$5.83–6.0 = -0.17, 5.83–7.0 = -1.17, 5.83–8.0 = -2.17, 5.83–9.0 = -3.17, \ldots, \text{etc.}$$

The sum of the 12 negative deviations equals –32.0; the sum of the 18 positive deviations is 32.0. The sum of the deviations of the mean from the 30 indices is zero. When the mean of the set of indices, 5.83, is used to mark the location of the center of the distribution of the pain indices, it has the property that the aggregated distance between the mean (5.83) and the smaller indices on its left equals the aggregated distance between the mean and the larger scores on its right.

Example 3.2.1.2

The sum of the 50 at-rest heart rates displayed in Table 1.1 is 4000; the mean of the heart rates is *MEAN* = *80* bpm. The distribution of the 50 heart rates is symmetric (Fig. 1.2) The mean: 80 bpm is at the center of the distribution and an operative label of the location of its center.

The mean is slower than 21 heart rates and faster than 21 rates. The deviations of the mean from the slower rates are 80 – 56 = 24, 80 – 60 = 20, 80 – 64 = 16, and so on; the deviations of the mean from the faster rates are 80 – 84 = −4, 80 – 68 = −8, 80 – 91 = –12, and so on. The sum of the 21 positive deviations equals 224; the sum of the 21 negative deviations equals –224. The sum of the deviations of the mean from the 50 at-rest heart rates is zero.

When the mean of 80 bpm is used to label the center of the distribution of the heart rates, it has the property that the aggregated distance between it and the slower rates equals the aggregated distance between it and the faster rates.

Example 3.2.1.3

Figure 1.3 shows that the distribution of the 50 after-exercise heart rates displayed in Table 1.1 is skewed to the left. Only 24% of the heart rates were scattered sparsely in the lower half of the range of the distribution between 96 and 116 bpm, and as much as 76% of the rates were clustered in the higher half of the range of the distribution between 120 and 140 bpm. The location of the center of the distribution is not apparent.

The sum of the heart rates is 6,332 bpm: the mean of the 50 heart rates equals 126.64. The deviations of the mean from the rates are shown in Table 3.1. It reveals that there are 20 positive deviations and 30 negative deviations. The sum of the 20 positive deviations equals 252.8, and the sum of the 30 negative deviations equals −252.8. The sum of the deviations of the mean from the 30 after-exercise heart rates is zero. When the mean 126.6 is used to label the location of the center of the distribution of the heart rate, it has the property that the aggregated between it and the slower rates equals the aggregated distance between it and the faster rates.

When the mean of the heart rates 126.64 is used to mark the location of the center of their distribution, it has the property that the aggregated distance between the mean and the 20 slower rates and the aggregated distance between the mean and the 30 faster rates are equal.

Example 3.2.1.4

Figure 1.4 shows that the distribution of the at-rest systolic blood pressures displayed in Table 1.1 is skewed to the right. A markedly lower percentage of pressures (20%) scatter sparsely in its higher half between 150 mm and 200 mmHg, and a markedly higher percentage of pressures cluster (80%) cluster in its lower half between 100 mmHg and 150 mmHg. The location of the center of the distribution is not apparent.

The sum of the 50 pressures is 6650. The mean of the 50 pressures is 133 mmHg. The mean 133 mmHg is higher than 29 pressures and lower than 21 pressures. The sum of the deviations of the mean from the 29 lower pressures is 439, and the sum of the deviations of the mean from the 21 higher pressures equals −439. The sum of the deviations of the mean from the 50 pressures is zero. When the mean (133 mmHg) is used to mark the location of the center of the distribution of the pressures, the aggregated distance between the mean and the 29 lower pressures equals the aggregated distance between the mean and the 21 higher pressures.

Table 3.1 Frequencies of deviations of after-exercise heart rates from their mean (126.64)

Values:	96	100	104	108	112	116	120	124	128	132	136	140
Deviations:	30.36	26.36	22.64	18.64	14.64	10.64	6.64	2.64	−1.36	−5.36	−9.36	−13.36
Number:	1	1	2	2	3	3	4	4	5	7	8	10

- *Mean and Proportion*

When the value 1 is assigned to each YES observation and the value 0 to each NO observation of a set of dichotomous observations, the mean of the set of binary observations equals the proportion of 1 in the set. The mean of a binary data set is the proportion of 1s in the data set.

Example 3.2.1.5
If the value 0 is assigned to each M and the value 1 to is assigned each F shown in column 1 of Table 1.1, there are 30 0s and 20 1s. The sum of the set of 50 binary observations equals 20. The mean of the observations is 0.40 and equals the proportion of female subjects in the groups.

Example 3.2.1.6
Table 2 of DeBaun and Others (2014) (Table 1.4) used + and – to indicate whether the neurological finding of a patient was an enlarged new infarct. The neurological findings of four of the six patients in the transfusion group were +. The proportion of subjects whose neurological findings were enlarge infarcts is 4/6 = 0.67 among the six subjects.

When the value 1 is assigned to each + and the value 0 to each -, the resulting binary observations are 0, 1, 1, 1, 0, and 1. The sum of these six binary observations is 4, which yields that the mean of the six binary observations is 4/6 = 0.67. It equals the proportion of 1s.

3.2.2 Standard Deviation

A principal challenge of medical research is that subjects are in vastly different conditions and respond to treatments in distinctly diverse ways. The degree of difference among a set of observations is manifested by the distribution of the observations; it is called the variation, variability, or dispersion of the distribution. Distributions of observations of medical research often vary widely; distinction variation is frequently an important facet of difference among data sets.

The standard deviation of a set of observations is a frequently used measure of the variation of the distribution of the observations. It is a measure of absolute difference among observations in a technical way. The degree if difference among a set of observations indicated by the value of the standard deviation of the observations is unclear. The standard deviation of a set of observations is the positive square root of its variance.

Definition: Variance

The variance of a set of observations is the resulting value when the sum of the squares of the deviations of the mean of the observations from the observations is divided by one less the number of observations.

Definition: Standard Deviation

The standard deviation of a set of observations is the positive square root of the variance of the observations.

Remark *Number of observations minus one?*

Using "number of observations minus one" to compute variance and standard deviation is now a standard practice. The variance and standard deviation of a set of observations may also be computed by using the number of observations as their denominators. In this book, standard deviation is computed by using number of observations minus one as denominator. Number of observations is used only on some special occasions.

- *Symbols for Variance and Standard Deviation*

The variance and standard deviation of a set of observations are written in this book as SD^2 and SD, respectively. When it is needed for clarity, SD_1, SD_2, SD_3, etc., are used to denote the standard deviations of several sets of observations on the same variable; SD_X, SD_Y, SD_Z, etc., are used to denote the standard deviations of sets of observations on difference variables. Similarly, $SD^2{}_1$, $SD^2{}_2$, $SD^2{}_3$, etc. are used to denote the variances of several sets of observations on the same variable; $SD^2{}_X$, $SD^2{}_Y$, $SD^2{}_Z$, *etc.*, are used to denote the variances of sets of observations on different variables. The standard deviation and variance of a set of observations are denoted by s and s^2 or S and S^2 in many texts of statistics.

Example 3.2.2.1

Figure 3.1 suggests that the four sets of pain indices feature distinct degrees of difference. The ranges of the four data sets are identically {0 to 9}. They do not accurately indicate the distinction in degrees of difference among the four sets of indices.

The mean of the scores of Set 3.1 is $MEAN_{3.1} = 4.5$. The sum of the squares of the deviations of the mean from the indices is:

$$(0–4.5)^2 + (1–4.5)^2 + (2–4.5)^2 + \ \dots \ + (7–4.5)^2 + (8–4.5)^2 + (9–4.5)^2 + \dots = 147.5$$

The variance of the set of indices is $SD^2{}_{3.1} = 147.5/29 = 5.09$. The standard deviation is the positive square root of the variance; it equals $SD_{3.1} = \sqrt{5.09} = 2.55$.

The mean of the indices of Set 3.2 is $MEAN_{3.2} = 4.5$. The sum of the squares of the deviations of the mean from the indices is:

$$(0–4.5)^2 + (1–4.5)^2 + (2–4.5)^2 + \dots + (7–4.5)^2 + (8–4.5)^2 + (9–4.5)^2 + \dots = 247.5$$

The variance of the set of indices is $SD^2{}_{3.2} = 247.5/29 = 8.53$. The standard deviation is the positive square root of the variances; it equals $SD_{3.2} = \sqrt{8.53} = 2.92$.

The mean of the indices of Set 3.3 is $MEAN_{3.3} = 3.17$. The sum of the squares of the deviations of the mean from the indices is:

$$(0\text{–}3.17)^2 + (1\text{–}3.17)^2 + (2\text{–}3.17)^2 + \ldots + (7\text{–}3.17)^2 + (8\text{–}3.17)^2 + (9\text{–}3.17)^2 + \ldots = 194.17$$

The variance of the set of indices is $SD^2{}_{3.3} = 194.2/29 = 6.70$. The standard deviation is the positive square root of the variance; it equals $SD_{3.3} = \sqrt{6.70} = 2.59$.

The mean of the indices in Set 3.4 is $MEAN_{3.4} = 5.83$. The sum of the squares of the deviations of the mean from the indices is:

$$(0\text{–}5.83)^2 + (1\text{–}5.83)^2 + (2\text{–}5.83)^2 + \ \ldots\ + (7\text{–}5.83)^2 + (8\text{–}5.3)^2 + (9\text{–}5.83)^2 + \ \ldots\ = 194.17$$

The variance of the set of indices is $SD^2{}_{3.4} = 194.2/29 = 6.70$. The standard deviation is the positive square root of the variance; it equals $SD_{3.4} = \sqrt{6.70} = 2.59$.

$SD_{3.1}$ (2.55) < $SD_{3.3}$ (2.59) = $SD_{3.4}$ (2.59) < $SD_{3.2}$ (2.92). Measured by standard deviations, the degree of difference among the indices of Set 3.1 is the smallest, and the degree of difference among the indices of Set 3.2 is the greatest. The degree of difference among the indices of Set 3.3 is the same as that among the indices in Set 3.4. Measured by standard deviations, the degree of difference among the indices of Set 3.3 and Set 3.4 are larger than that of Set 3.1 but smaller than that of Set 3.2.

- *Shortcomings of Standard Deviation*

As a measure of the degree of difference among a set of quantitative observations, standard deviation has several optimal mathematical properties. Nevertheless, it also has several shortcomings.

One critical shortcoming is that its indication is intangible. It is unclear what degree of difference among a set of observations is indicated by the value of its standard deviation. A small standard deviation indicates that the observations are close to their mean, and a large standard deviation indicates that many observations are distant from their mean. However, it is unclear how close or how distant the observations are from their mean. The standard deviation also has the following shortcomings:

1. The standard deviation of a set of observations is a measure of the absolute difference among observations; its magnitude is affected by the magnitudes of the observations.
2. The standard deviation of the same set of observations differs when the observations are expressed in different units.
3. The magnitude of the standard deviation of a set of observations is affected by one or a few exceptionally small or exceptionally large observations.

Table 3.2 Two sets of body weights

Data Set 3.2.2.2A: Birth weights (in pounds) of nine infants: 4, 5, 6, 7, 8, 9, 10, 11, 12
Data Set 3.2.2.2B: Weights (in pounds) of nine football players: 266, 267, 268, 269, 270, 271, 272, 27

Table 3.3 Heart rates of ten individuals

Individual ID	1	2	3	4	5	6	7	8	9	10
Set A (beats per 15 s)	18	19	20	21	22	19	20	21	20	20
Set B (beats per minute)	72	76	80	84	88	86	80	84	80	80

Example 3.2.2.2

Table 3.2 shows two data sets. Data Set 3.2.2.2A consists of birth weights of nine newborns, and Data Set 3.2.2.2B consists of body weights of nine professional football players. A newborn is considered exceedingly small when its weight is 4 pounds, and exceedingly large when its weight is 12 pounds. The degree of difference among the nine birth weights is enormous. The weights of the nine football players are close to 270 pounds; their degree of difference is trivial.

The standard deviations of the two sets of weights are identically 2.74 lbs. They do not realistically reflect the fact that the degree of difference among the nine birth weights is enormous and that among the weights of nine football players is negligible.

Example 3.2.2.3

Table 3.3 exhibits the heart rates of ten individuals. Set A shows the heart rates in beats per 15 seconds, and set B displays the same ten heart rates in beats per minute. The standard deviation of the heart rates of set A is $SD_A = 1.15$; the standard deviation of set B is $SD_B = 4.60$. The standard deviation of set B is four times that of set A despite the fact that the heart rates of the two sets are the same rates expressed in different units.

- *Coefficient of Variation*

The coefficient of variation is a measure of the variation of the distribution of quantitative observations. It is a measure of relative difference among observations and is unaffected when observations are recorded in different units. It, however, is rarely used.

Definition: Coefficient of Variation

The coefficient of variation of a set of observations is the resulting value when the standard deviation of the observations is divided by the mean of the observations.

When the mean, standard deviation, and coefficient of variation of a set of observations are denoted by

MEAN, *SD*, and *CV,* respectively, the coefficient of variation of the set of observations is:

$$CV = SD/MEAN \tag{3.2.2}$$

The coefficient of variation is often expressed as a percentage and may be computed as:

$$CV = (SD/MEAN) \times 100\% \tag{3.2.3}$$

Example 3.2.2.4

The mean and standard deviation of the nine birth weights of Data Set 3.2.2.2A are $MEAN_A = 8$ lbs and $SD_A = 2.7$ lbs. They yield that the coefficient of deviation of the nine birth weights is:

$$CV_A = SD_A/MEAN_{A.} = 2.7 \text{ lbs}/80 \text{ lbs} = 0.34.$$

The mean and standard deviation of the weights of the nine football players of data set 3.2.2.2B are $MEAN_B = 270$ lbs and $SD_B = 2.7$ lbs. They yield that the coefficient of variation of the body weights of the nine football players is:

$$CV_B = SD_B/MEAN_B = 2.7 \text{ lbs}/270 \text{ lbs} = 0.01.$$

The two coefficients of variation differ markedly and correctly reflect the distinction between the degrees of difference among the birth weights of nine infants and the body weights of nine football players. $CV_A = 0.34$ indicates that the standard deviation of the birth weights is 34% of the mean of the weights. Many birth weights differ from the mean substantially. $CV_B = 0.01$ indicates that the standard deviation of the weights of the football players is only 1% of the mean of the weights. The weights of the football players are close to their mean.

Example 3.2.2.5

Heart rates of the same ten individuals recorded in beats per 15 s and beats per minute are shown in Table 3.3 as set A and set B. The mean and standard deviation of set A are $MEAN_A = 20$ beats per 15 s and $SD_A = 1.15$ beats per 15 s; the mean and standard deviation of the heart rates of set B are $MEAN_B = 80$ beats per minute and $SD_B = 4.6$ beats per minute. The coefficients of variation of the two sets of heart rates are:

$$CV_A = SD_A/MEAN_A = 1.15/20 = 0.06 \text{ and } CV_B = SD_B/MEAN_B = 4.6/80 = 0.06.$$

The coefficient of variation of the ten heart rates remains the same when the heart rates are expressed as beats per minute and beats per 15 s. The standard deviation of the heart rates is 6% of their mean.

3.2.3 Mean and Standard Deviation

The pair of mean and standard deviation is probably the most frequently used synoptic description of quantitative observations. The mean of a set of observations labels the location of the center of the distribution of the observations; the standard deviation signals the degree of difference among the observations. However, the indication of the standard deviation is intangible. It is unclear whether a standard deviation is an indication of a great or a little difference among observations.

One crude way to probe the indication of the standard deviation of a set of observations is to compare it with the mean of the observations. Roughly, if the standard deviation of a set of observations is substantially smaller than the mean of the observations, it is deemed small and implies that the distribution of the observations does not vary widely and that the observations are relatively close to their mean. If the standard deviation of a set of observations is close to or larger than the mean of the observations, it is deemed large and implies that the distribution of the observations varies widely with many observations distant from the mean of the observations. However, this is vague.

- *Presentation of Mean and Standard Deviation*

Values of the mean and standard deviation of a set of observations are often presented by using the "±" sign as the mean±SD. They may also be presented as MEAN (SD). The value before the parenthesis is the mean and that in the parenthesis is the standard deviation.

Example 3.2.3.1 Anavekar (351, 13)

Anavekar and Others (2018) (Example 1.3.2.5) used 70.3 ± 21.3 ml per minute per 1.73 m^2 to denote the mean and standard deviation of baseline estimates of glomerular filtration rate (GFR) of 14,527 subjects. The indications of the mean and standard deviation are limited. The mean indicates that the center of the distribution of the GFR values is in the vicinity of 70.3 ml per minute per 1.73 m^2. However, it is unclear what the standard deviation (21.3) indicates. Does it suggest that there were many GFR estimates much smaller or much larger than the mean?

How baseline GFR estimates of the 14,527 subjects vary is informatively shown by the histogram of Figure 1 (Fig. 1.6) which shows that the distribution of the GRF estimates varies between 16 and 140 ml per minute per 1.73 m^2. There are many estimates much smaller than as well as many much larger than the mean.

Example 3.2.3.2

Table 1 of Walker and Others (2012) (Example 1.2.7) uses 5.4±2.1 and 5.3 (2.3) to depict baseline cigarette dependence scores of the subjects in the cytisine group and the nicotine replacement group, respectively. The values: 5.4±2.1 denote the mean and standard deviation of the scores of the subjects in the cytisine group; the values: 5.3 (2.3) denote the mean and standard deviation of the scores of the subjects in the nicotine replacement group.

Indications of the means and standard deviations are limited. The means suggest that the centers of the distributions of baseline cigarette dependence scores of the two treatment groups are in vicinities of 5.4 and 5.3. However, it is unclear what the standard deviations (2.1 and 2.3) indicate. It is uncertain how widely the baseline cigarette dependence scores of the subjects of the two treatment groups vary.

- *MEAN±SD or MEAN±SEM*

The "±" sign is often used to denote values of mean and standard deviation. However, the value following the "±" sign is sometimes not that of a standard deviation but that of the standard error of the mean. The standard error of the mean of a set of observations is an improvised assessment of the degree of difference among means of replicates of the study if the study is replicated a score of times (Chap. 10). It is not a measure of the degree of difference among the observations. It is smaller than the standard deviation and equals the standard deviation of the observations divided by the square root of the number of observations.

3.2.4 Speculated 95% Observation-Region

The pair of mean and standard deviation are often the only descriptions of quantitative data sets in addition to the number of observations. They yield limited useful information. One way to garner some more useful information from the mean and standard deviation of a set of observations is to use them to determine a region that might include a large percentage of the observations. The region is based on the speculation that the distribution of the observations is adequately characterized by a Gaussian distribution. The speculation is dubbed the Gaussian model for observations; the region is dubbed speculated 95% observation-region or Gaussian model speculated 95% observation-region.

- *Gaussian (Normal) Distribution*

The family of Gaussian distributions, which are often referred to as the family of normal, or Normal distributions, plays a vital role in statistics. Elaborations of statistical methods often assume that distributions of data are adequately characterized by Gaussian distributions implicitly.

Properties of Gaussian distributions are specified by a mathematical equation called density function. A graphical display of the density function of a Gaussian distribution is a smooth symmetric curve with a unique peak in its center and resembles the cross section of a bell. It is called a Gaussian curve, normal curve, Normal curve, or bell-shaped curve. Technically, Gaussian distributions do not have finite ranges. The left and right tails of Gaussian curves extend as far as one can imagine and never touch the horizontal axis.

The location of the center and the degree of variation of a Gaussian distribution are specified by two quantities known as its mean and standard deviation. The mean is called the location parameter. It marks the location of the peak at its center. The

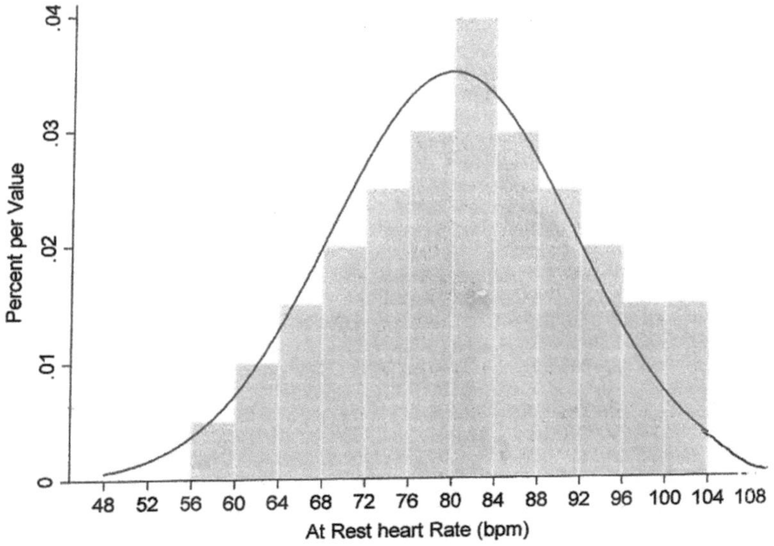

Fig. 3.2 Distribution of at-rest heart rates, curve of Gaussian model, and speculated regions

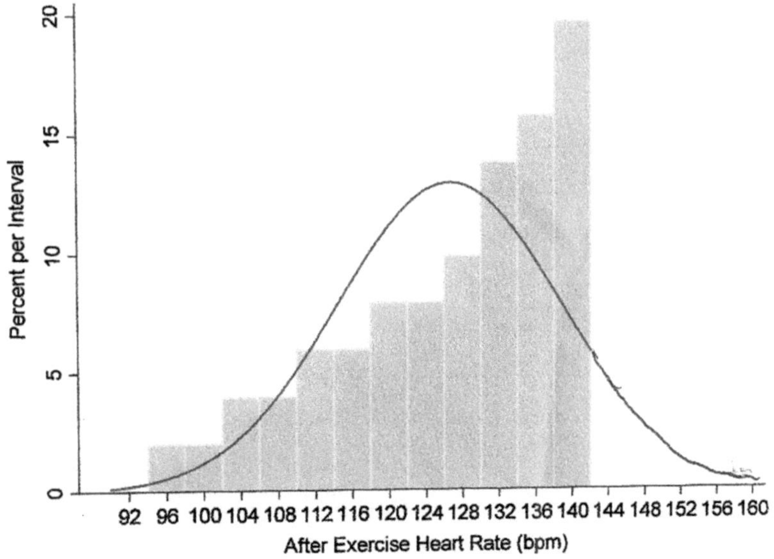

Fig. 3.3 Distribution of after-exercise heart rates and speculated Gaussian curve and regions

standard deviation is called the shape parameter. It is a measure of its variation and signifies the rate by which the curve of its density function ascends to and descends from its peak in its center. Examples of Gaussian curves are shown in Figs. 3.2 and 3.3, 3.4, 3.5.

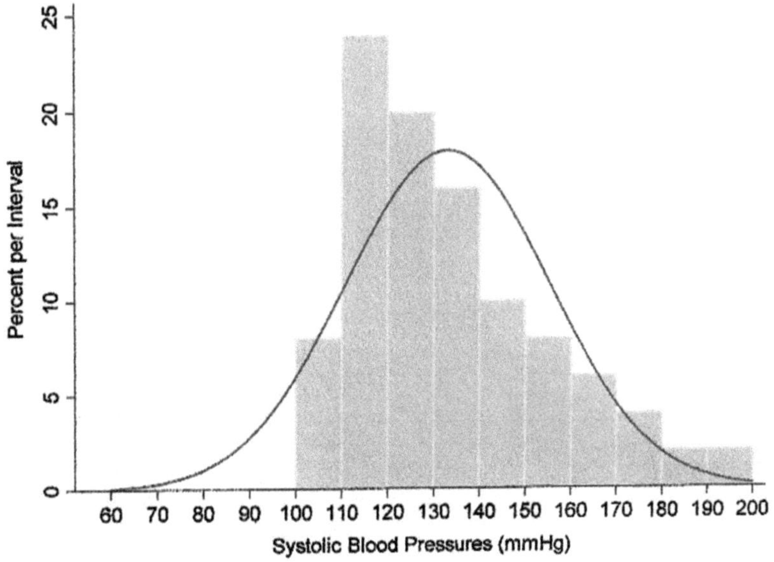

Fig. 3.4 Distribution of systolic blood pressures and the speculated observation-regions

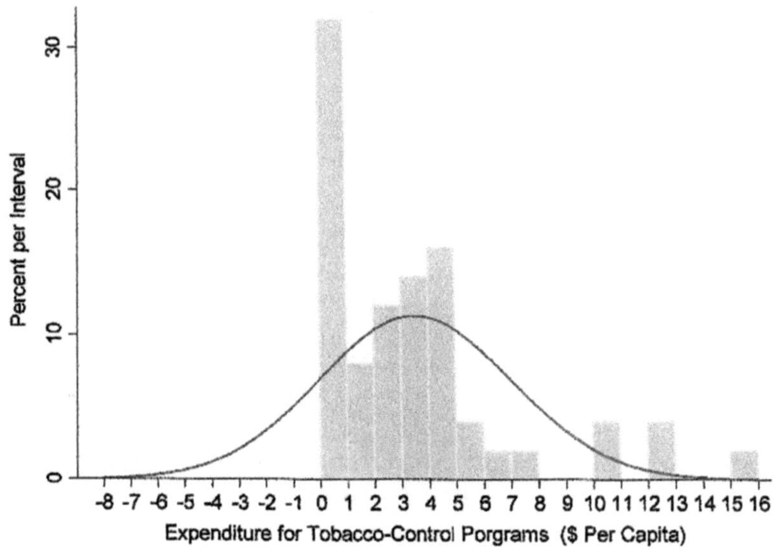

Fig. 3.5 Distribution of estimates of state expenditure on tobacco control programs and curve of the speculated Gaussian distribution

Table 3.4 Areas under the Gaussian curve in regions between mean plus and minus numbers of standard deviations

Region	Area in region
Between *MEAN* – 0.67*SD and MEAN* + 0.67*SD*	50%
Between *MEAN* – 1.00*SD and MEAN +1.00SD*	68%
Between *MEAN* – 1.28*SD and MEAN +1.28SD*	80%
Between *MEAN* – 1.65*SD and MEAN +1.65SD*	90%
Between *MEAN* – 1.96*SD and MEAN +1.96SD*	95%
Between *MEAN* – 2.58*SD and MEAN +2.58SD*	99%

Remark Gaussian or Normal distributions?

Gaussian distributions are frequently referred to as normal or Normal distributions. However, normal or Normal distributions may be interpreted as distributions of measurements of normal individuals. Distributions of measurements of normal individuals are often noticeably skewed and disagree with the symmetric Gaussian curves. For this reason, the term "Gaussian distribution" is used in this book.

- *Areas Under Gaussian Curves*

Tables displaying areas under Gaussian curves in regions are readily available. The total area under a Gaussian curve and above its horizontal axis is set as 1.0 or 100%. Areas in selected regions are presented in Table 3.4 as examples. This table uses *MEAN* and *SD* to denote the mean and standard deviation of a Gaussian distribution and shows areas under Gaussian curves in regions specified by mean minus and plus number of standard deviations.

Table 3.4 shows, for instance:

- The area under a Gaussian curve above its horizontal axis in the region between *MEAN – 0.67 SD* and *MEAN + 0.67 SD* is 50% of the total area.
- The area under a Gaussian curve above its horizontal axis in the region between *MEAN – 1.00 SD* and *MEAN + 1.00 SD* is 68% of the total area.
- The area under a Gaussian curve above its horizontal axis in the region between *MEAN – 1.65 SD* and *MEAN + 1.65 SD* is 90% of the total area.
- The area under a Gaussian curve above its horizontal axis in the region between *MEAN – 1.96 SD* and *MEAN + 1.96 SD* is 95% of the total area.

Gaussian curves are symmetric. Table 3.4 may also be used to determine areas outside and below or above the regions shown in the table. It suggests, for instance:

- The area under a Gaussian curve above its horizontal axis in the region on the left of *MEAN – 1.00 SD* is

  16%, and the area in the region on the right of *MEAN + 1. 00 SD* is 16%.
- The area under a Gaussian curve above its horizontal axis in the region on the left of *MEAN – 1.65 SD* is

  5%, and the area in the region on the right of *MEAN + 1.65 SD* is 5%.

- The area under a Gaussian curve above its horizontal axis in the region on the left of *MEAN – 1.96 SD* is 2.5%, and the area in the region on the right of *MEAN + 1.96 SD* is 2.5%.

Definition: Gaussian Model for Observations

The Gaussian model for observations is the speculation that the distribution of a set of observations is characterized by the density curve of a Gaussian distribution and that the mean and standard deviation of the Gaussian distribution equal the mean and standard deviation of the observations.

If the distribution of a set of observations is basically symmetric and features a prominent cluster of observations in its middle, the Gaussian model for observations is realistic. When the mean and standard deviation of a set of observations are *MEAN* and *SD*, the following observation-regions speculated by the Gaussian model for observations are useful.

- The region between *MEAN – 0.67 SD and MEAN + 0.*67 SD contains approximately 50% of the observations.
- The region between *MEAN – 1.65 SD and MEAN + 1.65 SD* contains approximately 90% of the observations.
- The region between *MEAN – 1.96 SD and MEAN + 1.*96 SD contains approximately 95% of the observations.
- The region between *MEAN – 2.58 SD and MEAN + 2.*58 SD contains approximately 99% of the observations.

The region speculated to contain 95% of the observations is particularly useful. The percentage of observations contained in the region (95%) is sufficiently high and 2.00 may be used in place of 1.96 for convenience. The 90% and 99% speculated observations also include sufficiently high percentages of observations. However, computations of their boundaries require more effort.

Definition: Speculated 95% Observation-Region

When MEAN and SD are the mean and standard deviation of a set of observations, the region bounded by the two values MEAN – 2SD and MEAN + 2SD is the speculated 95% observation region of the set of observations.

The speculated 95% observation-region of a set of observations would include about 95% of the middle observations if the distribution of the observations is relatively symmetric and features a cluster of observations in its middle. When the mean and standard deviation of a set of observations are the only descriptions of observations, the speculated 95% observation-region may be used to make some useful conjectures.

Example 3.2.4.1

The mean and standard deviation of the at-rest heart rates listed in Table 1.1 are *MEAN* = 80 bpm and *SD* = 11 bpm. The Gaussian model for observations speculates that the distribution of the heart rates is characterized by a Gaussian distribution with *MEAN* = 80 bpm and *SD* = 11 bpm. The distribution of the heart

Table 3.5 Percentages of resting heart rates in speculated observation-regions

Region	Boundaries	% Included[a]
Speculated 50% region:	$80 \mp 0.67 \times 11$ = [73 to 87 bpm]	40%
Speculated 90% region:	$80 \mp 1.65 \times 11$ = [62 to 98 bpm]	88%
Speculated 95% region:	$80 \mp 2.00 \times 11$ = [58 to 102 bpm]	96%
Speculated 99% region:	$80 \mp 2.58 \times 11$ = [52 to 108 bpm]	100%

[a]Based on Table 1.6

rates features a prominent cluster of rates in its middle and is symmetric. Figure 3.2 shows that it is fittingly characterized by the curve of the Gaussian distribution speculated by the Gaussian for observations. The Gaussian model is realistic.

Four observation-regions speculated by the Gaussian model are shown in Table 3.5 and schematically displayed in Fig. 3.2. The table shows:

- The speculated 50% observation-region is in the middle of the distribution but includes only 40% of the heart rates.
- The speculated 90% observation-region is in the middle of the distribution and includes 88% of the heart rates.
- The speculated 95% observation-region is in the middle of the distribution and includes 96% of the heart rates.
- The speculated 99% observation-region is noticeably wider than the range of the observations.

Example 3.2.4.2 Hays (348, 19)

Table 2 of Hays and Others (2003) (Example 2.5.1) uses -0.6 ± 13.6 to depict the mean and standard deviation of changes from baseline to year 1 in the physical functioning score in the estrogen plus progestin group. The mean: −0.6 suggests that the center of the distribution of the changes is in the vicinity of −0.6, and the standard deviation suggests that the changes might vary widely. It, however, is unknown how widely.

Figure 2A of the article (Fig. 2.14) shows that the distribution of the changes in the physical functioning score is basically symmetric, with a cluster of changes in its middle. The histogram is fittingly characterized by the bell-shaped curve of a Gaussian distribution; the Gaussian model for observations is credible.

The mean and standard deviation yield that the boundaries of the speculated 95% observation-region are $-0.6 \mp 2.00 \times 13.6$ = [−27.8 to 26.6]. It is in the middle of the distribution of changes and includes close to 95% of the changes. The speculated 95% observation-region is operative.

Example 3.2.4.3

Anavekar and Others (2018) (Example 1.3.2.5) reports: "*The baseline estimated GRF for the 14,527 patients was normally distributed (Fig. 1). The mean (±SD) estimated GFR was 70.2±21.3 ml per minute per 1.73 m*^{2} *(range, 7.6 to 139.8).*"

Figure 1 (Fig. 1.6) shows that the distribution is basically symmetric with a cluster of estimates in its middle. The Gaussian model for observations is realistic.

The mean and standard deviation yield that the boundaries of the speculated 95% observation-region are $70.2 \mp 2.00 \times 21.3$ = [27.6 to 112.8]. They speculate that approximately 95% of the estimates vary between 27.6 and 112.8 ml/min/1.73 m^2.

Figure 1 (Fig. 2.14) suggests that the speculated 95% observation-region is in the middle of the distribution approximately and includes close to 95% of the estimates. Although the speculated 95% observation-region is inexact, it would be useful if a comprehensive description of the distribution were not available.

3.2.5 *Speculated 95% Observation-Regions of Skewed Data Distributions*

The distributions of medical research data are often conspicuously skewed and suggest that the Gaussian model for observations is not realistic. In such instances, speculated 95% observation-regions are not in the middle of the data distributions. They extend below the smallest observation if the distribution is skewed to the right and beyond the greatest observation if the distribution is skewed to the left. It is astute to use speculated observation-regions with care when it is unknown whether the distribution of a data set is basically symmetric and features a prominent cluster of observations in its middle.

Example 3.2.5.1
Figure 1.3 shows that the distribution of the after-exercise heart rates listed in Table 1.1 is left skewed.

There is a smaller percentage of heart rates dispersed in its left half and a higher percentage of heart rates clustered in it right half. The mean and standard deviation of the heart rates are 126.6 bpm and 12.0 bpm, respectively. The Gaussian model for observations speculates that the distribution is characterized by the Gaussian distribution with $MEAN = 12.3$ bpm and $SD = 12.0$ bpm.

Figure 3.3 shows the symmetric curve of the Gaussian distribution speculated by the Gaussian model and a histogram that is a precise delineation of the distribution of the set of heart rates. Apparently, the symmetric Gaussian curve is not a fitting characterization of the left-skewed distribution. The Gaussian distribution is not a realistic model of this set of heart rates.

Three observation-regions speculated by the Gaussian model are shown in Table 3.6 and displayed in Fig. 3.3. The table shows that percentages of heart rates included in the speculated regions are close to their nominal values, but the regions are not in the middle of the distribution. The speculated observation-regions extend beyond the fastest rate (140 bpm) and miss some slower rates. For instance, the speculated 95% observation-region [102 to 150.6 bpm] extends far beyond the fastest rate (140 bpm) and misses slower rates, such as 100 and 96 bpm.

Table 3.6 Speculated observation-regions and percentages of after-exercise heart rates

Region	Boundaries	% Included[a]
Speculated 90% region:	$126.6 \mp 1.65 \times 12$ = [106.8 to 146.4 bpm]	92%
Speculated 95% region:	$126.6 \mp 2.00 \times 12$ = [102.6 to 150.6 bpm]	96%
Speculated 99% region:	$126.6 \mp 2.58 \times 12$ = [95.6 to 157.6 bpm]	100%

[a]Based on Table 1.7

Table 3.7 Speculated observation-regions and percentages of systolic pressure

Region	Boundaries	% Included[a]
Speculated 90% region:	$133 \mp 1.65 \times 22$ = [97 to 169 mmHg]	92%
Speculated 95% region:	$133 \mp 2.00 \times 22$ = [89 to 177 mmHg]	96%
Speculated 99% region:	$133 \mp 2.58 \times 22$ = [76 to 190 mmHg]	98%

[a]Based on Table 1.9

Example 3.2.5.2
Figure 1.4 shows that the distribution of the systolic blood pressures listed in Table 1.1 is right skewed with a smaller percentage of pressures disperse in its right half. The mean and standard deviation of the pressures are 133 Hg and 22 mmHg, respectively. The Gaussian model for observations speculates that the distribution is characterized by the Gaussian distribution with $MEAN = 133$ mmHg and $SD = 22.0$ mmHg.

Figure 3.4 shows the symmetric curve of the Gaussian distribution speculated by the Gaussian model and a histogram that is an expressive description of the distribution of the set of pressures. Apparently, the symmetric Gaussian curve is not a fitting characterization of the right-skewed distribution. The Gaussian distribution is not a realistic model of this set of systolic blood pressures.

Three observation-regions speculated by the Gaussian model are shown in Table 3.7 and displayed schematically in Fig. 3.4. The table shows that the percentages of heart rates included in the speculated regions are close to their nominal values, but the regions are not in the middle of the distribution. The speculated observation-regions extend below the lowest pressure and miss some higher pressures. For instance, the speculated 95% observation-region [89 to 177 mmHg] extends well below the lowest pressure (102 mmHg) and misses pressures higher than 177 mmHg.

Example 3.2.5.3
Figure 1.4 shows that the distribution of the estimates of 2001 state expenditure on tobacco control programs compiled by Gross and Others (2002) is right skewed. There is a smaller percentage of estimates dispersed in its right half. The mean and standard deviation of the estimates are $3.5 per capita and $3.5 per capita, respectively. The Gaussian model for observations speculates that the distribution of the estimates is characterized by the Gaussian distribution with *MEAN* = $3.5 per capita and *SD* = $3.5 per capita.

Table 3.8 Speculated observation-regions and percentages of estimates included in regions

Region	Boundaries	% Included[a]
Speculated 90% region:	$3.5 \mp 1.65 \times 3.5 = [-\$2.2 \text{ to } \$9.2]$	90%
Speculated 95% region:	$3.5 \mp 2.00 \times 3.5 = [-\$3.5 \text{ to } \$10.5]$	92%
Speculated 99% region:	$3.5 \mp 2.58 \times 3.5 = [-\$5.5 \text{ to } \$12.5]$	94%

[a]Based on Tables 1.10 and 1.11

Figure 3.5 shows the symmetric curve of the Gaussian distribution speculated by the Gaussian model for observations and a histogram that is an expressive description of the distribution of the estimates. Apparently, the symmetric Gaussian curve is not a fitting characterization of the right-skewed distribution. The Gaussian distribution is not a credible model of this set of estimates.

Three speculated observation-regions are shown in Table 3.8 and displayed schematically in Fig. 3.5. The table reveals that the percentages of estimates included in the speculated observation-regions are close to their nominal values. However, the regions are not in the middle. The speculated 90%, 95%, and 99% observation-regions extend below zero dollar per capita. For instance, the speculated 95% observation-region [-$3.5 to $10.5 per capita] includes negative expenditures and missed expenditures over $10.5 per capita.

3.2.6 *Speculated 95% Observation-Region and Skewness of Data Distribution*

Speculated 95% observation-regions yield some useful clues about skewness of data distributions if the smallest and greatest observations or the smallest and greatest possible values of the observations are known. The following are two examples:

1. ***Right skewness****: Right skewness is suggested if the lower boundary of the speculated 95% observation-region is noticeably smaller than the smallest observation or the smallest possible value of the observations.*
2. ***Left skewness****: Left skewness is suggested if the upper boundary of the speculated 95% observation-region is noticeably larger than the greatest observation or the greatest possible value of the observations.*

Example 3.2.6.1

Alboni and Others (2004) presented results of a study that evaluated effects of out-of-hospital self-administration of flecainide or propafenone in patients with mild heart disease or none who came to the emergency room with atrial fibrillation or recent onset that was hemodynamically well tolerated. It stated: "Treatment was successful in 534 episodes (94 percent); the time to resolution of symptoms was 113 ±84 min." The mean suggests that the center of the distribution of the elapsed times is in the vicinity of 113 min. The standard deviation is not small relative to the mean. It suggests that the distribution of the elapsed times of the 534 episodes varied widely. However, it is unclear how widely. Were there episodes shorter than 10 min or longer than 4 h?

To garner some pointers from the mean and standard deviation, they were used to determine the speculated 95% observation-region. $MEAN \mp 2SD$ yields that the speculated observation-region is [−55 to 281 min]. As elapse times may not be negative, the speculated 95% observation-region suggests that the distribution of the elapse times is skewed to the right and conjectures that approximately 95% of the elapse times varied from 0 to longer than 281 min. The majority of the elapse times clustered below 113 min, and there were elapse times longer than four hours.

Percentages of short or long elapse times are more forthright and constructive descriptions of elapsed times of episodes of arrhythmia than mean and standard deviation. For instance, percentages of elapse times shorter than 30 and those longer than 180 min or percentages of elapse times shorter than 60 and those longer than 240 min are relevant and valuable.

Example 3.2.6.2

Cooper and Others (2014) presented the results of a study evaluating the effect of renal artery stenting on the incidence of important cardiovascular and renal adverse events. A total of 947 subjects who had atherosclerotic renal artery stenosis and either systolic hypertension while taking two or more antihypertensive drugs or chronic kidney disease were randomly assigned to medical therapy plus renal artery stenting or medial therapy alone. The article affirms:

> At baseline, subjects were taking a mean of 2.1±1.6 antihypertensive medications.

The mean and standard deviation yield limited tangible information. The mean 2.1 suggested that the center of the distribution of numbers of medications is in the vicinity of 2.1. The standard deviation of 1.6 is relatively close to the mean and suggests that the distribution of the numbers might vary widely. However, it is unclear how widely. Were there many subjects who took four antihypertensive medications?

To garner more tips from the mean and standard deviation, they were used to determine the speculated 95% observation-region: [−1.1 to 5.3].

As taking two or more antihypertensive drugs was an inclusion criterion of the study, the lower boundary of the speculated 95% observation-region suggests that the distribution of the numbers is skewed to the right. There is a sizable percentage of subjects who took two antihypertensive drugs, and there might be some subjects who took five or more medications.

An alternative is to use percentages of subjects who took 2, 3, 4, 5, or more antihypertensive drugs. Indications of these percentages are more useful compared with indications of the mean and standard deviation.

Example 3.2.6.3 Cohen (364,11)

Cohen and Others (2011) presented the results of a study that randomly assigned 1800 patients with three vessel or left main coronary artery disease to undergo either

PCI Group:	[--------------▲----}----------]
92.4∓2 × 15.6	*61.2* *92.46* *100* *123.6.*
CABG group:	[---------------▲---}--------]
93.8 ∓2 × 14.2	*65.4* *93.8* *100* *122.2.*

Fig. 3.6 Speculated 95% regions for SAQ scores at 12 months

coronary artery bypass grafting (CABG, 903 patients) or percutaneous coronary intervention (PCI, 897 patients). The primary outcome was the score on the angina frequency subscale of the Seattle Angina Questionnaire (SAQ), which ranges from 0 to 100, with higher scores indicating better health status. Table 2 of the article uses 92.4±15.9 and 93.8±14.2 to denote means and standard deviations of the SAQ scores in the PCI and CABG groups at 12 months. The means suggest that the center of the distributions of the scores are in vicinities of 92.4 and 93.8; the standard deviations suggest that the distributions may vary widely. It, however, is unclear how widely the distributions vary and whether they are skewed.

To garner more information from the means and standard deviations, they were used to determine speculated 95% observation-regions displayed schematically in Fig. 3.6. As the SAQ score ranges from 0 to 100, the schematic displays suggest that the distributions of the scores of the two groups are skewed to the left with long left tails. They speculate that in both groups, the bulk of the scores clustered in the vicinity of 90 and that a few scores scattered below 70. It is more informative to present graphical displays of the highly left skewed distributions and use percentages of large scores, say 80 or more, to depict the two sets of SAQ scores synoptically.

It is more forthright and relevant to use percentages of high SAQ scores to depict the scores in the two treatment groups. For instance, percentages of scores as large or larger than 80 would be interesting.

3.3 Median, Interquartile Range, and Range

Median, interquartile range, and range are often used to describe quantitative data synoptically. They are specified by percentiles and are more palpable than mean and standard deviation. The following is a simple definition of percentile:

- *Percentile*

The Pth percentile of a set of observations is a value that is greater than or equal to P percent of the observations.

It follows that the Pth percentile of a set of observations is also a value that is smaller than or equal to (100% – P%) of the observations.

This definition is not rigorous and may not yield unique percentiles when the number of observations is small. The exact percentage of observations smaller than or equal to the Pth percentile of a set of observations is higher than P% if there are several observations equaling the percentile. Similarly, the exact percentage of observations larger than or equal to the Pth percentile is higher than (100% – P%) if there are several observations equaling the percentile.

- *Quartile, Decile, and Quintile*

The 25th, 50th, and 75th percentiles are called quartiles; the 10th, 20th,. . . , 80th, and 90th percentiles are called deciles, and the 20th, 40th, 60th, and 80th percentiles are called quintiles.

Median

> The median of a set of observations is the 50th percentile of the observations. It is greater than or equal to 50% of the observations and is smaller than or equal to 50% of the observations.

Range

> The range of a set of observations is specified by the 1st and the 100th percentiles of the observations—the smallest and the largest observations. It includes 100% of the observations.

Interquartile Range

> The interquartile range of a set of observations is the sector between the 25th and 75th percentiles of the observations. It includes the middle 50% of the observations when the observations are arranged in an ordered sequence.

Remark Indications of percentiles may be imprecise when observations are recorded in coarse values and there are arrays of observations with identical values. Suppose that a set of 100 observations are ratings on a 1 to 10 scale and are recorded as integers. The median is 3, which indicates that 50% of the ratings are lower than or as low as 3. The exact percentage of ratings as low as 3 or lower is larger than 50% if there is more than on observation equaling 3. It may be substantially higher than 50%. If the 75th percentile is 5, it indicates that 75% of the ratings are lower than or as low as 5. The exact percentage of rating as low as 5 or lower is larger than 5 if there is more than on observation equaling 5. It may be substantially higher than 75%.

Example 3.3.1

Cunningham and Others (2014) analyzed data from the Early Childhood Longitudinal Study, Kindergarten Class of 1988–1999 to evaluate the incidence of childhood obesity. The article states:

> We used the 2000 Centers of Disease Control and Prevention (CDC) Growth Charts to calculate each child's BMI, standardized to the reference population for the child's age and sex. We determined cutoffs for normal weight, overweight, and obesity using the CDC's standard thresholds of the 85th percentile for overweight and 95th percentile for obesity.

This suggests that the boys' BMI values were compared with a reference set consisting of the BMI values of many boys of the same age. The weight of a boy is rated overweight if his BMI was between the 85th percentile and the 95th percentile, and obese if his BMI was larger than the 95th percentile of the reference set. In other words, a boy is rated overweight if his BMI was larger than 85% but smaller than 95% of the values in the reference set, and obese if his BMI was larger than the 95% of the values of the reference set.

Example 3.3.2

Soria and Others (2018) reported the results of a study that randomly assigned 556 patients with previously untreated epidermal growth factor mutation-positive advanced non-small cell lung cancer to receive either osimertinib or standard epidermal growth factor receptor tyrosine kinase inhibitor (EGFR-TKI). A description of the primary end point of the study—the duration of progression-free survival—was presented in the article as follows:

> The median progression-free survival was 18.9 months (95% confidence interval [CI], 15.2 to 21.4) in the osimertinib group and 10.2 months (95% CI, 9.6 to 11.1) in the standard EGFR-TK1 group (Fig. 1A).

The medians unveil that the progression-free survival times of 50% of the subjects in the osimertinib group were shorter than or equal to 18.9 months, and those of 50% of the subjects in the standard EGFR-TKI group were shorter than or equal to 10.2 months.

If the progression-free survival times of more than one subject in the osimertinib group were 18.9 min, the percentage of progression-free survival times shorter than or as long as 18.9 months in the group would be slightly higher than 50%. Similarly, if the progression-free survival times of more than one subject in the standard EGFR-TKI group were 20.2 months, the percentage of progression-free survival times shorter than or as long as 10.2 months in the group would be slightly higher than 50%.

Compared with the medians, percentage of 10 months or longer and percentage of and 20 months or longer would be more forthright synoptic descriptions of the progression-free survival times of the subjects of the two treatment groups and the distinction between the two treatment groups.

Example 3.3.3

Weintraub and Others (2014) (Example 1.3.2.6) used the following account to relate CABG propensity scores:

> As expected, patients in the PCI group had a lower probability of being selected for CABG than those in the CABG group (Fig. 1), with the median and interquartile range of the propensity scores for CABG reflecting the difference (PCI group: median, 20.3%; interquartile range, 9.9 to 44.7; CABG group: median, 71.3%; interquartile range, 50.1 to 85.1).

The medians and interquartile ranges unveil the following:

- In the PCI group, 25% or more of the propensity scores were smaller than or equal to 9.9 percentage points, 50% or more were smaller or equal to 20.3 percentage points, 75% or more were smaller or equal to 44.7 percentage points, and the middle 50% of the scores were between 9.9 and 44.7 percentage points.

- In the CABG group, 25% or more of the propensity scores were smaller than or equal to 50.1 percentage points, 50% or more were smaller or equal to 71.3 percentage points, 75% or more were smaller or equal to 85.1 percentage point, and the middle 50% of the scores were between 50.1 and 85.1 percentage points.

An alternative is to use percentages of scores as low as 25 percentage points or lower or percentages of scores as low as 50 percentage points or lower to corroborate the assertion that the PCI group had a lower probability of being selected for CABG than did those in the CABG group.

- *Five-Number Summary and Box Plot*

Quantitative data are depicted at times by five number summaries consisted of the 25th, 50th, and 75th percentiles and two other numbers. The two other numbers may be the 1st and 100th percentiles, the 5th and 95th percentiles, the 10th and 90th percentiles, or other numbers. The use of five-number summaries comprised of percentiles is reviewed here.

Five-number summaries are often depicted graphically. A vertical box bordered by the 25th and 75th percentiles denotes the interquartile range. A symbol is shown in the box to denote the median. The other two numbers are often shown by short horizontal bars below and above the box and are connected by vertical lines. The short bars below and above the box and the vertical lines connecting them to the box are dubbed whiskers. When the whiskers of a box plot are not the smallest and the largest observations, observations smaller and larger than the two numbers are shown outside the whiskers. Such a graph is called a box plot or a box-and-whiskers plot.

Box plots use labels marked along a vertical line, the vertical axis (y-axis) of the graph, to denote values signified by heights of bars and other symbols.

Example 3.3.5

A brief report by Stengaard-Pedersen and Others (2003) described a case of inherited deficiency of mannan-binding lectin-associated serine protease 2 (MASP-2). Figure 3 of the report (Fig. 3.7) uses a dot to denote the MASP-2 level of this patient and box plots to depict the distributions of those of two groups of controls, homozygous for the wild type (D120/D120) and heterozygous (D120/G120). Each box plot uses a box to denote the interquartile range, a horizontal line inside the box to indicate the mean, and two short horizontal lines, one below and one above the box, to signal the 10th and 90th percentiles. Open circles are used to denote MASP-2 levels below the 10th and those above the 90th percentile.

The figure submits that the MASP-2 level of the patient is close to 0 and lower than those of both groups of controls. The box plots suggest the following:

- Subjects homozygous for wild type (D120/D120):
  - Plasma MASP-2 levels vary in a wide range from approximately 600 to 3900 mU/ml.

Fig. 3.7 Figure 3 of Stengaard-Pedersen and Others (2003)

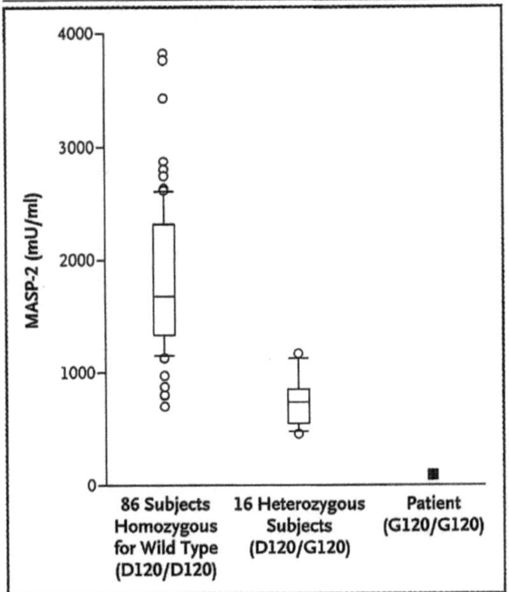

Figure 3. **Mannan-Binding Lectin–Associated Serine Protease 2 (MASP-2) Levels in Plasma from 86 Control Subjects Who Were Homozygous for the Wild Type (D120/D120), 11 Heterozygous (D120/G120) Control Subjects and the 5 Heterozygous Members of the Patient's Family, and the Patient, Who Was Homozygous for the Mutant Sequence (G120/G120).**

The levels of MASP-2 were estimated by means of a double-antibody assay. Standard curves were constructed with the use of a pool of normal plasma arbitrarily assigned the value of 1 U of MASP-2 per milliliter. The mean levels (horizontal lines), the 10th and 90th percentiles (I bars), and outliers (open circles) are shown. $P<0.001$ for the difference in MASP-2 values between the patient and the other two groups.

- The middle 50% of the levels vary between 1200 and 2200 mU/ml.
- The mean plasma MASP-2 level is approximately 1500 mU/ml.
- The lowest 10% vary from approximately 600 to 1100 mU/ml.
- The highest 10% of the levels vary from approximately 2600 to 3800 mU/ml.

- Heterozygous subjects (D120/G120):
  - The plasma MASP-2 levels of the heterozygous controls vary in a narrow low range between 500 to 1100 mU/ml approximately and are comparable with the lower 10% of the homozygous controls.

  - The mean MASP-2 levels of the heterozygous controls are distinctly lower than the mean of the homozygous controls (approximately 800 vs. 1500 mU/ml).

- *Percentile Rank*

Percentile rank is a useful indicator of the position of an observation relative to a set of observations that are used as reference. For instance, if it is known that the percentile rank of an observation is 10, it means that the observation equals the tenth percentile of a reference set; it is larger than or equal to 10% and is smaller than or equal to 90% of the observations in the reference set. If the percentile rank of an observation is 95, it means that the observation equals the 95th percentile of a reference set; it is larger than or equal to 95% and is smaller than or equal to 5% of the observations in the reference set.

Example 3.3.6
It is known that the percentile rank of the IQ score of a girl is 95. The girl is deemed smart. Her IQ score equals the 95th percentile of the scores in a reference set composed of IQ scores of a number of girls of the same age. She is considered smart because her score is higher than or equal to 95% of the scores in the reference set.

The percentile rank of the IQ score of a boy is 55. His IQ is considered average. His IQ score equals the 55th percentile of the scores in a reference set composed of IQ scores of a large number of boys of the same age. His IQ score is higher or equal to the scores of 55% and is smaller than or equal to 45% of the boys of the same age in the reference set.

Example 3.3.7
It is known that the percentile rank of the height of a girl was 90. Her height equals the 90th percentile of a reference set consisting of heights of a number of girls of the same age. She is taller than or equal to as much as 90% of the girls of the same age whose heights were included in the reference set.

The percentile rank of the height of a boy is 15. His height equals the 15th percentile of the heights of the boys of the same age in a reference set. He is shorter than 85% of the boys of the same age whose heights were included in the reference set.

Example 3.3.8
Gross and others (2002) (Example 1.1.2) referred to the six states of Georgia, Kentucky, North Carolina, South Carolina, Tennessee, and Virginia as tobacco-producing states. The six states accounted for approximately 94 percent of the US tobacco output of 1999.

One way to show the statuses of the tobacco-producing states among the 50 states with respect to expenditure on tobacco control programs is to use their percentile ranks. Table 1 of Gross and Others (2002) reveals that the percentile ranks of the estimates of the six tobacco-producing states are 6 (Tennessee), 12 (North Caroline), 28 (South Carolina), 32 (Kentucky), 42 (Georgia), and 52 (Virginia). They submit that the 2001 expenditures on tobacco control programs of the tobacco-producing states are not high relative to the other states.

The percentile rank of the most tight-fisted state (Tennessee) is 6. It is the third largest in the ascending sequence and is larger than or equal to only 6% (3) of the states. The percentile rank of the most generous state, Virginia, is 52. It is the 26th in the ascending sequence and is higher than or equal to 52% (26) of the states. In other words, the expenditure on tobacco control programs of Tennessee is lower than or equal to 94% (47) of the states, and that of Virginia is lower than or equal to 48% (24) of the states.

3.4 Percentage of Germane Observations

Means and standard deviations yield limited tangible information. Medians, interquartile ranges, and ranges are frequently imprecise. Percentages of observations in germane categories are simple and exact. They are often relevant precis of data revelation. Examples 3.2.6.1, 3.2.6.2, and 3.2.6.3 suggest that the percentages of germane observations are more telling than the means and standard deviations. Examples 3.3.2 and 3.3.3 suggested that the percentages of germane observations are more telling than the median, interquartile range, and range.

Example 3.4.1
A 2001 study asked nurses and social workers who cared for patients in hospice programs in Oregon, which legalized physician-assisted suicide in 1997, to provide information about those who had made an explicit request for a lethal prescription and subsequently died. The importance of reasons for requesting physician-assisted suicide given in actual conversations with the patients or their families was quizzed. Each reason was scored on a 5-point scale with 1 denoting not at all important and 5 denoting very important. One description of the results was given in a special article by Ganzini and Others (2002) as follows:

> According to the hospice nurses, the most important reasons for requesting assistance with suicide among patients who received prescription for lethal medications were a desire to control the circumstances of death, a desire to die at home, the belief that continuing to live was pointless, and being ready to die (Table 2). Depression and other psychiatric disorders, lack of social support, and concern about being a financial drain were, according to nurses, relatively unimportant.

Table 2 of the article uses medians and interquartile ranges to depict ratings. As ratings of importance have only five possible values, there are many identical ratings. Indications of the medians and interquartile ranges are imprecise. It would be precise and more informative if percentages of scores of 1, 2, 3, 4, and 5 were displayed in place of the medians and interquartile ranges. The following are two examples.

Desire to control circumstances of death
Table 2 shows that 5.0 and 5.0 to 5.0 are the median and interquartile range of ratings of the reason: Desire to control circumstances of death. They disclose that the 25th,

50th, and 75th percentiles of the set of ratings are identically 5 (very important) and that the percentage of 5 is 75% or higher. However, it is unknown whether it is 90% or even 100%. It would be precise and useful if the percentage of 5 were presented.

Lack of social support
The median and interquartile range of the ratings of the reason lack of social support are 1.0 and 1.0 to 2.0, respectively. They disclose that the 25th and 50th percentiles of the set of ratings are identically 1 (not at all important) and that the 75th percentile is 2. The percentage of 1s is 50% or higher, and the percentage of 1s or 2s is 75% or higher. The exact percentages are unknown. The percentage of 1s may be close to 75%, and the percentage of 1s or 2s may be 90% or higher. It would be precise and useful if the percentage of 1s and 2s were presented.

Example 3.4.2
A study interviewed officials of 108 US medical schools about provisions in their institutions' agreements with industry sponsors of multicenter clinical trials. Respondents were asked to estimate the percentage of their agreements with industry sponsors in the previous year that addressed specific items. The reported percentages were referred to as the institution's compliance scores. A description of the compliance scores is presented in a special article by Shulman and Others (2002) as:

> Site agreements rarely needed the presence of an independent executive committee or data safety monitoring board as a condition of the institution's participation in multicenter trials (Table 1). For example, with regard to the percentage of agreements that needed a data safety monitoring board, the median compliance score was 1 percent (interquartile range, 0 to 13). Additionally, agreements infrequently addressed the collection and monitoring of data or the analysis and interpretation of data.

Table 1 of the article uses median and interquartile range to depict compliance scores. The following are two examples.

Agreement Requiring an Independent Data and Safety Monitoring Board
The median and interquartile range of this agreement are 1 and [0 to 13]. They unveil the following:

- The 25th percentile (0) reveals that 25% or more of institutions did not include this item in any of their agreements with industry sponsors.
- The median (1) reveals that 50% or more institutions included this item in 1% or less of their agreements with industry sponsors.
- The 75th percentile (13) reveals that 75% or more of institutions included this item in 13% or less of their agreements with industry sponsors.

The exact percentage of institutions that included this item in 0%, 1% or less, and 13% or less of their agreements with industry sponsors are unknown. They might be noticeably higher than 25%, 50%, and 75%. It is more informative to cite the exact percentages of institutions that include this item in 0%, 1%, and 19% of their agreements with industry sponsors.

Agreement Allows Use of Site Data for Other Educational or Research Purposes
The median and interquartile range of this item are 85 and [35–100].

- The 25th percentile (35) reveals that 25% or more institutions included this item in 35% or less of their agreements with industry sponsors.
- The median (85) reveals that 50% or more institutions included this item in 85% or less of their agreements with industry sponsors.
- The 75th percentile (100) reveals that 75% or more institutions included this item in 100% or less of their agreements with industry sponsors.

The exact value of the percentage of institutions that included this item in 35% or less, 85% or less, and 100% or less of their agreements with industry sponsors are unknown. It is more informative to cite the exact percentages of institutions that included this item in 35%, 85%, and 100% of their agreements with industry sponsors.

Example 3.4.3
Self and Others (2018) presents the results of a study comparing balance crystalloids with salient crystalloids among adults who were treated in the emergency department and were subsequently hospitalized outside an ICU. Table 2 of the article uses 1608±1095, 1089 (1000–2000), and 2207 (32.9) and 1597±1105, 1071 (1000–2000), and 2150 (32.4) to depict volumes of balanced crystalloids received by subjects in the balanced crystalloids group and the saline group. These are mean ± standard deviation, median (interquartile range), and number (percent) of subjects whose volumes were ≥2000 ml.

The means, standard deviations, medians, and interquartile ranges are technical and yield limited palpable information. They suggest the following:

- In the balanced crystalloids group, the mean: 1608 suggests that the center of the distribution of the transfusions is in the vicinity of 1608 ml. The standard deviation 1059 suggests that the distribution varies widely. However, it is unclear how widely. The median 1086 suggests that 50% of the transfusions are smaller or equal to 1089 ml. The interquartile range (1000–2000) suggests that the middle 50% of the transfusions vary from 1000 to 2000 ml.
- In the saline group, the mean: 1597 suggests that the center of the distribution of the transfusions is in the vicinity of 1597 ml. The standard deviation of 1105 suggests that the distribution varies widely. It, however, is unclear how widely. The median 1071 suggests that 50% of the transfusions were smaller than or equal to 10871 ml. The interquartile range (1000–2000) suggests that the middle 50% of the transfusions varied from 1000 to 2000 ml.

The percentages of transfusions ≥2000 ml 32.9% and 32.4% are simple and forthright. They summarize the indications of the means, standard deviations, medians, and interquartile ranges coherently.

It would be informative and easier to appreciate if the volumes received by the two groups of subjects were depicted by percentages of transfusions ≥1000 ml, ≥2000 ml, and ≥3000 ml.

Example 3.4.4
Fradin and Days (2002) presented the results of a study that assessed the relative efficacy of insect repellents against mosquito bites. A batch of ten disease-free, laboratory-reared female mosquitoes of the same species between 7 and 24 days old that had not been exposed to the repellents being tested was placed into a test cage for each test. Fifteen volunteers participated. Each participant inserted their treated arm into the test cage according to protocol. The elapse time to the first bite was recorded as the "complete protection time." The article uses means to compare complete protection times of repellents. For instance, it states:

> The formulation containing 4.75% DEET protected an average of 88.4 minutes of complete protection time; the formulation containing 23.8% DEET protected for an average of 301.5 minutes.

The difference in means of complete protection times (23.8 vs. 301.5 min) is enormous. It seems that the repellent containing 23.8% DEET (N,N-diethyl-3-methylbenzamide) was much more effective than the repellent containing 4.75% DEET. However, it is unknown whether the protection times of the formulation containing 23.8 percent DEET were all longer than those of the formulation containing 4.75 percent DEET and by how much.

Table 1 shows that the mean, standard deviation, and range of the protection times of the repellent containing 23.8% DEET were 301.5±37.6 and 200 – 360, respectively, and those of the repellent containing 4.75% DEET were 88.4±21.4 and 45 – 104, respectively. The ranges reveal clearly that the protection times of the repellent containing 23.8% DEET are longer than those of the repellent containing 4.75% DEET by at least 96 min. This is one example that the simpler ranges are more telling than the means and standard deviations.

3.5 Mode and Geometric Mean

Mode is a useful label of the center of the distribution of a set of observations if the distribution features a single prominent cluster of observations. Geometric means are often used to label centers of distributions of data sets when the distributions are highly skewed to right, particularly if the statistical significance of the difference between data sets is assessed by testing the statistical significance of the difference in the means of logarithms of observations.

3.5.1 Mode

Mode is often discussed in statistical texts but is rarely used in medical research. When the distribution of a set of observations is depicted by percentages or numbers of observations equaling distinct values and features a single prominent cluster of observations, the mode of the distribution is the most frequent value if there is a unique one and the mean of the most frequent values if there are two or more most frequent values that are nearby. When the distribution is depicted by percentages or numbers of observations in intervals and features a single prominent cluster of observations, the midpoint of the most frequent interval is used as the mode of the distribution if there is a unique most frequent interval, and the mean of the midpoints of most frequent intervals is used as the mode of the distribution if there are two or more frequent intervals that are adjoining.

Example 3.5.1.1
The distributions of data sets 3.1, 3.3, and 3.4 feature prominent clusters of observations. The locations of clusters of observations are operatively labeled by their modes.

Data set 3.1 has two most frequent scores 4 and 5. Their mean 4.5 may be used as the mode of the distribution of the set of scores. Data set 3.3 has two most frequent scores 0 and 1. Their mean 0.5 may be used as the mode of the distribution of the set of scores. Data set 3.4 has two most frequent scores 8 and 9. Their mean 8.5 may be used as the mode of the distribution of the set of scores. The modes of these data sets are operative labels of the clusters of observation.

Data set 3.2 does not have a prominent cluster of observations; there is not a unique mode.

Example 3.5.1.2
The histogram of Fig. 1.2 shows that the distribution of the at-rest heart rates displayed in Table 1.1 features one prominent cluster of heart rates and a unique most frequent distinct value 80 bpm. The mode of the distribution of the 50 heart rates is 80 bpm; it is an operative label of the cluster of heart rates.

The histogram of Fig. 1.3 shows that the distribution of the after-exercise-rest heart rates displayed in Table 1.1 features a single prominent cluster of heart rates and a unique most frequent distinct value 140 bpm. The mode of the distribution of the heart rates is 140 bpm. It is an operative indicator of the location of the cluster of heart ration but not an operative label of the location of the center of the distribution of the heart rates.

Table 1.9 presents an expressive description of the distribution of the systolic blood pressures listed in Table 1.1. It shows that $\geq$110 to $<$120 mmHg is the most frequent class interval and includes 24% of the pressures. The midpoint of the interval 115 mmHg may be used as the mode of the distribution. It is an operative indicator of the location of the cluster of pressures but not an operative indicator of the location of the center of the distribution of the of pressures.

Example 3.5.1.3 Gross (347, 14)

Table 1.11 presents an expressive description of the distribution of estimates of 2001 state expenditures on tobacco-smoking control programs. It shows that ≥0 to < \$1.00 per capita is the most frequent interval and includes 32% of the estimates. The midpoint of the interval \$0.50 per capita is the mode of the distribution of the estimates. It is an operative indicator of the location of the cluster of estimates but not an operative indicator of the location of the center of the distribution of the estimates.

- *Averages*

The median, mean, and mode are often referred to as averages. The mean has the property that the aggregated distance between it and the smaller observations and the aggregated distance between it and the larger observations are equal. The median of a set of observations has the property that it is larger than or equal to 50 percent of the observations. When the distribution of a set of observations features a prominent cluster of observations, the mode of the distribution is an operative label of the location of the cluster of observations.

If the distribution of a set of observations is features a prominent cluster of observations in its middle and is symmetric, its mean, median, and mode are close. They are operative labels of the location of the center of the distribution. When the distribution of a set of observations features a prominent cluster of observations but is conspicuously skewed, its mean, median, and mode differ noticeably. When the mean, median, and mode of the distribution of a set of observations are written as *MEAN, MEDIAN, and MODE,* the following relationships among them hold generally.

- When the distribution of a set of observations features a single bulk of observations in its middle and is basically symmetric:

  MEAN ≈ MEDIAN ≈ MODE

- When the distribution of a set of observations is noticeably skewed to right and features a considerably lower percentage of larger observations in its right half and an evidently higher percentage of smaller observations in its left half:

  MEAN > MEDIAN > MODE

- When the distribution of a set of observations is noticeably skewed to left and features a considerably lower percentage of smaller observations in its left half and an evidently higher percentage of larger observations in its right half:

  MEAN < MEDIAN < MODE

- *Representative Values*

Mean, median, and mode are sometimes used as representative values. It is important to note that the mean, median, or mode are representative only if all observations are close. The distributions of observations obtained in medical research usually vary widely. The medians, means, and modes are not representative.

Example 3.5.1.4

The distribution of the at-rest heart rates in Table 1.1 is symmetric (Fig. 1.2). Its mean, median, and mode are identically 80 bpm. However, the distribution varies from 56 to 104 bpm; 80 bpm is hardly a representative value of the set of heart rates. There are many noticeably slower and noticeably faster rates.

The distribution of the after-exercise heart rates in Table 1.1 is skewed to left (Fig. 1.3). Its mean (126.64 bpm) is smaller than its median (130 bpm), which is smaller than its mode (140 bpm). The distribution varies from 96 to 140 bpm. The mean, median, and mode are hardly representative values of the set of heart rates.

There are many noticeably slower and noticeably faster rates.

The distribution of the systolic blood pressures in Table 1.1 is skewed to right (Fig. 1.4). Its mean (133 mmHg) is larger than its median (130 mmHg), which is larger than its mode (115 bpm). The distribution varies from approximately 100 to 200 mmHg. The mean, median, and mode are hardly representative values of the set of pressures. There are many noticeably lower and noticeably higher pressures.

The distribution of the estimates of 2001 state expenditures on tobacco-smoking control programs reported by Gross and Others (2002) is highly skewed to right (Fig. 1.5). Its mean ($3.50 per capita) is larger than its median ($2.71 per capita), which is larger than its mode ($0.50 per capita). The distribution varies widely from $0.10 to 15.47 per capita. The mean, median, and mode are hardly representative values of the 50 estimates. There are many markedly higher estimates.

Example 3.5.1.5

Anavekar and Others (2018) (Example 1.3.2.5) reported that the mean of the GFR estimates of 14,527 patients with acute myocardial infarction is 70.2 ml per minute per 1.73 m^2. The histogram depicted in Figure 1 of the article (Fig. 1.6) is a cogent description of the distribution of the estimates. It features two most frequent intervals. The midpoints of these two intervals are 66 and 72 ml per minute per 1.73m^2. Their average 68 ml per minute per 1.73m^2 may be used as the mode of the distribution of GFR estimates. The histogram suggests that the distribution is relatively symmetric; the mean and mode are close.

The histogram suggests that the distribution varies widely from 20 to 140 ml per minute per 1.73 m^2. The mean (70.2 ml per minute per 1.73 m^2) and mode (68 ml per minute per 1.73 m^2) are hardly representative.

Example 3.5.1.6

Weintraub and Others (2014) (Example 1.3.2.6) reported that the medians of the propensity scores of the PCI and CABG groups are 0.20 and 0.50, respectively. Figure 1 of the article (Fig. 1.7) suggests that 0.08 is the midpoint of the most frequent interval of the histogram depicting the distribution of the propensity scores of the PCI group, and 0.92 is the midpoint of the most frequent interval of the histogram depicting the distribution of the propensity scores of the CABG group. They are the modes of the distributions.

The distribution of the propensity scores of the PCI group is skewed to right, and its median (0.20) is greater than its mode (0.08). The distribution varies widely from

0 to 0.96. The median and mode are hardly representative. The distribution of the propensity scores of the CABG group is skewed to left, and its median (0.50) is smaller than its mode (0.92). The distribution varies widely from 0.02 to as large as 0.98. The median and mode are hardly representative.

3.5.2 Geometric Mean

When the distributions of two sets of observations are highly right skewed, the statistical significance of distinction between the two data sets is often evaluated by testing the statistical significance of the difference between the means of logarithms of observations. In this case, the geometric means of the observations are usually presented to depict the data sets synoptically.

Definition: Geometric Mean

> The geometric mean of a set of **n** observations is the **n**th root of the product of the observations.

It is more convenient to compute geometric means by using logarithms of observations. First, the mean of the logarithms of the observations is computed. The antilogarithm of the resulting value is the geometric mean of the observations.

Geometric mean of a set of observations
= The antilogarithm of the mean of the logarithms of the observations. (3.5.2.1)

More specifically:

Geometric mean of a set of observations
= 10 to the power of the mean of the logarithms (base 10) of the observations.
= 2 to the power of the mean of the logarithms (base 2) of observations.
= The natural number ($e = 2.71828$) to the power of the mean of the natural logarithms of the observations. (3.5.2.2)

One shortcoming of the geometric mean is that its indication is not clear.

Example 3.5.2.1
Suppose that endotoxin levels determined from surfaces of five mattresses are 10, 100, 1,000, 10,000, and 100,000 endotoxin units per square meter. The geometric mean of these five endotoxin levels is the fifth root of their product. It can be computed as follows:

$$GEOMETRIC\ MEAN = (10 \times 100 \times 1000 \times 10000 \times 100000)^{(1/5)}$$
$$= 1000 \text{ endotoxin per units per square meter.}$$

The logarithms (base 10) of the five endotoxin levels are $\log_{10}(10) = 1$, $\log_{10}(100) = 2$, $\log_{10}(1000) = 3$,

$\log_{10}(10000) = 4$, and $\log_{10}(100000) = 5$. Their mean is 3. The geometric mean of the five endotoxin levels equals

$$GEOMETIC\ MEAN$$
$$= 10 \text{ to the power of the mean of the logarithms (base 10) of the levels}$$
$$= 10^3 = 1000 \text{ endotoxin units per square meter.}$$

The median and mean of the five endotoxin levels are:

$$MEDIAN = 1000 \text{ endotoxin units per square meter and}$$
$$MEAN = 22,222 \text{ endotoxin units per square meter.}$$

The mean is larger than four of the five endotoxin levels. It is not an operative label for the location of the center of the distribution of the endotoxin levels. The median 1000 endotoxin units is in the middle of the five endotoxin levels and an operative label of the location of the center of their distribution. The geometric equals the median; it is also an operative label for the location of the center of the distribution.

Example 3.5.2.2
The lengths of hospital stay of seven patients are 2, 4, 8, 16, 32, 64, and 128 days. The geometric mean of the seven hospital stays is the seventh root of their product and can be computed as:

$$GEOMETRIC\ MEAN = (2 \times 4 \times 8 \times 16 \times 32 \times 64 \times 128)^{(1/7)} = 16 \text{ days.}$$

The logarithms (base 2) of the five observations are $\log_2(2) = 1$, $\log_2(4) = 2$, $\log_2(8) = 3$, $\log_2(16) = 4$, $\log_2(32) = 5$, $\log_2(64) = 6$, and $\log_2(128) = 7$. Their mean is 4. The geometric mean of the seven hospital stays can be computed as:

$$\text{Geometric Mean of the set of the seven hospital days}$$
$$= 2 \text{ to the power of the mean of the logarithms (base 2) of the hospital days}$$
$$= 2 \text{ to the power of } 4$$
$$= 16 \text{ days.}$$

The mean and median of the seven hospital days are MEAN = 36.2 days and MEDIAN = 16 days. The mean is larger than five of the seven hospital days; it is not an operative label of the location of the center of their distribution. The median is in

Table 3.9 Geometric means of egg counts of children positive for *T. trichiura* (no. of eggs per g of stool)

	Oxantel pamoate–albendazole		Oxantel pamoate		Albendazole		Mebendazole	
Treatment group	Before	After	Before	After	Before	After	Before	After
Number of children	112	77	114	84	114	111	110	97
Geometric mean	796	31	874	59	853	469	813	203

the middle of the seven hospital stays and an operative label for the location of the center of their distribution. In this case, the geometric mean equals the median. It is an operative label for the location of the center of the distribution.

Remark The geometric mean of a set of observations is often relatively close to the median of the observations. One way to assess the indication of a geometric mean of a set of observations is to note that it may be close to the median of the observations.

Example 3.5.2.3
The results of a study assessing the efficacy and safety of a combination of oxantel pamoate and albendazole in children infected with *T. trichiura* are presented in Speich and Others (2014). Children 6 to 14 years of age were randomly assigned to receive one of four treatments: oxantel pamoate at a dose of 20 mg per kilogram of body weight, plus 400 mg of albendazole administered on consecutive days; oxantel pamoate at a single dose of 20 mg per kilogram of body weight; albendazole at a single dose of 400 mg; or mebendazole at a single dose of 500 mg. Table 2 of the article used geometric means to depict egg counts (no. of eggs/g of stool). The geometric mean egg counts of children positive for *T. trichiura* are shown in Table 3.9.

The geometric means yield limited useful information. For instance, the before-treatment geometric mean of the oxantel pamoate–albendazole group (796) is the 112th root of the product of the egg counts of 112 children; the after-treatment geometric mean of the group (31) is the 77th root of the product of the egg counts of the 77 children. It is unclear what they reveal. It is likely that they are close to the medians of the distributions, and the centers of the distributions are in the vicinities of 769 eggs per g of stool and the vicinity of 31 eggs per g of stool. However, it is not sure. It is unknown how widely the distributions of egg counts are dispersed. It is expected that the distributions are skewed to right, but the degrees of right skewness are unknown.

Example 3.5.2.4 DiazGranados (371,7)
DiazGranados and Others (2014) presented the results of a study that randomly assigned 31989 adults 65 years of age or older to receive either IIV3-HD (60 μg of hemagglutinin per strain) or IIV3-SD (15 μg of hemagglutinin per strain). The subjects were enrolled during two periods: September 6 through October 9, 2011

(Year 1) and from October 9 through October 21, 2012 (Year 2). Hemagglutination inhibition (HAI) titers determined in a subset of subjects 28 days after vaccination are depicted as follows:

> HAI antibody geometric mean titers and seroprotective rates 28 days after vaccination were significantly higher after vaccination with IIV3-HD than with IIV3-SD for all three vaccine strains (Table 4).

Table 4 uses geometric means to depict HAI titers. It shows, for instance, that the geometric means of HAI titers of the 2375 year 1 subjects who received IIV3-HD is 481.8 and that of the 2382 year 1 subjects who received IIV3-SD is 271.8. Here, 481.8 is the 2375th root of the product of 2375 titers, and 271.8 is the 2382nd root of the product of 2382 titers.

It is unclear what the geometric means suggest. It is likely that the medians of the two sets of titers were close to 481.8 and 271.8 and the center of the distribution of the titers of the subjects who received IIV3-HD is in the vicinity of 481.8 and distantly higher than the center of the distribution of the titers of the subjects who received IIV3-SD, which is in the vicinity of 271.8. However, it is unknown whether the two distributions vary widely and overlap extensively. It is unknown whether either group has HAI titers close to zero or higher than 1000 or even 2000.

3.6 Measures of Skewness

The distributions of observations of medical research are often skewed and feature noticeably unequal percentages of large and small observations. However, the skewness of data distributions is rarely addressed in descriptions of data. There are several measures of skewness. A few basic ones are reviewed here for the sake of completeness.

- *Simple Coefficients of Skewness*

  There are several simple coefficients of skewness.

SK_{Half}

The distribution of a set of observations is symmetric when the percentages of observations in its left and right halves are equal. It is right (positively) skewed when the percentage of larger observations in the right half of its range is noticeably lower than the percentage of smaller observations in the left half of its range. It is left (negatively) skewed when the percentage of smaller observations in the left half of its range is noticeably lower than the percentage of larger observations in the right half of its range. When the percentages of observations in the lower half and the higher half of the range of the distribution of the observations are written as *Percent in Lower Half and Percent in Higher Half,* a simple coefficient of skewness is:

$$SK_{\text{Half}} = \textit{Percent} \text{ in } \textit{Lower Half} - \textit{Percent} \text{ in } \textit{Higher Half} \tag{3.6.1}$$

SK_{Mean}

When the distribution of a set of observations is symmetric, the mean of the observations is in its middle. The percentage of observations smaller than and the percentage of observations larger than the mean of the observations are equal. Generally, the percentage of observations larger than the mean of the observations is noticeably lower than the percentage of observations smaller than the mean if the distribution of a set of observations is right (positively) skewed, and the percentage of observations smaller than the mean of the observations is noticeably lower than the percentage of observations larger than the mean when the distribution of the observations is left (negatively) skewed. If the mean of set of observations is written as *MEAN* and the percentages of observations smaller than and larger than MEAN are written as *Percent* <*MEAN* and *Percent* >*MEAN,* a coefficient of skewness is:

$$SK_{\text{Mean}} = \textit{Percent} < \textit{MEAN} - \textit{Percent} > \textit{MEAN} \tag{3.6.2}$$

SK_{Median} and SK_{Mode}

The mean, median, and mode of a set of observations are equal when the distribution of the observations is symmetric. Generally, when the distribution of a set of observations is right (positively) skewed, the mean of the observations is larger than the median and mode of the observations; when the distribution of a set of observations is left (negatively) skewed, the mean of the observations is smaller than the median and mode of the observations. If the mean, median, mode, and standard deviation of a set of observations are written as *MEAN, MEDIAN, MODE,* and *SD*, two coefficients of skewness are determined as follows:

$$SK_{\text{Median}} = (MEAN - MEDIAN)/SD \tag{3.6.3}$$

$$SK_{\text{Mode}} = (MEAN - MODE)/SD \tag{3.6.4}$$

These four simple coefficients of skewness suggest the following:

- $SK \approx 0$ suggests that the distribution of a set of observations is basically symmetric.
- $SK > 0$ suggests that the distribution of a set of observations is right (positively) skewed. A larger value indicates a higher degree of right skewness.
- $SK < 0$ suggests that a distribution of a set of observations is left (negatively) skewed. A larger value indicates a higher degree of left skewness.

Example 3.6.1.1

Figure 1.2 shows that the distribution of the set of at-rest heart rates displayed in Table 1.1 is symmetric. The mean of the heart rates 80 bpm is in the middle of the distribution. Table 1.6 shows that the percentage of heart rates slower than 80 bpm and the percentage of heart rates faster than 80 bpm are both 42%.

$$SK_{\text{Half}} = Percent \text{ in } Lower\ Half - Percent \text{ in } Higher\ Half = 42\% - 42\% = 0.$$
$$SK_{\text{Mean}} = Percent < MEAN - Percent > MEAN = 42\% - 42\% = 0.$$

The mean, median, and mode of the heart rates are identically 80 bpm. The standard deviation of the heart rates is SD = 11. They yield:

$$SK_{\text{Median}} = (MEAN - MEDIAN)/SD = (80 - 80)/11 = 0.$$
$$SK_{\text{Mode}} = (MEAN - MODE)/SD = (80 - 80)/11 = 0.$$

The four coefficients of skewness suggest that the distribution of the heart rates is symmetric and agree with the indication of the histogram shown in Fig. 1.2.

Example 3.6.1.2
Figure 1.3 shows that the distribution of the after-exercise heart rates shown in Table 1.1 is left skewed. Table 1.7 shows that 24% of the heart rates are in the lower half of the range of the distribution on the left of 118 bpm, and 76% of the heart rates are in the higher half of the range of the distribution on the right of 118 bpm. They yield:

$$SK_{\text{Half}} = Percent \text{ in } Lower\ Half - Percent \text{ in } Higher\ Half = 24\% - 76\% = -52\%.$$

The mean of the heart rates is MEAN = 126.6 bpm. Table 1.7 shows that 40% of the after-heart rates are smaller than 126.6 bpm, and 60% of the after-heart rates are larger than 126.6 bpm. They yield:

$$SK_{\text{Mean}} = Percent < MEAN - Percent > MEAN = 40\% - 62\% = -22\%.$$

The median and mode of the heart rates are *MEDIAN* = 130 bpm and *MODE* = 140 bpm. They yield:

$$SK_{\text{Median}} = (MEAN - MEDIAN)/SD = (120.6 - 130)/12.2 = -0.28.$$
$$SK_{\text{Mode}} = (MEAN - MODE)/SD = (120.6 - 140)/12.2 = -1.10.$$

The four coefficients are negative and suggest that the distribution is left skewed. $SK_{\text{Half}} = -52\%$ reveals that the percentage of heart rates in the lower half of the range of the distribution on the left of 118 bpm is 52 percentage points lower than the percentage of rates in the higher half of the range of the distribution. $SK_{\text{Mean}} = -20\%$ reveals that the percentage of heart rates slower than the mean of the 50 heart rates (126.6 bpm) is 20 percentage points lower than the percentage of rates faster than the mean of the 50 heart rates. $SK_{\text{Median}} = -0.28$ reveals that the mean of the heart rates is smaller than the median by approximately one third of the standard deviation. $SK_{\text{Mode}} = -1.08$ reveals that the mean of the heart rates is smaller than the mode by approximately one standard deviation.

Example 3.6.1.3

Figure 1.4 shows that the distribution of the systolic blood pressures shown in Table 1.1 is right skewed. Table 1.8 shows that 78% of the pressure is in the lower half of the range of the distribution on the left of 150 mmHg, and 22% of the pressure is in the higher half of the range of the distribution on the right of 150 mmHg. It follows:

$$SK_{\text{Half}} = \textit{Percent} \text{ in } \textit{Lower Half} - \textit{Percent} \text{ in } \textit{Higher Half} = 78\% - 22\% = 56\%.$$

The mean of the pressures is 133 mmHg. Table 1.8 shows that 58% of the pressures are lower and 42% of the pressures are higher.

$$SK_{\text{Mean}} = \textit{Percent} < \textit{MEAN} - \textit{Percent} > \textit{MEAN} = 58\% - 42\% = 16\%.$$

The mean, median and mode of the distribution are 133, 127, and 115 mmHg, respectively. The standard deviation is 22. It follows that

$$SK_{\text{Median}} = (MEAN - MEDIAN)/SD = (133 - 127)/22 = 0.27.$$
$$SK_{\text{Mode}} = (MEAN - MODE)/SD = (133 - 115)/22 = 0.82.$$

The four coefficients are positive. Each suggests that the distribution is right skewed. $SK_{\text{Half}} = 56\%$ indicates that the percentage of pressures in the lower half of the range of the distribution is 56 percentage points higher than the percentage of pressures in the higher half of the range of the distribution. $SK_{\text{Mean}} = 16\%$ reveals that the percentage of pressures smaller than the mean of the pressures (133 mmHg) is 16 percentage points higher than the percentage of pressures larger than the mean. $SK_{\text{Median}} = 0.27$ reveals that the mean of the pressures is larger than the median by approximately one third of the standard deviation. $SK_{\text{Mode}} = 0.36$ reveals that the mean of the pressures is larger than the mode by approximately four eight tenths of standard deviation.

Example 3.6.1.4

Figure 1.5 shows that the distribution of the estimates of 2001 state expenditures on tobacco control programs compiled by Gross and Others (2002) is highly right skewed. Table 1.10 shows that 90% of the estimate rates are in the lower half of the range of distribution of the estimates on the left of \$8.00 per capita, and only 10% of the estimates are in the higher half of the range of the distribution on the right of \$8.00 per capita.

$$SK_{\text{Half}} = \textit{Percent} \text{ in } \textit{Lower Half} - \textit{Percent} \text{ in } \textit{Higher Half} = 90\% - 10\% = 80\%.$$

The mean of the estimates is \$3.50 per capita. Table 1.10 shows that 62% of estimates are smaller than \$3.50 per capita, and 38% are larger.

$$SK_{\text{Mean}} = Percent < MEAN - Percent > MEAN = 62\% - 38\% = +24\%$$

The mean, median, and mode of the distribution are \$3.50, \$2.80, and 0.5 per capita, respectively. The standard deviation is \$3.50 per capita. Table 1.1 suggests that the mode of the estimates is 0.5. It follows that:

$$SK_{\text{Median}} = (MEAN - MEDIAN)/SD = (3.5 - 2.8)/3.5 = 0.20.$$
$$SK_{\text{Mode}} = (MEAN - MODE)/SD = (3.5 - 0.5)/3.5 = 0.86.$$

The four coefficients are positive and suggest that the distribution of the estimates is right skewed. $SK_{\text{Half}} = 80\%$ reveals that the percentage of estimates in the left half of the distribution is 80 percentage points higher than the percentage of estimates in the right half of the distribution. $SK_{\text{Mean}} = 24\%$ reveals that the percentage of estimates smaller than the mean of the estimates (\$3.50 per capita) is 24 percentage points higher than the percentage of estimates larger than the mean. $SK_{\text{Median}} = 0.20$ reveals that the mean of the estimates is larger than the median by about two tenths of the standard deviation. $SK_{\text{Mode}} = 0.86$ reveals that the mean of the estimates is larger than the mode by more than eight tenths of the standard deviation.

3.6.1 Skewness Measures Based on Third Powers of Deviations

Many statistical software packages print values of coefficients of skewness that are functions of the third powers of the deviations of the observations from their mean. For example, values of the following coefficients of skewness or their minor variations are printed by some statistical software packages.

$$SK_1 = \left\{\frac{1}{n}\right\} \times \left\{\frac{\text{Sum of the 3rd Powers of Deviations}}{(\text{Standard Deviation})^3}\right\} \tag{3.6.2.1}$$

$$SK_2 = \left\{\frac{(\text{Sum of the 3rd Powers of Deviations})}{(\text{Number of observations})}\right\} / \left\{\frac{\text{Sum of the 2nd Powers of Deviations}}{(\text{Number of Observations})}\right\}^{3/2} \tag{3.6.2.2}$$

The skewness coefficients SK_1 and SK_2 of a data set are zero when the distribution of the data set is symmetric, positive when the distribution of the data set is skewed to the right, and negative when the data distribution is skewed to the left. A larger value indicates a higher degree of skewness. It, however, is difficult to use their values to arrive at a palpable assessment of the degree of skewness.

Example 3.6.2.1
Statistical software was used to compute the coefficient of skewness SK_1 of the data sets shown in Table 1.1. It yields the following results:

- At-rest exercise heart rate: $SK_1 = 0$. This agrees with the indication of Fig. 1.2 that the distribution is symmetric.
- After-exercise heart rate: $SK_1 = -0.76$. This agrees with the indication of Fig. 1.3 that the distribution is skewed to left. It, however, is unclear what degree of left skewness is indicated by $SK_1 = -0.76$.
- At-rest systolic blood pressure: $SK_1 = +0.93$. This agrees with the indication of Fig. 1.4 that the distribution is skewed to right. It, however, is unclear what degree of right skewness is indicated by $SK_1 = 0.93$.

Computed from estimates of 2002 state expenditure on tobacco control programs, $SK_1 = 1.67$. This agrees with the indication of Fig. 1.5 that the distribution is skewed to the right. It, however, is unclear what degree of right skewness is indicated by $SK_1 = 1.67$.

Review Questions

1. How do percentage of observations and percentage of observational units differ?
2. What do the mean and standard deviation of a set of observations suggest?
3. What do the median, interquartile range, and range of a set of observations suggest?
4. When is a percentage of germane observations more useful than the mean and standard deviation of the observations?
5. What are the key properties of Gaussian distributions?
6. Under what conditions is the Gaussian model for observations plausible?
7. When are conjectured by speculated 95% observation-regions?
8. When does a speculated 95% observation-region suggest that the distribution of a set of observations might be skewed?
9. Under what condition is the mode of a data distribution uniquely determined and useful?
10. How do percentiles and percentile ranks differ?
11. Is it important to know how wide the distribution of a set of observations varies and whether the distribution is symmetric?
12. If the percentage of observations in the right half of the distribution of a set of observations is conspicuously smaller than the percentage of observations in the left half of the distribution, is the distribution skewed to right or left?

Exercise

3.E.1 Review the urine outputs of patients who did and did not survive hypovolemic shock shown in Table 1.E.1.

(a) Compute the values of the means, standard deviations, medians, interquartile ranges, and ranges of the two sets of urine outputs.

(b) Elaborate the limitations of using the means and standard deviations to depict the revelation of the urine outputs.
(c) Elaborate the limitations of using the medians, interquartile ranges, and ranges to depict the revelation of the urine outputs.
(d) Elaborate the limitations of using a percentage of germane observations to depict the revelation of the urine outputs.
(e) Display the distributions of the two sets of urine outputs graphically and elaborate the limitations of using manifestations of the graphical display to articulate the revelation of the urine outputs.

3.E.2 Review the ratings of the severity of pain before and after treatment with a pain reliever are shown in Table 1.E.2.

(a) Compute the values of the means, standard deviations, medians, interquartile ranges, and ranges of each set of ratings.
(b) Elaborate the limitations of using the means and standard deviations to depict the revelation of the ratings.
(c) Elaborate the limitations of using the medians, interquartile ranges, and ranges to depict the revelation of the ratings.
(d) Elaborate the limitations of using a percentage of germane observations to depict the revelation of the urine outputs.
(e) Display the distributions of the before- and after-treatment ratings graphically and elaborate the limitations of using manifestations of the graphical display to depict the revelations of the urine outputs.

3.E.3 Three punters were evaluated by a football team. Each was asked to punt 10 times. The results are shown in Table 3.E.3.

(a) Determine the mean, median, and range of the punting distances by each punter. The values of each of the three descriptive statistics are used to rate the punters.
(b) Use means and standard deviations to rate the punters.
(c) Use median and range to rate the punters.
(d) Use percentage of long punts to rate the punters.
(e) Depict the distributions of the three sets of punting distances graphically; use indications of the graphs to rate the punters.
(f) Discuss the relative advantages of these ratings.

Table 3.E.3 Punting distance in yards

Player 1: 20, 60, 30, 50, 36, 54, 40, 44, 46, 47
Player 2: 56, 20, 54, 30, 52, 35, 50, 40, 46, 44
Player 3: 60, 30, 52, 30, 50, 32, 48, 35, 46, 44

3.E.4 Review fractions of CDC recommendations that were spent for tobacco control programs computed for Problem 1.E.4.

(a) Use mean and standard deviation to relate the revelation of the fractions.
(b) Use median, interquartile range, and range to relate the revelation of the fractions.
(c) Use percentages of small fractions to relate the revelation of the fractions.
(d) Use manifestations of a graph to display the distribution of the fractions to relate the revelation of the fractions.
(e) Discuss the relative advantages of the four narratives.
(f) For each of the six tobacco-producing states Georgia, Kentucky, North Carolina, South Carolina, Tennessee, and Virginia, find the percentile ranks of their fractions and discuss their suggestions.

3.E.5 Figure 2.8 presents a stem-and-leaf display of the first plasma aluminum concentrations of the premature infants exhibited in Table 1 of Sedman and Others (1985) (Table 1.5).

(a) Suggest a narrative of the revelation of the concentrations using mean and standard deviation.
(b) Suggest a narrative of the revelation of the concentrations using median and range.
(c) Suggest a narrative of the revelation of the concentrations using a percentage of high concentrations.
(d) Suggest a narrative of the revelation of the concentrations citing indications of the stem-and-leaf display.

3.E.6 Table 2 of Hays and Others (2003) (Example 3.2.4.2) uses -1.4 ± 13.6 and -1.8 ± 20.9 to depict means and standard deviations of changes from baseline to year 1 in scores of physical functioning and bodily pain in the placebo group.

(a) Elaborate what the means and standard deviation suggest.
(b) Determine the speculated 95% observation-regions.
(c) Review Figure 2 of the article (Fig. 2.14) and discuss how credible the regions are.

3.E.7 Table 1 of Walker and Others (2012) (Example 3.2.3.2) used 19.3 ± 11.9 and 19.0 (10.0) to depict the means and standard deviations of the numbers of cigarettes smoked per day in the cytisine and the nicotine replacement groups at baseline. Elaborate what they suggest.

3.E.8 Alboni and Others (2004) (Example 3.2.6.1) reported that the mean time from the onset of symptoms to treatment was 36±93 min, and the median was 10 min.

(a) Elaborate what 36±93 min suggest.
(b) Determine the speculated 95% observation-region and discuss what the region insinuates.
(c) Elaborate what the median (10 min) suggests.
(d) Discuss whether the distribution of the elapse times is highly right skewed.
(e) Suggest a way to depict the elapse times that is straightforward and informative.

3.E.9 Ganzini and Others (2002) (Example 3.4.1) reported that a desire to die at home is one of the most important reasons to request assistance with suicide. Table 2 shows that the median and interquartile range of the ratings of the reason: Desire to die at home are 5.0 (3.0–5.0), and those of reason: Depression or other psychiatric disorders are 2.0 (1.0–3.0).

(a) Elaborate the suggestions of the medians and interquartile ranges.
(b) Suggest an alternative way to depict the ratings. (Ratings range between 1 and 5.)

3.E.10 Table 1 of Shulman and Others (2002) (Example 3.4.2) uses 2 (0–10) and 40 (5–95), to depict the compliance score of the item: Agreement requires an independent steering or executive committee and the item: Agreement addresses editorial control of reports on the trial results. These are medians and interquartile ranges.

(a) Elaborate the indications of 2 (0–10) and suggest an alternative way to depict the compliance scores.
(b) Elaborate the indications of 40 (5–95) and suggest an alternative way to depict the compliance scores.

3.E.11 Table 3.9 shows that the geometric means of egg counts of the oxantel-pamoate group are 879 before treatment and 59 after treatment. Elaborate their suggestions.

References

Albers, G. W., et al. (2018). Thrombectomy for stroke at 6 to 16 hours with selection by perfusion imaging. *The New England Journal of Medicine, 378*, 708–718.

Alboni, P., et al. (2004). Outpatient treatment of recent-onset atrial fibrillation with the "pill-in-the-pocket" approach. *The New England Journal of Medicine, 351*, 2384–2391.

Anavekar, N., et al. (2018). Relation between renal dysfunction and cardiovascular outcomes after myocardial infarction. *The New England Journal of Medicine, 378*(8), 1285–1295.
Chosidow, O., et al. (2010). Oral ivermectin versus malathion lotion for difficult-to-treat head lice. *The New England Journal of Medicine, 362*, 896–905.
Cohen, D. J., et al. (2011). Quality of life after PCI with drug-eluting stents of coronary-artery bypass surgery. *The New England Journal of Medicine, 364*, 1016–1026.
Cooper, C. J., et al. (2014). Stenting and Medical therapy for atherosclerotic renal-artery stenosis. *The New England Journal of Medicine, 370*, 13–22.
Cunningham, S. A., et al. (2014). Incidence of childhood obesity in the United States. *The New England Journal of Medicine, 370*(5), 403–411.
DeBaun, M. R., et al. (2014). Controlled trial of transfusions for silent cerebral infarcts in sickle cell anemia. *The New England Journal of Medicine, 371*, 699–710.
DiazGranados, C. A., et al. (2014). Efficacy of high-dose versus standard-dose influenza vaccine in adults. *The New England Journal of Medicine, 371*(7), 635–645.
Fradin, M. S., & Day, J. F. (2002). Comparative efficacy of insect repellents against mosquito bites. *The New England Journal of Medicine, 347*(1), 13–18.
Ganzini, L., et al. (2002). Experiences of Oregon nurses and social workers with hospice patients who requested assistance with suicide. *The New England Journal of Medicine, 347*(8), 582–588.
Gross, C. P., et al. (2002). State expenditure for tobacco-control programs and the tobacco settlement. *The New England Journal of Medicine, 347*(14), 1080–1086.
Hays, J., et al. (2003). Effects of estrogen plus progestin on health-related quality of life. *The New England Journal of Medicine, 348*(19), 1839–1854.
Sedman, A. B., et al. (1985). Evidence of aluminum loading in infants receiving intravenous therapy. *The New England Journal of Medicine, 312*(21), 1337–1343.
Self, W. H., et al. (2018). Balanced crystalloids versus saline in noncritically ill adults. *The New England Journal of Medicine, 378*(9), 819–828.
Shulman, K. A., et al. (2002). A national survey of provisions in clinical-trial agreements between medical schools and industry sponsors. *The New England Journal of Medicine, 347*, 1335–1341.
Soria, J.-C., et al. (2018). Osimertinib in untreated EGFR-mutated advanced non-small-cell lung cancer. *The New England Journal of Medicine, 378*(2), 113–125.
Speich, B., et al. (2014). Oxantel pamoate-albendazole for Trichuris trichiura. *The New England Journal of Medicine, 370*(7), 610–620.
Stengaard-Pedersen, K., et al. (2003). Brief report: Inherited deficiency of mannan-binding lectin-associated serine protease 2. *The New England Journal of Medicine, 349*(6), 554–560.
Walker, N., et al. (2012). Cytisine versus nicotine for smoking cessation. *The New England Journal of Medicine, 366*, 16.
Weintraub, W. S., et al. (2014). Comparative effectiveness of revascularization strategies. *The New England Journal of Medicine, 371*(25), 2353–2362.
Zheng, M.-X., et al. (2018). Trial of contralateral seventh cervical nerve transfer for spastic arm paralysis. *The New England Journal of Medicine, 378*(1), 22–34.

Part II
Intelligent Reading and Informative Reporting

This part (Chaps. 4 to 9) demonstrates intelligent reading and informative reporting of results of data analysis. Articles published in the New England Journal of Medicine are used as examples. Intelligent reading and informative reporting of revelations of unpaired and paired quantitative data sets are demonstrated in Chaps. 4 and 5. The cases of unpaired and paired qualitative data sets are illustrated in Chaps. 6 and 7. Descriptions of relationships between two quantitative and two qualitative data sets are probed in Chaps. 8 and 9.

- *Statistical Significance and 95% Confidence Interval*

P-values of statistical significance tests are regularly presented to corroborate descriptions of data revelations. Data revelations are declared "significant" when *P*-values are smaller than 0.05. The statistics portraying data revelations are not identified, and the revelations are not candidly described. Narratives of "significant" data revelations are stylish but hyperbolic. Indeed, distinctions between two unpaired quantitative data sets are declared "significant" when the distributions of the data sets overlap extensively and demonstrate germane similarities. Relationships between two quantitative variables are declared "significant" when scatterplots demonstrate that the relationships are trivial. To read intelligently such descriptions of data revelations, it is critical to put statistical significance in perspective.

Examples of this book show that declaration of statistical significance is not a certification of clinical importance. Small *P*-values insinuate that data revelations would be unlikely if chance were the explanation. Declaration of a data revelation "significant" when the *P*-value is small is a declaration that the data revelation would be particularly unlikely if chance were the explanation. The concern that the data revelations are incidental may be dismissed. Suggestions of "significant" data revelations are scrutinized by identifying the statistic that is declared statistically significant and examining instructive descriptions of the observations.

95% confidence intervals are frequently presented alongside *P*-values of statistical significance tests. *P*-values are smaller than 0.05 when the null values of the statistics portraying data revelations, 0 if a difference and 1.0 if a ratio, are excluded from the intervals and are larger than 0.05 otherwise. However, suggestions of the intervals are rarely commented on. This book uses 95% confidence intervals as assessments of reproducibility. Narrow 95% confidence intervals are used as suggestions of adequate reproducibility, and wide intervals are used as suggestions of inadequate reproducibility. When it is not evident whether a 95% confidence interval suggests adequate reproducibility, the following improvised scheme is used:

1. *Adequate reproducibility*: A revelation of data is considered adequately reproducible if the boundaries of its 95% confidence interval are between 90% and 110% of the statistic portraying the revelation. The revelation may be used to make inference.
2. *Moderate reproducibility*: A revelation of data is considered moderately reproducible if the boundaries of the 95% confidence interval are between 75% and 90% or between 110% and 125% of the statistics portraying the revelation. It is astute to be tentative when the revelation is generalized.
3. *Inadequate reproducibility*: A revelation of data is considered inadequately reproducible if the boundaries of its 95% confidence interval are less than 75% or more than 125% of the statistic portraying the revelation. It is astute to limit the revelation to the subjects of the study and use it as a preliminary clue.

- *Intention-to-Treat Analysis*

An inherent difficulty of clinical studies is that there are often protocol violations. There may be subjects who did not receive assigned treatment, crossed over to another treatment group, received additional treatment, or did not complete outcome evaluation. Revelations of data presented in medical articles are often the results of intention-to-treat analyses that used data from all subjects assigned to treatment groups regardless of protocol violation. These revelations are not indisputable assessments of treatment effects but more credible assessments of the effects of being assigned to treatment groups. The results of per-protocol analyses that used data from subjects who received only assigned treatment and completed outcome evaluation without protocol violation are sometimes reported. These revelations are more credible assessments of treatment effects.

To read intelligently descriptions of revelation of data, it is essential to ascertain whether revelations of data are assessments of effects of treatments or effects of treatment assignment. To report informatively, it is critical to make clear whether revelations of data are results of intention-to-treat analyses or per-protocol analyses.

- *Paired and Unpaired Data Sets*

Two sets of observations are paired if there is a one-to-one pairing between every observation of one set and a specific observation of the other set. Two sets of observations are unpaired if there is not such one-to-one pairing. Sets of observations may be matched but unpaired. Sets of observations are matched if the observations form subsets and each subset of one data set is matched with a specific subset of the other set with respect to some traits; they are unmatched otherwise. If the numbers of observations in subsets are larger than the number of data sets, the data sets are matched but unpaired. If the numbers of observations in subsets are identical to the number of data sets, the data sets are paired. It is a common practice to analyze matched data sets as unpaired.

Whether data sets of medical studies are unpaired or paired is determined by study design.

– Randomized Clinical Trials

An important type of study is a randomized clinical trial that assigns subjects to treatment groups by a random allocation procedure. Whether the groups of subjects of a randomized clinical trial are unpaired, paired, or matched depends on the random allocation procedure. There are two basic types of random allocation procedures. They are known as complete randomized designs and randomized block designs.

A completely randomized design assigns eligible subjects to treatment groups in a way such that every eligible subject has the same chance of being assigned to each group. A randomized block design stratifies subjects into blocks and then uses a completely randomized design to assign the subjects within each block to treatment groups. Groups of subjects that are results of a completely randomized design are unpaired; their data sets are unpaired. Groups of subjects that are the results of a randomized block design are matched with respect to the criterion used to stratify subjects into blocks. The groups of subjects and their data sets are matched but unpaired if the numbers of subjects in the blocks are larger than the number of treatment groups; they are paired if the number of subjects in the blocks is equal to the number of treatment groups. Matched but unpaired data sets are usually analyzed as unpaired data sets.

– Cohort Studies

A cohort study is one that enrolls one or more groups of subjects with specific traits to evaluate the presence or occurrence of conditions. If the subjects of two groups are identified separately according to specific criteria and enrollment of subjects in one group is not based on a match with a specific subject in the other group, the two groups of subjects and their data sets are unpaired. If each subject of a group is identified by matching with a specific subject of the other group, the two groups of subjects and their data sets are paired.

– Case–Control Studies

A case–control study is a special type of cohort study. It enrolls a group of patients with a disease, and one or more groups of individuals free of the disease. The patients with the disease are called cases, and the individuals free of the disease are dubbed controls. Controls of case–control studies are also dubbed referrers; case–control studies are also dubbed case-referrer studies. The presence of risk factors for the disease, concurrent or historical, is assessed to evaluate the association between the risk of the disease and the risk factors.

The group of cases and a group of controls of a case–control study and their data sets are paired if each control is identified by matching with a specific case; they are unpaired if the group of cases and the group of controls are enrolled separately without individual matching.

Chapter 4
Unpaired Quantitative Data Sets

Observations of medical studies are often quantitative. Revelations of quantitative data sets are cogently manifested by the respective distributions of the observations in the data sets if the data sets are unpaired.

Descriptions of revelations of unpaired quantitative data sets are ambiguous and hyperbolic frequently. Distinctions between unpaired quantitative data sets are often dubbed "significant" despite the fact that their distributions overlap extensively and demonstrate important similarities.

This chapter demonstrates that to read intelligently descriptions of revelations of unpaired quantitative data sets, it is productive to explore manifestations of their distributions, and that revelations of unpaired quantitative data sets are informatively reported by articulating the manifestations of data distributions.

Section 4.1 uses examples to identify five archetypes of distinctions between unpaired quantitative data sets. Section 4.2 illustrates that "significantly" distinct unpaired quantitative data sets often overlap extensively and demonstrate relevant similarities. Examples of intelligent reading and informative reporting are presented in Sect. 4.3.

4.1 Archetypes of Distinctions

Revelations of quantitative observations are manifested by their respective distributions when they are unpaired. The distributions may differ in many ways and suggest different types of distinctions. Examples of this section exemplify five archetypes.

Example 4.1.1 (All larger)

Zile and Gaasch (2004) (Example 2.4.1) used the following narrative to depict chamber stiffness constants in subjects with and without diastolic heart failure:

> As shown in Figure 3, the chamber-stiffness constant was higher in the patients with diastolic heart failure than in the controls.

P. C. Chang, *Data Analysis of Medical Studies*,
https://doi.org/10.1007/978-3-031-49984-5_4

Chamber stiffness constants are quantitative observations. The two groups of subjects were enrolled separately; enrollment of subjects in one group was not based on a match with a specific subject of the other group. There is not a one-to-one pairing of the subjects in the two groups. The two groups of subjects and their data sets are unpaired. Revelations of the unpaired data sets are informatively manifested by their respective distributions.

The dot diagrams of Figure 3 (Fig. 2.9) are informative descriptions of the distributions of the chamber stiffness constants of the two groups of subjects. It unveils that the distribution of the group of subjects with diastolic heart failure varies in a wide range from 0.015 to 0.075 approximately; the distribution of the constants of the group of subjects without diastolic heart failure varies in a low and narrow range between 0.002 and 0.015 approximately. The distributions of the two sets of chamber stiffness constants are completely separated. The most prominent facet of the distinction between the two groups is that the chamber stiffness constants of all subjects with heart failure are higher than those of all controls.

Example 4.1.2 (All smaller)

Figure 1 of Perrine and Others (1985) (Fig. 2.10) used dot diagrams to depict ratios of β-globin synthesis to total non-α-globin in 10 infants of diabetic mothers and those in 11 infants of normal mothers. The ratios are quantitative observations. The two groups of infants were identified separately; enrollment of an infant in one group was not based on a match with a specific infant in the other group. There is not a one-to-one pairing of the infants in one group with specific infants in the other group. The two groups of infants and their data sets are unpaired. Revelations of the two unpaired data sets are informatively manifested by their distributions.

The dot diagrams unveil that the distributions of the ratios of the two groups of infants are totally separated. The distribution of the infants of diabetic mothers varies in a low and narrow range extending from 10 to 25 approximately; the distribution of the ratios of the infants of normal mothers varies in a higher and wider range extending from 30 to 65 approximately. The distributions of the two sets of ratios of β-globin synthesis to total non-α-globin values are totally separated. The most salient aspect of the distinction between the two groups of infants is that the ratios of β-globin synthesis to total non-α-globin of all infants of diabetic mothers are lower than those of the infants of normal mothers.

Example 4.1.3 (Smaller than many)

Figure 1A of Petersen and Others (2010) (Fig. 2.11) uses dot diagrams to depict liver triglyceride contents of two groups of Asian Indian men. One consisted of Asian Indian men who are APOC3 variant allele carriers and the other Asian Indian men who are APOC3 wild-type homozygotes.

Liver triglyceride contents are quantitative observations. The two groups of Asian Indian men were identified separately according to genotypes. Identification of a subject in one group was not based on a match with a specific subject of the other group. The two groups of subjects are unpaired, so are the two sets of liver triglyceride contents. Revelations of the unpaired data sets are eloquently manifested by their distributions.

The dot diagram on the right of Fig. 1A shows that one salient aspect of the distinction between the two groups of subjects is that the distribution of the APOC3 variant allele carriers varies widely from close to 0 to as high as nearly 50%, and that the distribution of the liver triglyceride contents of the wild-type homozygotes varies in a conspicuously narrower and lower range and overlaps the lower end of the distribution of the APOC3 variant allele carriers.

One feature of the figure is that it shows the liver triglyceride contents of the subjects who had nonalcoholic fatty liver disease in a box. The figure unveils that nonalcoholic fatty liver diseases were found only in APOC3 variant allele carriers and not in any of the wild-type homozygotes. The liver triglyceride contents of APOC3 variant allele carriers with nonalcoholic fatty liver disease are high and vary widely from 5% to as high as 50%; the contents of APOC3 variant allele carriers without the disease are all below 5% and are comparable with those of the wild-type homozygotes who are all free of nonalcoholic fatty disease.

Example 4.1.4 (Smaller than many)

Figure 3 of Stengaard-Pedersen and Others (2003) (Fig. 3.7) suggests that the distribution of plasma mannan-binding lectin-associated serine protease 2 (MASP-2) levels of the subjects homozygous for wild type (D120/D120) varies in a wide range from 600 to 3900 mU/ml approximately. The distribution of the heterozygous controls, on the other hand, varies in a narrow range from 500 to 1100 mU/ml approximately and overlaps the lower 10% of the distribution of the subjects homozygous for wild type (D120/D120). It is clear that the plasma MASP-2 levels of the heterozygous controls were lower than those of about 90% of the subjects homozygous for wild type (D120/D120).

Example 4.1.5 (Many comparable)

Figure 2 of Urbano-Marquez and Others (1989) (Fig. 2.12) depicts measurements of muscular strength of asymptomatic alcoholic men and nonalcoholic men. The measurements are quantitative observations. The group of asymptomatic alcoholic men and the group of nonalcoholic men were unrolled separately. Enrollment of the subjects in one group was not based on a match with a specific subject in the other group. The two groups are unpaired, so are the two sets of muscular-strength measurements.

The dot diagrams are informative descriptions of the distributions of the two sets of observations. They indicate that the distribution of the measurements of the asymptomatic alcoholic men varies widely from as low as 10 kg to almost 30 kg, and the distribution of the nonalcoholic men varies in a higher and narrower range from 23 kg to 34 kg approximately. The higher portion of the distribution of the alcoholic men overlaps the lower portion of the distribution of the nonalcoholic men. One forceful way to relate the distinction between the two groups of men is that the stronger nonalcoholic men were stronger than those of the alcoholic men, and the weaker alcoholic men were weaker than the nonalcoholic men.

Example 4.1.6 (Many comparable)

Figure 1 of Monath and Others (2011) (Fig. 2.13) shows that the day 42 $PRNT_{50}$ titers of the low-dose group vary from 5 to 160, and those of the high-dose group vary from 20 to 640. The higher portion of the distribution of the low-dose group overlaps the lower portion of the distribution of the high-dose group. The two groups are similar in that the smaller titers of the high-dose group are comparable with the larger titers of the low-dose group. One way to articulate the distinction between the two groups is to stress that the titers of all subjects in the high-dose group are larger than 20, and those of only 46% of the low-dose group are larger than 20.

Example 4.1.7 Weintraub (366, 16) (More larger)

Figure 1 of Weintraub and Others (2014) (Fig. 1.7) uses histograms to depict coronary artery bypass grafting (CABG) propensity scores—estimates of probability of being selected for coronary artery bypass grafting (CABG)—of a group of subjects who underwent CABG and a group who underwent percutaneous coronary intervention (PCI). CABG propensity scores are quantitative. The two groups of subjects were identified separately. There is not a one-to-one match of the subjects in one group with a specific subject in the other group. The two groups as well as their data sets are unpaired. The revelations of the two sets of unpaired quantitative observations are cogently manifested by their distributions.

The histograms submit that the distribution of the propensity scores of the two groups of subjects vary widely from close to 0 to close to 100 and are nearly totally overlapped. The distribution of the scores of the CABG group is skewed to the left with a notably smaller percentage of scores below 50 as compared with the percentage of scores above 50; the distribution of the PCI group is skewed to the right with a notably smaller percentage of propensity scores above 50 as compared with the percentage of scores below 50. In other words, the CABG group has a substantially higher percentage of scores about 50 than the PCI group.

Example 4.1.8 (More larger)

Figure 2 of Albers and Others (2018) (Fig. 1.1) shows the distributions of scores on the modified Rankin scale of the endovascular therapy group and the medical therapy group. The two groups of subjects are results of a randomized block design; they and their data sets are unpaired though matched. The scores are quantitative observations; revelations of the unpaired quantitative data sets are informatively manifested by their distributions.

The two distributions overlap completely. A salient distinction between the two sets of scores is that their distributions are skewed in different directions. The endovascular therapy group had a noticeably higher percentage of low scores (0, 1, or 2) and a noticeably low percentage of high scores (5 or 6). The medical therapy group, on the other hand, had a noticeably lower percentage of low scores (0, 1, or 2) and a noticeably higher percentage of high scores (5 or 6). One way to characterize their distinction is to underscore that the percentage of low scores (0, 1, or 2) is noticeably higher in the endovascular therapy group than in the medical group (44% vs. 20%).

Example 4.1.9 (Little difference – nearly identical)

Figure 2A of Hays and Others (2003) (Fig. 2.14) uses overlaid histograms to depict distributions of changes in measurements of physical functioning from baseline to year 1 in subjects of the estrogen plus progestin group and the placebo group. Changes in measurements of physical functioning are quantitative observations. The two groups of subjects were formed by random allocation. They and their data sets are unpaired. Revelations of the two sets of changes are cogently manifested by their distributions.

The histograms suggest that the distributions of changes in physical functioning of subjects in the two groups are nearly totally overlapped. They vary from decreases of 50 points to increases of 50 points approximately and are relatively symmetric with prominent clusters in the middle. The red and blue top sections of the bars are short and suggest that there is little difference between the distributions of the two groups of subjects. A subtle difference is that the estrogen plus progestin group had slightly higher percentages of increases (red sections) compared with the placebo group (blue sections).

- *Types of Distinction Between Unpaired Quantitative Data Sets*

The above examples demonstrate that unpaired quantitative data sets may differ in many ways. When distinction between unpaired quantitative data sets is evaluated, it is vital to assess how their distributions differ. The examples demonstrate five archetypes of distinctions. The five types are useful references when unpaired quantitative data sets are analyzed. To stress their pivotal features, the five types are dubbed in this book as all larger (smaller), many larger (smaller), many comparable, more small and more large, and little difference. Each type has variations, and there are other types.

1. *All larger* (No overlap)

This is the highest level of distinction between two unpaired quantitative data sets. The distributions of the data sets are completely separated and suggest that all observations in one data set are larger than all observations in the other set. The variation and skewness of the distributions may or may not differ. (Examples 4.1.1 and 4.1.2.)

2. *Smaller (larger) than many* (One distribution overlaps one end of the other)

The distribution of one data set varies in a narrow range and overlaps the lower or higher portion of the distribution of the other set, which varies widely. In other words, observations of one set are smaller or larger than many observations of the other set (Examples 4.1.3 and 4.1.4.).

3. *Many comparable* (Higher portion of one distribution overlaps the lower portion of the other)

The higher portion of the distribution of one data set overlaps the lower portion of the distribution of the other data set. A salient distinction between the data sets is that the smaller observations of one data set are comparable with the larger observations of the other set (Examples 4.1.5 and 4.1.6).

4. *More larger* (Complete overlap but distinct skewness)

Distributions of data sets are nearly totally overlapped but skewed in different directions. One data set has more smaller observations and fewer larger observations and the other set has more larger observations and fewer smaller observations (Examples 4.1.7 and 4.1.8).

5. *Little difference* (Complete overlap and similar shape)

Distributions of data sets overlap nearly completely and demonstrate similar shapes (Example 4.1.9).

Example 4.1.10
An article by van Bon and Others (2014) presents the results of a study that isolated plasmacytoid dendritic cells from healthy persons and from patients with systemic sclerosis and distinct phenotypes. Proteome-wide analysis showed that CXCL4 is the predominant protein secreted by plasmacytoid dendritic cells in systemic sclerosis, in both circulation and skin. One account of CXCL4 in circulation asserted: *"In the identification cohort, levels of circulation CXCL4 were markedly higher in patients with systemic sclerosis than in healthy controls and were particularly high in patients with early diffuse disease (P < 0.001 for both comparisons) (Fig. 2A)."*

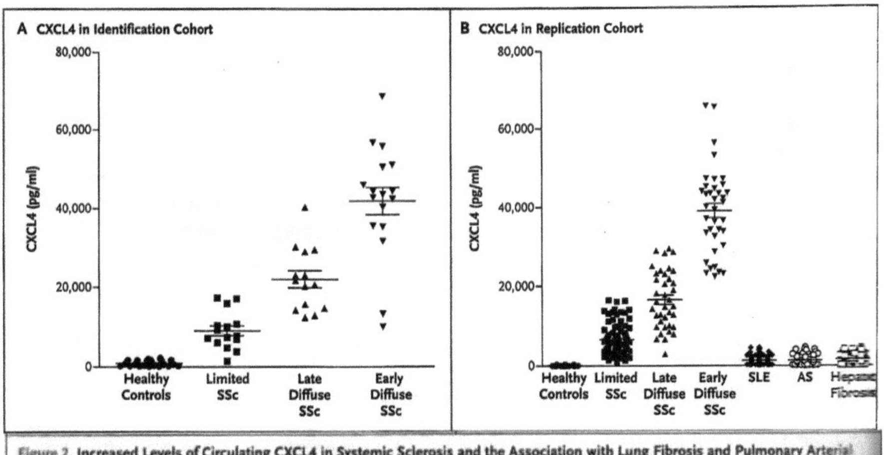

Figure 2. Increased Levels of Circulating CXCL4 in Systemic Sclerosis and the Association with Lung Fibrosis and Pulmonary Arterial Hypertension.
High levels of CXCL4 were observed in the circulation of patients with limited systemic sclerosis (SSc), late diffuse SSc, and early diffuse SSc in the identification cohort at Boston University (Panel A) and in 161 patients with corresponding subtypes of systemic sclerosis in two independent (Dutch and Swedish) replication cohorts, as compared with 129 age- and sex-matched healthy controls, 109 patients with systemic lupus erythematosus (SLE), 93 with ankylosing spondylitis (AS), and 93 with hepatic fibrosis (Panel B). The horizontal lines indicate means, and I bars standard deviations. Shown are the estimated times until the development of lung fibrosis (Panel C) and pulmonary arterial hypertension (PAH) (Panel D) within the first 24 months after the diagnosis of systemic sclerosis among patients with a high circulating CXCL4 level (≥10 ng per milliliter) and among those with a low CXCL4 level (<10 ng per milliliter).

Fig. 4.1 Figure 2A and B of van Bon and Others (2014)

Figure 2A (Fig. 4.1) uses dot diagrams to depict the distributions of CXCL4 in circulations in three groups of subjects with systemic sclerosis and a group of controls without the disease. The three groups of subjects with systemic sclerosis (limited, late diffuse, and early diffuse systemic sclerosis) and the group of healthy controls were identified separately. Identification of the subjects in one group was not based on a match with specific subjects in another group. There is not a one-to-one pairing of any subject in one group with a specific subject in another group. The four groups and the four sets of CXCL4 levels are unpaired. Revelations of the four sets of CXCL4 levels are informatively manifested by their respective distributions. The dot diagrams suggest that the CXCL4 levels of the four groups of subjects differed in several ways. For instance:

- All larger: With only one exception, the CXCL4 levels of the three group of subjects with systemic sclerosis were larger than those of the group of healthy controls. The one exception is a subject with limited systemic sclerosis.
- Many larger: The CXCL4 levels of the group of subjects with early diffuse systemic sclerosis are larger than those of many subjects with late diffuse systemic sclerosis and many subjects with early diffuse systemic sclerosis.
- Many smaller: The CXCL4 levels of the group of subjects with limited systemic sclerosis are smaller than those of many subjects with late diffuse systemic sclerosis and many subjects with early diffuse systemic sclerosis.

4.2 Significant Distinctions

Distinctions between unpaired quantitative data sets are often declared "significant." The modifier "significantly" means that the statistics gauging the distinctions, e.g., difference in means or medians, may be declared statistically significant. The distributions of the data sets may overlap extensively and be comparable in some pertinent ways. The differences in means or medians may also be slight.

Example 4.2.1 Hays and Others (2003) (Example 4.19) stated:

> When the change in measures of health-related quality of life between baseline and year 1 were examined, a few differences were observed between the estrogen-plus-progestin group and the placebo group (Table 2). There were small but statistically significant positive effects of estrogen plus progestin, relative to placebo, on physical functioning, ($P < 0.001$), bodily pain ($P < 0.001$), and sleep disturbance ($P < 0.001$). For example, the mean benefit in terms of physical functioning was 0.8 point on the 100-point scale.

The assertion that there were small but statistically significant effects of estrogen plus progestin is corroborated by small *P*-values. The small but statistically significant positive effects of estrogen plus progestin, relative to placebo, alludes to distinctions in the means of change between the two treatment groups.

The mean benefit of physical functioning 0.8 points was cited as an example. It is miniscule. The score on physical functioning was measured on a 0–100 scale. Figure 2A (Fig. 2.14) shows that the distributions of the changes in scores of physical functioning of the two groups are completely overlapped and vary from − 50 to 50 approximately. Table 2 shows that the means of changes from baseline to year 1 in scores of physical functioning in the estrogen plus progestin group and the placebo group are −0.6 and −1.4, respectively. They and their distinction are minute.

$P < 0.001$ suggested only that the minute difference in means of changes would be particularly unlikely if chance were the only explanation. The distinction in the means of changes may be declared statistically significant, and the concern that the miniscule distinction in the means of changes is incidental may be dismissed. $P < 0.001$ and declaration of statistical significance are not certifications of clinically importance.

The effects of the two treatment groups are informatively manifested by the distributions of the changes. Figure 2A (Fig. 2.14) shows that the distributions of the changes in scores of physical functioning of the two groups are totally overlapped and have similar shapes. The changes in the score on physical functioning of the two treatment groups are comparable and are hardly a demonstration that estrogen plus progestin was more effective than the placebo.

One feature of the study reported by Hays and Others (2003) is that a large number of subjects were studied. The means of changes in scores on physical functioning are the means of 7503 changes in the estrogen plus progestin group and 7106 changes in the placebo group. The asserted small but statistically significant positive effect of estrogen plus progestin on physical functioning alludes to the miniscule distinction in the means of changes. The small *P*-value and statistical significance, to a large extent, are results of the large numbers of changes.

Instead of asserting that there were small but statistically significant positive effects of estrogen plus progestin, it is more constructive to stress the indication of Fig. 2A that most changes in the two treatment groups are comparable. They differ only in that the estrogen plus progestin group had a slightly higher percentage of improvements than the placebo group.

Example 4.2.2 Lange and Others (2004) (Example 2.7.1) asserted:

> The primary angiographic end point – minimal luminal diameter – was significantly smaller in the folate group than in the placebo group at follow-up (1.59 ± 0.62 vs. 1.74 ± 0.64 mm, $P = 0.008$).

The assertion that the minimal luminal diameter was significantly smaller in the folate group than in the placebo group at follow-up is corroborated by means and standard deviations and *P*-value (*1.59 ± 0.62 vs. 1.74 ± 0.64 mm, P = 0.008*). $P = 0.008$ suggests that the distinction between the means of the two treatment groups (1.74 – 1.59 = 0.15 mm) may be declared statistically significant and the concern that it is incidental may be dismissed. It is the distance between the centers of the distributions of the minimal luminal diameter of the two groups that was declared statistically significant. It is unknown whether the distributions overlap extensively or are comparable in some pertinent ways.

The standard deviations of minimal luminal diameters of the two groups are not small relative to the means. The means and standard deviations (1.59 ± 0.62 and 1.74 ± 0.64 mm) suggest that the distributions of the minimal luminal diameters of the two treatment groups overlap extensively. Probably, the minimal luminal diameters of many subjects in the two groups were comparable.

The extent of overlap of the two distributions is indicated by the cumulative distribution curves of Fig. 1 (Fig. 2.20). The two curves in the middle submit that the distributions of the minimal luminal diameters of the two groups vary in comparable ranges from close to 0.5 to close to 3.0 mm approximately and overlap completely. Although the distinction between their means (1.74 vs. 1.59) may be declared statistically significant, the minimal luminal diameters of most subjects in the two treatment groups are comparable. A subtle difference is that the folate group had a slightly larger percentage of small minimal luminal diameters. For instance, the percentage of follow-up minimal luminal diameters less than 1.0 mm is about 30% in the folate group and about 20% in the placebo group.

It is more constructive to accentuate the indication of the cumulative distribution curves that the minimal luminal diameters at follow-up of many subjects in the two treatment groups are comparable, and that a subtle difference is that the folate group had a slightly larger percentage of small minimal luminal diameters at follow-up.

Example 4.2.3

Results of a study that randomly assigned 872 subjects with adenocarcinoma of the colon to undergo open or laparoscopically assisted colectomy are presented in an article by The Clinical Outcomes of Surgical Therapy Study Group (2004). The article states:

> Operation times were significantly longer in the laparoscopic-surgery group than in the open colectomy group (150 minutes vs. 95 minutes, $P < 0.001$).

This is impressive. The values: 150 minutes and 95 minutes are the medians of operation times of the two groups. $P < 0.001$ suggests that the distinction between the two medians may be declared statistically significant. It is the median of the laparoscopic surgery group that was "significantly" greater than that of the open colectomy group, not the operation times of all subjects in the group.

Table 2 shows the ranges of the operation times are 35–450 minutes and 27–435 minutes. The medians and ranges are shown schematically in Fig. 4.2. The figure suggests that the distributions of operation times of the two groups overlap extensively and are highly skewed to the right. To read intelligently, it is critical to note that although the distinction in medians may be declared statistically significant,

```
Laparoscopic-surgery group:   {----------▼-----------------------------}
                              35        150                          450

Open-colectomy group:         {-----▼---------------------------------}
                              27    95                              425
```

Fig. 4.2 Mediums and ranges of operation times in minutes the distributions of operation times of the two groups overlap extensively and the operation times of most subjects in the two groups are comparable.

To report informatively, it is productive to present comprehensive descriptions of the distributions of operation times and use percentages of short or long operation times to highlight the distinction between the two treatment groups. Percentages of operation times shorter than 90 minutes or 120 minutes may be used.

Example 4.2.4 Buehler and Others (1990) (Example 2.5.2) stated:

> The results of the enzyme determination suggest that the mean epoxide hydrolase activity in patients with the fetal hydantoin syndrome is significantly lower than that in a random sample of amniocytes as determined by a two-tailed t-test for samples of different sizes and populations with unequal variances (P <0.001). This suggests that it is possible to recognize fetuses at risk on the basis of their microsomal epoxide hydrolase activity.

The t-test is a procedure for testing the statistical significance of distinction between means. $P < 0.001$ suggests that the difference between the means of the two sets of epoxide hydrolase activities would be unlikely if chance were the only explanation. It is the distinction in the means of epoxide activity between the patients with the fetal hydantoin syndrome and the random sample of amniocytes that was declared statistically significant. The statistical significance of the distinction in means is not an affirmation that the epoxide hydrolase activities of all or most patients with the fetal hydantoin syndrome were lower than those of random samples of amniocytes. The small *P*-value and statistical significance are not plausible evidence that it is possible to recognize fetuses at risk on the bases of their microsomal epoxide activity.

How the two sets of epoxide hydrolase activity determinations differed is informatively depicted by Fig. 1 of the article (Fig. 2.15). The figure discloses that the determinations of all 16 infants with fetal hydantoin syndrome were below 37.5% of the standard, and those of many pregnant women, but not all, were higher.

The indication of Fig. 1 is articulated by the following two narratives:

> The values for the samples ranged from a low of 8 percent of the standard to a high of 116 percent of the standard; the values were distributed as shown in Figure 1.
>
> And
>
> For the affected children, however, the range of enzymatic activity was quite limited; the lowest value was 9.6 percent of the standard, and the range extended only to 30 percent of the standard (Fig. 1).

These two narratives and Figure 1 present a candid description of the distinction between the two sets of enzymatic activity levels. They constitute a persuasive argument that epoxide hydrolase activity determinations may be used to recognize fetuses at risk of fetal hydantoin syndrome. Thirty percent of the standard could be used as a cutoff value.

4.3 Intelligent Reading and Informative Reporting

Revelations of quantitative data sets are often portrayed synoptically by values of descriptive statistics such as mean and standard deviation or median and range. Distinctions between unpaired quantitative data sets are frequently declared "significant" when their distributions overlap and demonstrate pertinent similarities. To read intelligently, it is critical to ascertain the suggestions of the statistics portraying the revelations and the manifestations of the distributions of the data sets. To report informatively, it is vital to stress salient indications of the distributions of data sets. The following suggestions are presented as a reference.

- Intelligent reading

  1. Find out whether revelations of data are the results of intention-to-treat analysis or per-protocol analysis and determine whether revelations of data pertain to effects of treatments or effects of being assigned to treatment groups. Assume that revelations pertain to effects of assignment to treatment groups instead of effects of treatments when in doubt.
  2. Read descriptions of "significant" differences between data sets with caution. Keep in mind that the elegant modifier "significant" is used in the sense of statistical significance and is only a declaration that it is alright to dismiss the concern that the statistic portraying the revelation is incidental. It is critical to assess the indications of the statistic portraying the revelations and the distributions of the data sets. Declaration of statistical significance is not an affirmation that all or most observations in one data set are larger than all those in the other set. The distributions of the data sets may overlap extensively and demonstrate relevant similarities.
  3. Whether the distinction between data sets is or is not "significant," scrutinize how the distributions of the data sets differ, particularly whether distributions overlap extensively or are skewed in the same direction. Use the archetypes of distinction identified in Sect. 4.1 as reference. It is constructive to find out whether all, many, or just a few of the observations in one set are larger than those in the other set.
  4. When means and standard deviations are the only available descriptions of data, use speculated 95% observation-regions to reap some provisional pointers regarding ranges and skewness of distributions of observations.
  5. When data are depicted synoptically by median, interquartile range, and range, keep in mind that they are imprecise if there are arrays of observations with identical magnitudes.

- Informative reporting

  Clarity and simplicity are more important than sophistication and eloquence. The following comments are presented here as a reference.

1. Indicate clearly whether revelations of data pertain to the effects of being in treatment groups or effects of treatments. Indicate the numbers and characteristics of subjects whose data were used in analysis.
2. Use graphical displays or tables to depict comprehensively how observations distribute and how distributions differ.
3. Do not simply assert whether distinctions between data sets are or are not "significant." Use manifestations of the distributions of the data sets to articulate how the data sets differ.
4. Use percentages of observations in germane categories to underline revelations of data sets and distinctions between data sets synoptically.
5. Median and range are more informative than mean and standard deviation if the distributions of observations are notably skewed. Percentages of observations in germane categories are more direct than median and range particularly when there are arrays of identical observations.

Example 4.3.1 Amiel (316, 22)
Amiel and Others (1987) presented the results of a study that infused small doses of insulin for 3 hours in 8 subjects without diabetes, 11 subjects with well-controlled diabetes, and 10 subjects with poorly controlled diabetes to simulate the mild peripheral hyperinsulinemia observed during insulin treatment. One outcome is related as follows:

> There was a clear separation between the glucose nadirs in the participants with good control (all <45 mg per deciliter, or 2.5 mmol per liter) and those in the other groups (all >55 mg per deciliter, or 3.1 mmol per liter).

This is simple and clear.

Example 4.3.2
The distinction between subjects with diastolic heart failure and those without evidence of cardiovascular diseases with respect to chamber stiffness constants is recounted in the abstract of Zile and Gaasch (2004) (Example 4.1.1) as follows:

> The corrected left ventricular passive stiffness constant was significantly higher in the group with diastolic heart failure than in the control group (0.03 ± 0.01 vs. 0.01 ± 0.01, $P < 0.001$).

The article states: *Differences between the group with diastolic heart failure and the control group were examined with the use of an unpaired t-test. A P-value of less than 0.05 was considered to indicate statistical significance.* The unpaired t-test is a procedure for testing statistical significance of distinction between the means of two unpaired quantitative data sets. $P < 0.001$ suggests that the distinction between the means of the two groups of subjects (0.03 vs. 0.01) may be declared statistically significant. It is the mean of the corrected left ventricular passive stiffness constants of the group of subjects with diastolic heart failure that is statistically significantly higher than the mean of the control group. It is unknown whether the distributions of the passive stiffness constants of the two groups overlap extensively and suggests that the constants of many subjects in the two groups are comparable.

The narrative cited in Example 4.1.1: "*As shown in Figure 3, the chamber-stiffness constant was higher in the patients with diastolic heart failure than in the controls.*" is a more illuminating description compared with the one asserting that the ventricular passive stiffness constant was significantly higher in the group with diastolic heart failure than in the control group.

Example 4.3.3
The following is a description of *globin synthesis* levels of 11 infants of normal mothers and 10 infants of diabetic mothers presented in Perrine and Others (1985) (Example 4.12).

> Globin synthesis in the study infants and their controls is shown in Figure 1. The mean β-globin synthesis in 11 normal infants at 36 to 39 weeks of gestation was 44.6 per cent of the amount of non-α-globin; this finding is consistent with previous data in normal infants. The mean β-globin synthesis in the 10 infants of diabetic mother was 14.8 per cent. The difference between the two groups was statistically significant ($P < 0.001$, Student's t-test).

$P < 0.001$ is the ground of the assertion that the difference between the two groups was statistically significant. It is a result of using the Student's t-test to test the statistical significance of the distinction between the means of β-globin synthesis levels of the two groups of infants. It suggests that the distinction between the means of β-globin synthesis levels of the two groups of infants as large as 29.8 (44.6 vs. 14.8) or larger would be particularly unlikely if chance were the only explanation. The assertion that the difference between the two groups was statistically significant affirms only that the distinction between means may be declared statistically significant and the concern that the distinction in means is incidental may be dismissed. It is not an affirmation that the globin synthesis of the study infants were all larger than those of the controls.

To report informatively, it is more telling to refer to Fig. 1 (Fig. 2.10) and stress its indication that the β-globin synthesis levels of all infants of diabetic mothers were lower than those of normal infants.

Example 4.3.4
The primary outcome of the study reported by Zheng and Others (2018) (Example 3.1.5) is change in total score on the Fugl–Meyer upper extremity scale between baseline and the end of month 12. The article stated:

> The mean changes in the total Fugl-Meyer score from baseline to month 12 was 17.7 ± 5.6 in the surgery group versus 2.6 ± 2.0 in the control group, showing significant greater improvement in the surgery group (difference, 15.1; 95% confidence interval [CI], 12.2 to 17.9; $P < 0.001$) (Table 2).

The values 17.7 ± 5.6 and 2.6 ± 2.0 are the means and standard deviations of changes in the total Fugl–Meyer score from baseline to month 12. The 95% confidence interval excludes 0. It and $P < 0.001$ suggest that the distinction in means $(17.7 - 2.3 = 15.1)$ may be declared statistically significant.

The "significant greater improvement in the surgery group" refers to the statistical significance of the distinction in means of changes in the total Fugl–Meyer score from baseline to month 12 (17.7 vs. 2.6). It is not an affirmation that all or most

Control Group: [--0---▲------]
2.6∓2 × 2.0   *- 1.4   2.6   6.6.*

Surgery group: [--------------▲-------------------]
17.7 ∓2 × 5.6   *6.5   17.7   28.9.*

Fig. 4.3 Speculated 95% regions for changes in Fugl–Meyer score

changes of the surgery group were greater improvements as compared with the changes of the control group. To read intelligently, it is critical to find out how the changes of the two groups differed. As comprehensive descriptions of the distributions of changes are not available, the means and standard deviations of the changes were used to determine speculated 95% observation-regions.

Figure 4.3 shows schematically the speculated 95% observation-regions for the changes in total Fugl–Meyer score. The regions speculate the following:

- The changes in the surgery group were all improvements and those in the control group included some small improvements and some small deteriorations.
- Nearly all the improvements in the surgery group were larger than the improvements in the control group.

This is a rare special case. The distinction between the means of two data sets is larger than two times the sum of the standard deviations of the data sets. The speculated 95% observation-regions do not overlap and conjecture that the distributions of the data sets do not overlap. This occurs rarely.

To report informatively, it is more informative to present comprehensive descriptions of the distributions of changes in the two treatment groups and accentuate the indications of the distributions. The distributions would indicate clearly how the changes in the two treatment groups differed. Revelations of the two data sets may be highlighted by percentages of noteworthy improvements in the two treatment groups.

Example 4.3.5

Petersen and Others (2010) (Example 4.1.3) used the following account to depict hepatic triglyceride contents:

> The average hepatic triglyceride content was markedly higher in the APOC3 variant-allele carriers than in the wild-type homozygotes (mean, 7.5 ± 10.3% [median, 3.2%] vs. 1.5 ± 1.3% [median, 1.1%]; $P < 0.001$) (Fig. 1A).

The means of the hepatic triglyceride contents of the APOC3 variant allele carriers is indeed markedly greater than that of the wild-type homozygotes (7.5% vs. 1.5%); the median is also larger (3.2% vs. 1.1%). $P<0.001$ suggests that the distinction between means and mediums may be declared statistically significant.

To read intelligently, it is astute to note that Fig. 1A (Fig. 2.11) suggests that the distinction in hepatic triglyceride contents between the two groups is much more than just the difference between means and the difference between medians. The liver triglyceride contents of the APOC3 variant allele carriers who had nonalcoholic fatty liver disease vary in a wide range from close to 5% to 45% and are higher than those of the APOC3 variant allele carriers who did not have nonalcoholic fatty liver disease, which vary between 0% and 5%. The contents of the wild-type homozygotes, similar to the contents of the APOC3 variant allele carriers who did not have nonalcoholic fatty liver disease, vary in a narrow range between 0% and 5%.

To report informatively, it is more captivating to stress the indication of Fig. 1 that the hepatic triglyceride contents of the APOC3 variant-allele carriers with nonalcoholic fatty disease vary from 5% to 45% and are higher than those of the APOC3 variant-allele carriers without nonalcoholic fatty disease, which are all below 5% and are comparable with the hepatic triglyceride contents of the wild-type homozygotes.

Example 4.3.6

Maisel and Others (2002) reported the results of a study evaluating the use of B-type natriuretic peptide level in the diagnosis of congestive heart failure; 1586 patients who went to emergency departments with acute dyspnea were evaluated. The final diagnosis was congestive heart failure in 744 subjects, dyspnea due to noncardiac causes in 72 subjects with a history of left ventricular dysfunction, and no finding of congestive heart failure in 770 subjects. The B-type natriuretic peptide levels of the three groups of subjects were related as follows:

> Figure 1 presents a box plot of B-type natriuretic peptide values for the three groups of patients. The difference among groups was significant (P $<$ 0.001 for each pairwise comparison.) Patients with a diagnosis of acute congestive heart failure had mean (±SD) B-type natriuretic peptide levels of 675 ± 450 pg per milliliter, whereas those without congestive heart failure had B-type natriuretic peptide levels of 110 ± 225 pg per milliliter.

The article stated: "*Comparisons of B-type natriuretic peptide levels values among diagnostic groups were performed by the t-test for independent samples and analysis of variance.*" The t-test is a procedure for testing statistical significance of distinction between means of two unpaired quantitative data sets, and analysis of variance is a procedure for testing statistical significance of distinction among means of two or more unpaired quantitative data sets. They are closely related and yield the same *P*-value.

$P < 0.001$ suggests that the distinction among the means of the three groups would be particularly unlikely if chance were the explanation. The distinction between means may be declared statistically significant.

The suggestions of the box plot of Fig. 1 (Fig. 4.4) though not noted, are much more valuable than the suggestions of the means and standard deviations and the statistical significance of the distinction between the means. It suggests:

- The percentage of B-type natriuretic peptide levels below 300 pg/ml was close to 100% among the subjects without congestive heart failure, more than 50% among the subjects who had a history of left ventricular dysfunction and dyspnea due to noncardiac causes, and about 75% among the subjects with congestive heart failure.

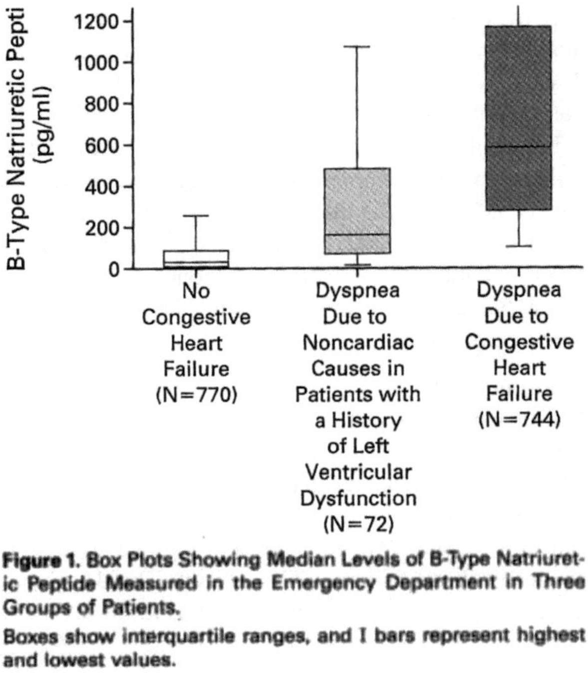

Fig. 4.4 Figure 1 of Maisel and Others (2002)

- The percentage of B-type natriuretic peptide levels higher than 500 pg/ml was 0% among the subjects without congestive heart failure, about 25% among the subjects who had a history of left ventricular dysfunction and dyspnea due to noncardiac causes, but higher than 50% among the subjects with congestive heart failure.

To report informatively, it is more constructive to stress the indications of the box plots as compared to citing the means and standard deviations and declare the distinction between means statistically significant.

Example 4.3.7

The article by the SUPPORT Study Group of the Eunice Kennedy Shriver NICH Neonatal Research Network (2010) (Example 2.6.2) stated:

> "The median levels of oxygen saturation in infants who were receiving oxygen supplementation in the two treatment groups differed substantially but as expected, there was considerable overlap (Fig. 3). The actual median levels of oxygen saturation were slightly higher than targeted levels in both treatment groups.

To read intelligently, it is critical to review Fig. 3 (Fig. 2.18). The figure shows that the distributions of the actual levels of oxygen saturation in the infants of the two treatment groups differ substantially. A footnote of Fig. 3 states: "*The medians of the distributions were significantly different on the basis of a rank-sum test ($P < 0.001$).*"

Figure 3 shows that, in the high target range group, the actual levels of oxygen saturation of about 90% of the infants were in the target range, and those of about 10% were higher than the target range. But in the low target range group, the actual levels of oxygen saturation of nearly all infants were higher than the target range (85–89%), and those of close to 50% were in the high target range (91–95%).

The actual levels of oxygen saturation are descriptions of the treatments received by the infants. It is critical whether the actual levels of oxygen saturation of the two groups of infants are within target ranges. Whether the distinction between the two groups is statistically significant is unimportant. To report informatively, it is important to report the percentages of infants whose actual levels of oxygen saturation were in the target ranges. The percentage of infants in the low target range group whose actual levels of oxygen saturation were higher than the target range is particularly important.

Review Questions

1. What does the statistical significance of the distinction between data sets suggest?
2. Why are distinctions between data sets declared "significant" without a plain description?
3. Do "significant" distinct means or medians suggest that all observations in one data set are larger than those of the other set?
4. What are the limitations of mean and standard deviation when they are only descriptions of quantitative data sets?
5. What are the limitations of medium and range when they are the only description of quantitative observations?
6. What are the characteristics of the five archetypes of distinctions between quantitative data sets identified in Sect. 4.1?
7. Are the five archetypes of distinctions between quantitative data sets signaled by their means and standard deviations or medians and ranges?
8. Could the distinction between two quantitative data sets be statistically significant when their distributions overlap extensively and are comparable in some pertinent ways?
9. As measures of the degree of distinction between two quantitative data sets, what are the relative advantages of the difference in means, difference in medians, and difference in the percentage of germane observations?
10. What does a small *P*-value of a distinction between two means suggest?
11. Is the statistical significance of the distinction between means and between medians affirmations that all or most observations in one data set are larger or smaller than those in another data set?
12. Is statistical significance a certification of clinical importance?
13. Why are graphical displays of data distributions often mentioned in passing and their indications are not commented on in descriptions of distinctions between quantitative data sets.
14. Are the mean and standard deviation, medium and range, or percentage of germane observations more informative?

Exercise

4.E.1. One result of Hays and Others (2003) is that there were small but statistically significant positive effects of estrogen plus progestin, relative to placebo, on bodily pain (Example 4.1.9). Table 2 uses 77.6 ± 22.4 and 75.6 ± 23.1 to depict the means and standard deviations of the changes from baseline to year 1 and 1.9 ± 0.3 to depict the standard error of distinction between the means of changes of the two groups.

(a) Examine Fig. 2B of the article (Fig. 2.14) and elaborate how the changes in body pain of the subjects in the two treatment groups differed.
(b) Discuss whether it is correct to interpret the "small but statistically significant positive effect of estrogen plus progestin" an assertion that the changes in body pain of all subjects in the estrogen plus progestin group were significant improvements as compared with the changes of all subjects in the placebo group.

4.E.2. Table 2 of the article by The Clinical Outcomes of Surgical Therapy Study Group (2004) (Example 4.2.3) uses 18 and 3–35 cm and 6 and 2–35 cm to denote medians and ranges of length of incision in the open colectomy group and the laparoscopic surgery group, respectively. It also shows $P = 0.001$.

(a) Discuss what $P = 0.001$ suggests and whether it is an affirmation that the incisions of all subjects in the laparoscopic surgery group were shorter than those of the subjects in the open colectomy group.
(b) Use the suggestions of the medians and ranges to recap the distinction between the two groups with respect to length of incision.
(c) Suggest a way to depict informatively the distinction between the two groups with respect to length of incision cogently.

4.E.3. Table 2 of Zheng and Others (2018) (Example 4.3.4) uses 18.4 ± 2.9 and 3.3 ± 1.1 to depict means and standard deviations of changes in total Fugl–Meyer score from baseline to month 12 of the surgery group and the control group when the cause of paralysis was stroke. $P < 0.004$ is shown for the distinction between the two groups.

(a) Elaborate what $P < 0.004$ suggests, particularly whether it suggests that all changes in the surgery groups were greater improvements as compared with the changes in the control groups.
(b) Use speculated 95% observation-regions to assess how the changes in the two groups differ.
(c) Suggest a more informative description between the two groups.

4.E.4. Review Fig. 1B of Petersen and Others (2010) (Fig. 2.11) and relate how the liver triglyceride contents of the non-Asian Indian men who are wild-type homozygotes and those who are variant allele carriers differed.

4.E.5. Review Fig. 1 of Monath and Others (2011) (Fig. 2.13) and elaborate how the day 31 $PRNT_{50}$ titers of the low- and high-dose group differed.

References

Albers, G. W., et al. (2018). Thrombectomy for stroke at 6 to 16 hours with selection by perfusion imaging. *The New England Journal of Medicine, 378*(8), 708–718.

Amiel, S. A., et al. (1987). Defective glucose counterregulation after strict glycemic control of insulin-dependent diabetes mellitus. *The New England Journal of Medicine, 316*(22), 1376–1383.

Buehler, B. A., et al. (1990). Prenatal prediction of risk of the fetal hydantoin syndrome. *The New England Journal of Medicine, 322*(22), 1567–1572.

Hays, J., et al. (2003). Effects of estrogen plus progestin on health-related quality of life. *The New England Journal of Medicine, 348*(19), 1839–1854.

Lange, H., et al. (2004). Folate therapy and in-stent restenosis after coronary stenting. *The New England Journal of Medicine, 350*(26), 2673–2681.

Maisel, A. S., et al. (2002). Rapid measurement of B-type natriuretic peptide in the emergency diagnosis of heart failure. *The New England Journal of Medicine, 347*(3), 161–167.

Monath, T. P., et al. (2011). An inactivated cell-culture vaccine against yellow fever. *The New England Journal of Medicine, 364*(14), 1326–1333.

Perrine, S. P., et al. (1985). Delay in the fetal globin switch in infants of diabetic mothers. *The New England Journal of Medicine, 312*, 334–338.

Petersen, K. F., et al. (2010). Apolipoprotein C3 gene variants in nonalcoholic fatty liver disease. *The New England Journal of Medicine, 362*(12), 1082–1089.

Stengaard-Pedersen, K., et al. (2003). Brief report: Inherited deficiency of mannan-binding lectin-associated serine protease 2. *The New England Journal of Medicine, 349*(6), 554–560.

SUPPORT study Group of the Eunice Kennedy Shriver NICHD neonatal research network. (2010). Target ranges of oxygen saturation in extremely preterm infants. *The New England Journal of Medicine, 362*(21), 1959–1969.

The Clinical Outcomes of Surgical Therapy Study Group. (2004). A comparison of laparoscopically assisted and open colectomy for colon cancer. *The New England Journal of Medicine, 350*(20), 2050–2059.

Urbano-Marquez, A., et al. (1989). The effect of alcoholism on skeletal and cardiac muscle. *The New England Journal of Medicine, 320*(7), 409–415.

van Bone, L., et al. (2014). Proteome-wide analysis and EXCL4 as a biomarker in systemic sclerosis. *The New England Journal of Medicine, 370*(5), 433–443.

Weintraub, W. S., et al. (2014). Comparative effectiveness of revascularization strategies. *The New England Journal of Medicine, 366*(16), 1467–1476.

Zheng, M.-X., et al. (2018). Trial of contralateral seventh cervical nerve transfer for spastic arm paralysis. *The New England Journal of Medicine, 378*, 22–34.

Zile, M. R., & Gaasch, W. H. (2004). Diastolic heat failure-abnormalities in active relaxation and passive stiffness. *The New England Journal of Medicine, 350*(19), 1953–1959.

References

Chapter 5
Paired Quantitative Data Sets

Sets of observations obtained from a group of subjects on two occasions are paired data sets. The observations form observation-pairs. Unlike the case of unpaired data sets, revelations of the paired data sets are not manifested by comprehensive descriptions of the observations of the data sets but by comprehensive descriptions of the observation-pairs. If the observations are quantitative, revelations of the data sets are clearly manifested by the distribution of a pair index that characterizes the observation-pairs.

Revelations of paired quantitative data sets are often related by synoptic descriptions of the respective distributions of the two data sets, which yield limited useful information. The revelations are declared significant even if the observation-pairs suggest that the revelations are trivial.

This chapter demonstrates that to read descriptions of revelations of paired quantitative data sets intelligently, it is critical to review the distribution of a pair index that characterizes the observation-pairs. To report revelations of paired quantitative data sets, it is productive to articulate the manifestations of the distribution of the pair index.

Section 5.1 uses examples to demonstrate that revelations of paired quantitative data sets are manifested by the distribution of a pair index that characterizes observation-pairs. Section 5.2 reviews the properties of pair indices that are quantitative characterizations of observation-pairs. Section 5.3 presents examples of intelligent reading and informative reporting.

5.1 Examples

This section uses examples to demonstrate that revelations of paired quantitative data sets are instructively manifested by the distribution of a pair index that characterizes observation-pairs and that the respective distributions of the paired data sets

P. C. Chang, *Data Analysis of Medical Studies*,
https://doi.org/10.1007/978-3-031-49984-5_5

yield limited useful information. It is critical to examine the distribution of a pair index that characterizes the observation-pairs of the data sets.

Example 5.1.1

The study reported by Hillmen and Others (2004) (Example 1.1.3) used the following account to depict changes in transfusion rate between baseline and 3 months after eculizumab treatment:

> Before eculizumab treatment, the mean and median transfusion rates were 2.1 and 1.8 units per patient per month, respectively (Table 1). These transfusion rates decreased to 0.6 and 0.0 unit per patient per month, respectively, during the three months of treatment with eculizumab (P = 0.003).

Clearly, the mean transfusion rate declined 1.5 units per patient per month from 2.1 to 0.6 units per patient per month, and the median declined 1.8 units per patient per month from 1.8 to 0.0 units per patient per month. $P = 0.003$ is below 0.05, which suggests that the decline in means and the decline in medians could be declared statistically significant. The declines in means and medians and $P = 0.003$ did not unveil how the rates of the subjects changed individually. It is unknown whether the rates of all or only some subjects declined and by how much.

Table 1 of Hillmen and Others (2004) (Table 1.3) exhibits 12 months before and 3 months after treatment transfusion rates. The rates are depicted by stem-and-leaf displays in Fig. 5.1. The figure shows clearly that all subjects received 1.0 or more units per patient, per month before treatment and that the rates of two received more than 3 units per month. It is also clear that, three months after treatment, as many as six subjects did not require transfusion, but one needed as many as 2.9 units per month. Nonetheless, the 12 months before and 3 months after treatment transfusion rates do not unveil how the rates of the subjects changed individually.

There is a one-to-one pairing of the before-and-after treatment transfusion rates of each subject. The two rates constitute an observation-pair. How the rates of a subject changed is indicated by his observation-pair. One way to assess how the transfusion rates of the 11 subjects changed is to compute the difference between the before-and-after transfusion rates of each subject and examine the distribution of the differences.

Table 5.1 shows the 12 months before and 3 months after treatment transfusion rates of the 11 subjects and their differences.

Figure 5.2 uses a stem-and-leaf display to exhibit the distribution of the before-and-after differences. The display clearly shows that the rates of 10 of the 11 subjects declined. The before-treatment rates of the six subjects who did not require transfusion 3 months after treatment were all less than 3 units per month.

Before Treatment Rates	After Treatment Rates
|	|0.0 0.0 0.0 0.0 0.0 0.0 0.7 0.70
|1.0 1.2 1.2 1.6 1.7 1.8 1.9	|1.1 1.8
|2.3 2.8	|2.9
|3.4	|
|4.5	|

Fig. 5.1 Distributions of before-and-after treatment transfusions rates and their differences

Table 5.1 Transfusion rates 12 months before and 3 months after eculizumab treatment

Patient No.	1	2	3	4	5	6	7	8	9	10	11
12 months before treatment	1.8	1.9	1.6	2.3	1.0	1.2	2.8	1.7	4.5	3.4	1.2
3 months after treatment	0.7	2.9	0.0	0.0	0.7	0.0	0.0	0.0	1.1	1.8	0.0
Pair-difference	1.1	-1.0	1.6	2.3	0.3	1.2	2.8	1.7	3.4	1.6	1.2

Red indicates subjects who did not require transfusion 3 months after treatment

```
| -1
| 0.3
| 1.1 1.2 1.2 1.6 1.6 1.6 1.7
| 2.3 2.8
| 3.4
```

† Red indicates subjects who did not require transfusion 3 months after treatment.

Fig. 5.2 Differences of 12 months before and 3 months after treatment transfusion rates
Red indicates subjects who did not require transfusion 3 months after treatment

It is of interest to note that the mean of the pair differences 1.47 equals the difference between the before-and-after treatment means $2.12 - 0.65 = 1.47$. The median of the pair differences 1.6 does not equal, although close to, the difference between the before-and-after treatment medians $1.8 - 0 = 1.8$.

Example 5.1.2

Russell and Others (2014) (Example 2.5.3) used the mean glucose levels of each subject during a monitoring period as a summary measure of the glucose levels of the subject during the period. Mean glucose levels on days 2 through 5 of continuous monitoring are described by Russell and Others (2014) as follows:

> During the bionic-pancreas period, all the patients had a mean glucose level of less than 154 mg per deciliter (8.5 mmol per liter) on continuous monitoring, a level that corresponds to a glycated hemoglobin level of 7%, the therapeutic goal for adults recommended by the American Diabetes Association. In contrast, only 9 of 20 patients had a mean glucose level on continuous monitoring that was below this threshold during the control period (Fig. 3A and 4A).

Clearly, the mean glucose levels of all subjects were below the therapeutic goal for adults during the bionic pancreas period, and those of 9 subjects (45%) were below the therapeutic goal during the control period. However, it is unclear how the mean glucose levels of the subjects changed individually.

There is a one-to-one pairing of the mean glucose levels of each adult during the two monitoring periods. The two mean glucose levels of a subject form a pair. The set of mean glucose levels of the 20 adults during the bionic pancreas period and the set during the control period are paired; there are 20 observation-pairs. How the mean glucose levels of the adults changed between the two periods is indicated by

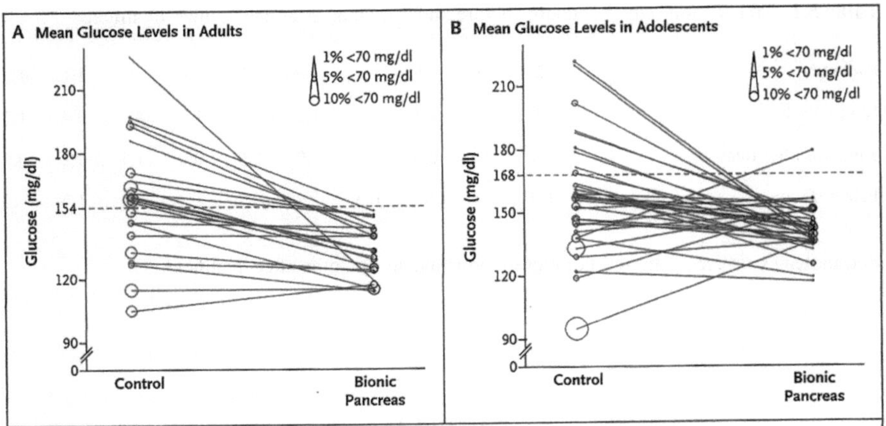

Figure 3. **Distributions of Mean Glucose Levels and Hypoglycemia among Adults and Adolescents.**
Panel A shows the mean glucose level in each adult on days 2 through 5 of the control period (red circles), which is connected to the corresponding mean glucose level during the bionic-pancreas period (black circles). The diameter of each circle is proportional to the percentage of time that the patient spent with a low glucose value (<70 mg per deciliter) on days 2 through 5. The dashed red line indicates a mean glucose threshold of 154 mg per deciliter, which corresponds to a glycated hemoglobin level of 7%, the upper limit of the therapeutic goal for adults as outlined by the American Diabetes Association. This goal was met in all patients during the bionic-pancreas period. Panel B shows a similar distribution for each of the adolescents, with a cutoff point for the mean glucose level of 168 mg per deciliter, which corresponds to a glycated hemoglobin level of 7.5%, as recommended for adolescents. The one patient in whom this level was not reached on days 2 through 5 had a mean glucose level of 148 mg per deciliter on days 3 through 5. In the two panels, the solid red line indicates the mean for all the patients in the study group. To convert the values for glucose to millimoles per liter, multiply by 0.05551.

Fig. 5.3 Figure 3 of Russell and Others (2014)

the 20 observation-pairs. The intermingled histograms of Figure 4A are descriptions of the mean levels during the two periods. Pairings of the mean levels of the adults were not accounted for; how the mean glucose levels of the adults changed between the two periods is not unveiled.

Figure 4A of the article (Fig. 2.16) shows that the mean glucose levels of the 20 adults during the bionic pancreas period were all below 154 mg/dl and were lower than the mean glucose levels of many adults during the control period. The mean glucose levels of the subjects whose mean glucose levels did not meet the therapeutic goal during the control period declined. However, the sizes of the declines are unknown. It is unknown how the mean glucose levels of the subjects who did not meet the therapeutic goal during the control period changed. Were there some increases?

Figure 3A of the article (Fig. 5.3) uses a line to connect the mean glucose levels of each adult during the two monitoring periods. Pairings of the mean glucose levels are explicitly indicated. The figure depicts how the mean glucose levels of subjects changed between the two monitoring periods. It shows:

1. Compared with their mean glucose levels during the control period, the mean glucose levels of 18 subjects declined during the bionic pancreas period, one remained approximately the same, and one was elevated.
2. The mean glucose levels of the adults whose mean glucose levels were larger than 154 mg/dl declined noticeably during the bionic pancreas period.
3. The mean glucose levels of the adults whose mean glucose levels were below 154 mg/dl during the control period declined slightly during the bionic pancreas period.
4. The mean glucose level of one adult whose mean glucose level was the highest during the control period was one of the lowest during the bionic period (approximately 105 mg/ml).

Example 5.1.3

Lockley and Others (2004) presented the results of a study that assessed work hours, sleep time, and attentional failures of 20 interns during a traditional rotation schedule and an intervention schedule. The traditional schedule included extended work shifts, and the intervention schedule limited work shifts to 16 or fewer consecutive hours. The article stated:

> Attentional failure occurred at more than double the rates during the night (from 11 p.m. to 7 a.m.) on the traditional schedule compared with the intervention schedule (P = 0.02) (Fig. 5) and 1.5 times the rate during the day (7 a.m. to 10 p.m.) (P = 0.07).

Figure 5 of the article (Fig. 5.4) uses the heights of bars to denote the mean of numbers of attentional failures per hour during the night (11 p.m. to 7 a.m.). The bars show that the mean of the numbers of attentional failures during the traditional schedule was approximately twice the mean of the numbers during the intervention schedule. The distinction between the means of numbers, however, does not unveil how the numbers of attentional failures of the interns changed between the two schedules individually.

There is a one-to-one pairing of the numbers of attentional failures of each intern on the two schedules. The two numbers constitute an observation-pair. How the numbers of the interns changed between the two schedules is indicated by the 20 observation-pairs. The right panel of Figure 5 (Fig. 5.3) uses lines to connect the two numbers of interns on the two schedules. The lines unveil that, compared to the traditional schedule, the numbers of attention failures of 15 of the 20 interns, not all, were lower during the intervention schedule. The numbers of 2 interns were markedly higher during the intervention schedule, and those of 3 stayed about the same.

It is constructive to refer to the right panel of Figure 5 and use the percentages of interns whose number of attentional failures were lower and higher during the intervention period to depict the distinction between the two schedules.

Note Figure 5 of Lockley and Others (2004) shows two vertical axes. Labels marked on the one on the left specify the numbers of attentional failures signified by heights of bars; labels marked on the one on the right specify the numbers of attentional failures signified by heights of dots.

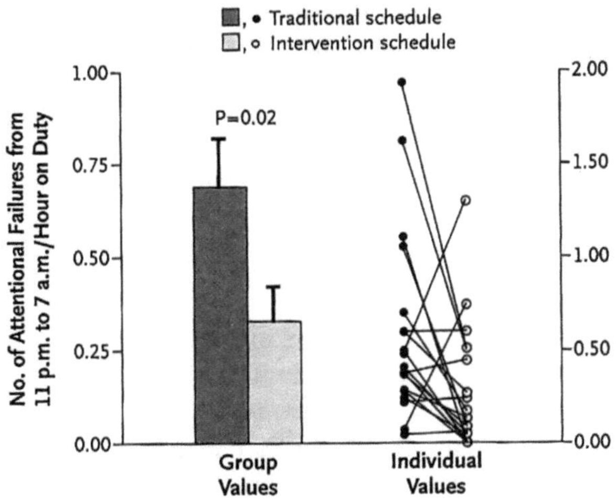

Figure 5. Mean (+SE) Number of Attentional Failures among the 20 Interns as a Group and Individually while Working Overnight (11 p.m. to 7 a.m.) during the Traditional Schedule and the Intervention Schedule.

The number of attentional failures was determined by the presence of at least one electrooculography-derived slow eye movement while the subject was awake and at work. The rate of attentional failures among interns who were working overnight (from 11 p.m. to 7 a.m.) during the intervention schedule (0.33 per hour, or 2.6 attentional failures per intern overnight) was less than half that during the corresponding times on the traditional schedule (0.69 per hour, or 5.5 attentional failures per intern overnight; P=0.02), and a trend (P=0.07) toward a reduction in attentional failures during day and evening call (7 a.m. to 10 p.m.) was also apparent (data not shown). Thirteen of the 20 interns had a decrease in the number of slow eye movements during overnight work on the intervention schedule as compared with the traditional schedule.

Fig. 5.4 Figure 5 of Lockley and Others (2004)

Example 5.1.4

Hsu and Others (2004) presented the results of a study evaluating the effect of catheter ablation for atrial fibrillation. Fifty-eight patients who had congestive heart failure and a left ventricular ejection fraction of less than 45%, and 58 who did not have congestive heart failure were studied. Changes in exercise time and capacity after ablation were related as follows:

> Exercise time and capacity also increased significantly in both groups. In the group with congestive heart failure, exercise time increased from 11±4 to 14±5 minutes (P<0.001) and maximal capacity from 123±44 to 144±55 W (P<0.001), whereas in the control group, the numbers increased from 14±4 to 16±5 minutes (P = 0.001) and from 145±44 to 158±52 W (P<0.001) during the follow-up period.

A: Subjects with Congestive Heart Failure		B: Subjects without Congestive Heart Failure	
Before ablation ($11 \mp 2\times 4$)	[--------▲--------] 3 11 19	Before ablation ($14 \mp 2\times 4$)	[--------▲--------] 6 14 22
During follow-up ($14 \mp 2\times 5$)	[----------▲----------] 4 14 24	During follow-up ($16 \mp 2\times 5$)	[----------▲----------] 6 16 26

Fig. 5.5 Speculated 95% observation-regions for exercise times before ablation and during follow-up

$P < 0.001$ suggests that the increases in the means of exercise time (11 to – 14 min) and the means of maximal capacity (123 to 144 W) in the group with congestive heart failure may be declared statistically significant. $P = 0.001$ suggests that the increases in the means of exercise time (14 to 16 min) and the means of maximal capacity (145 to 158 W) in the control group may be declared statistically significant. The increases in the means and the P-values are not certifications that the exercise times and maximal capacity of all subjects increased. It is unknown how the subjects changed.

To garner some clue regarding the changes in individual subjects, means and standard deviations of before-and-after ablation observations were used to determine the 95% observation-regions speculated by the Gaussian model for observations.

Figure 5.5 shoes schematically the speculated 95% observation-regions of the before and after ablation exercise times of the two groups of subjects. The speculated 95% observation-regions suggest that the before and after ablation exercise times of both groups overlap extensively. Although the distinctions between the means before and the means of after ablation exercise times were be declared statistically significant, the distributions of the before and the after ablation exercise times overlap extensively and suggest that there are both increases and decreases.

The means and standard deviations of the before and the after ablation observations yield limited information. Means and standard deviations of pair differences are more informative. It is more productive to use comprehensive descriptions of distributions of pair differences to depict how exercise time and capacity of the two groups of subjects changed. Narratives of indications of the distributions of pair differences are more revealing.

Example 5.1.5

The following is one result of Cooper and Others (2014) (Example 3.2.6.2):

> Stents were placed in 343 of the 459 patients in the stent group (94.6%) and resulted in a mean reduction of the stenosis from 68±11% to 16±8% (P<0.001).

Clearly, the mean stenosis was reduced markedly from 68% to 16%, and the reduction could be declared statistically significant. It, however, is unknown how the stenosis measure of the 343 subjects changed.

The standard deviations are rather small relative to the means. They suggest that the distributions of the stenosis before and after stents probably vary in narrow

```
Before Stenting:                              [----------▲-----------]
 (68%∓2×11%)                                  46        68         90
After Stenting:          [--------▲--------]
 (16%∓2×8%)              0       16       32
```

Fig. 5.6 Speculated 95% observation-regions for stenosis before and after stenting

ranges and do not overlap extensively. It, however, is unclear how narrowly the distributions varied and how little they overlapped. It is unknown how the stenosis of the subjects changed individually. Were they all decreases?

To garner some clues from the means and standard deviations, they were used to determine the 95% observation-regions speculated by the Gaussian model, which are displayed schematically in Fig. 5.6. The figure shows that the speculated 95% observation-regions are separated speculate that the stenosis measurements of most subjects reduced after stenting and that the reductions might be as small as 14 and as large as 90 percentage points.

This is a rare case. The standard deviations of the before-stenting and the after-stenting stenosis are exceedingly small relative to the means. The difference between the means of the before-stenting and the after-stenting measurements is larger than two times the sum of the two standard deviations. The speculated 95% observation-regions are totally separated. Nevertheless, the precise range of the deductions is unknown. It is unknown whether there were reductions as small as 14 percentage points or as large as 90 percentage points.

The set of before stenting and the set of after stenting stenosis are paired. There is a one-to-one pairing of the measurements of each subject. The two measurements constitute an observation-pair. A prolific way to assess how the stenosis measurements of the 343 subjects changed is to examine their pairs of measurements. If a difference between the two measurements of every subject was computed to document the change in the subject, how the measurements of the 343 subjects changed would be clearly manifested by the distribution of the pair differences. Percentages of clinically relevant reductions would be enlightening synoptic descriptions of the changes.

Example 5.1.6

A study followed 19 women with hypothyroidism before and throughout their pregnancies to identify the optimal timing and amount of levothyroxine adjustment during pregnancy. The results of the study are presented in Alexander and Others (2004). The article states:

> In subjects without a history of thyroid cancer who needed an increase in the dose of levothyroxine during pregnancy, the mean (±SD) thyrotropin concentration before pregnancy was 1.5±1.1 μU per milliliter, and at 38 weeks of gestation, it was 1.4±0.3 μU per milliliter (P = 0.92).

•

The values of 1.51 ± 1.1 μU per milliliter and 1.4 ± 0.3 μU per milliliter are descriptions of the thyrotropin concentrations of the subject before pregnancy and at 38 weeks of gestation. $P = 0.92$ suggests that the distinction in means would be

Before pregnancy: [-------0---------------▲-------------------------]
(1.5±1.1 μU per milliliter) -0.7 1.5 3.7

At 38 Weeks of Gestation: [------▲------]
(1.4±0.3 μU per milliliter) 0.8 1.4 2.0

Fig. 5.7 Speculated 95% observation-regions for thyrotropin concentrations in women without a history of thyroid cancer who required increase in thyroxine dose

likely if chance were the explanation. The distinction would *not* be declared statistically significant, and the concern that the distinction is incidental would not be dismissed.

The means and standard deviations of the thyrotropin concentrations before pregnancy and at 38 weeks of gestation yielded limited information. They do not unveil how the thyrotropin concentrations of the subjects changed. Were the changes all small? Did the changes include some large increases and some large decreases?

To expound what the means and standard deviations unveiled, they were used to determine 95% observation-regions speculated by the Gaussian model, which are schematically shown in Fig. 5.7. The regions suggest the following:

- Centers of the distributions of the thyrotropin concentrations before pregnancy and the distribution of concentrations at 38 weeks of gestation were close.
- The distribution of the thyrotropin concentrations before pregnancy varied widely from approximately 0 to 3.7 μU per milliliter. The distribution of the thyrotropin concentrations at 38 weeks of gestation, on the other hand, varied in a narrow range from approximately 0.8 to approximately 2.0 μU/ml.
- There were increases, as well as decreases at 38 weeks of gestation. The concentrations of the women whose concentrations before pregnancy were higher than 2.0 μU/ml decreased, and those of the women whose concentrations before pregnancy were lower than 0.8 μU/ml increased.
- There might be some declines as large as 2.9 μU/ml or elevations as large as 2.0 μU/ml.

This is a rare case. The mean before pregnancy and the mean at 38 weeks of gestation are close, and the standard deviation of the thyrotropin concentrations at 38 weeks of pregnancy is decidedly small. The speculated 95% observation-regions yield some clues regarding changes in thyrotropin concentration. Nevertheless, the numbers and magnitudes of declines and increases are unknown.

One feature of Alexander and Others (2004) is that Table 1 shows baseline thyrotropin levels. If thyrotropin levels at 38 weeks of gestation were also shown, numbers and magnitudes of increases and decreases would be known.

5.2 Pair Indices

There is a one-to-one pairing of the observations of paired data sets. The observations form observation-pairs. Revelations of paired data sets are comprehensively unveiled by the observation-pairs. The two sets of observations yield limited information and yield some useful deductions only on some special occasions.

One way to unravel revelations of paired quantitative data sets is to determine the value of a pair index that is a quantitative characterization of observation-pairs. The distribution of the pair index unveils the relations of the paired quantitative data sets candidly. Three pair indices: pair difference, pair ratio, and percent difference are often used.

- *Pair Difference*

Pair difference is the most frequently used pair index. When the observations are denoted by A and B, a pair difference may be D = A − B or D = B − A. If B and A are observations before and after a treatment, the pair difference is a quantitative measure of the change in the observations of a subject and is often computed in such a way that a positive difference is the type of change of interest. A pair difference may also be dubbed a before–after change or simply a change when it is a difference between observations obtained before and after a treatment.

One important property of pair difference is that the mean of pair differences of paired data sets equals the corresponding difference between the means of the before and the after data sets. The exact relationship between the standard deviation of the pair differences of two paired data sets and the standard deviations of the two data sets is known. It involves a third quantity, the correlation coefficient of the two data sets (Chapter 8). Pair difference in the only pair index with this convenient property.

- *Pair Ratio*

A pair ratio is a ratio of the observations of an observation-pair. When the observations are denoted by A and B, they may be computed as R = A/B or R = B/A. Descriptive statistics of the distribution of the pair ratios of paired data sets and the ratio of corresponding descriptive statistics of the respective distributions of the data sets are generally not equal.

- *Percent Difference*

A percent difference is a pair difference expressed as a percentage of one of the observations. When the two observations of an observation-pair are written as A and B, they may be computed as P = 100 × (B − A)/A or P = 100 × (A − B)/B. If the paired data sets consisted of before and after observations of the same group of subjects, a percent difference may be dubbed a percent change.

Like the pair ratio, descriptive statistics of the distribution of the percent differences of paired data sets and the corresponding percent difference of descriptive statistics of the data sets are generally not equal.

Table 5.2 Before-and-after BMI values of subjects in the two groups

Weight loss						Weight maintenance					
ID	B	A1	D1	R1	P1	ID	B	A2	D2	R2	P2
1	26	26	0	1.0	0%	26	26	30	−4	1.15	−15%
2	27	27	0	1.0	0%	27	27	32	−5	1.19	−19%
3	28	28	0	1.0	0%	28	28	34	−6	1.21	−21%
4	28	27	1	0.964	4%	29	28	31	−3	1.11	−11%
5	29	29	0	1.0	0%	30	29	27	2	0.93	7%
6	29	28	1	0.955	3%	31	29	31	−2	1.07	−7%
7	30	30	0	1.0	0%	32	30	29	1	0.97	3%
8	30	29	1	0.967	3%	33	30	29	1	0.97	3%
9	30	28	2	0.933	7%	34	30	28	2	0.93	7%
10	31	31	0	1.0	0%	35	31	26	5	0.84	16%
11	31	30	1	0.968	3%	36	31	29	2	0.94	6%
12	31	29	2	0.935	7%	37	31	30	1	0.97	3%
13	32	32	0	1.0	0%	38	32	32	0	1.00	0%
14	32	31	1	0.969	3%	39	32	28	4	0.88	13%
15	32	30	2	0.938	6%	40	32	33	−1	1.03	−3%
16	32	29	3	0.906	9%	41	32	32	0	1.00	0%
17	33	33	0	1.0	0%	42	33	33	0	1.00	0%
18	33	32	1	0.970	3%	43	33	27	6	0.82	18%
19	33	31	2	0.939	6%	44	33	28	5	0.85	15%
20	33	30	3	0.909	9%	45	33	30	3	0.91	9%
21	34	34	0	1.0	0%	46	34	30	4	0.88	12%
22	34	33	1	0.971	3%	47	34	31	3	0.91	9%
23	34	32	2	0.941	6%	48	34	31	3	0.91	9%
24	34	31	3	0.911	9%	49	34	30	4	0.88	12%
25	34	30	4	0.882	12%	50	34	29	5	0.85	15%

Example 5.2.1
Table 5.2 presents data from a fake study that determined BMI (body mass index) values of 50 participants of a camp who were randomly assigned to a weight loss group or weight maintenance group. The diet of the weight loss group was strictly controlled, and that of the other group was not. Distributions of the baseline and the end-of-camp BMI values are displayed in Fig. 5.8; distributions of the three pair indices are displayed in Figs. 5.9, 5.10, and 5.11. Descriptive statistics are shown in Table 5.3.

Figure 5.8 shows that the distributions of the baseline BMI values of the two groups are identical, and that the distributions of the end-of-camp values of the two groups are also identical. It seems that the effects of the two programs are identical.

```
                              Baseline
Weight-Loss                                    Weight-Maintenance
                         34                                                   34
                32 33 34                                                  33 34
        30 31 32 33 34                                      30 31 32 33 34
    28 29 30 31 32 33 34                              28 29 30 31 32 33 34
26 27 28 29 30 31 32 33 34                      26 27 28 29 30 31 32 33 34
----------------------------------              -----------------------------------
            BMI                                                 BMI
                          End-of-Camp
Weight loss                                     Weight maintenance
        30                                                30
    29 30 31                                          29 30 31
  28 29 30 31 32                                  28 29 30 31 32
27 28 29 30 31 32 33                          27 28 29 30 31 32 33
26 27 28 29 30 1 32 33 34                   26 27 28 29 30 31 32 33 34
----------------------------------          -----------------------------------
            BMI                                         BMI
```

Fig. 5.8 Distributions of baseline and end-of-camp BMI values

```
0
0       Weight-Loss                            Weight Maintenance
0 1
0 1
0 1 2
0 1 2
0 1 2 3                                          0 1 2 3 4 5
0 1 2 3                                          0 1 2 3 4 5
0 1 2 3 4                       -6 -5 -4 -3 -2 -1 0 1 2 3 4 5 6
----------------------          -----------------------------------------
Pair Difference                            Pair Difference
```

Fig. 5.9 Distributions of pair differences (D = B − E)

```
                                   1.00
                                   1.00
     Weight-Loss                   1.00                          Weight-Maintenance
                              0.97 1.00
                              0.97 1.00
          0.91      0.94      0.97 1.00                0.88 0.91           1.00
     0.88 0.91      0.94      0.97 1.00           0.85 0.88 0.91 0.93 0.97 1.00
0.84 0.85 0.88 0.91 0.93 0.94 0.96 0.97 1.00   0.82 0.84 0.85 0.88 0.91 0.93 0.94 0.97 1.00 1.03 1.07 1.11 1.15 1.18 1.19 1.21
--------------------------------------------||-----------------------------------------------------------------------------
              Pair-Ratio                                                  Pair-Ratio
```

Fig. 5.10 Distributions of pair ratio (R = E/B)

- *Distributions of Pair Indices*

The distributions of pair indices clearly show how the BMI values of the two groups of campers changed. The set of baseline values and the set of end-of-camp values of the group of campers are paired. The baseline and at end-of-camp BMI values of a camper form a pair. How the BMI values of a camper changed is indicated by the difference between pairs of BMI values of the camper. How the BMI values of a group of campers changed is indicated by the distribution of the pair

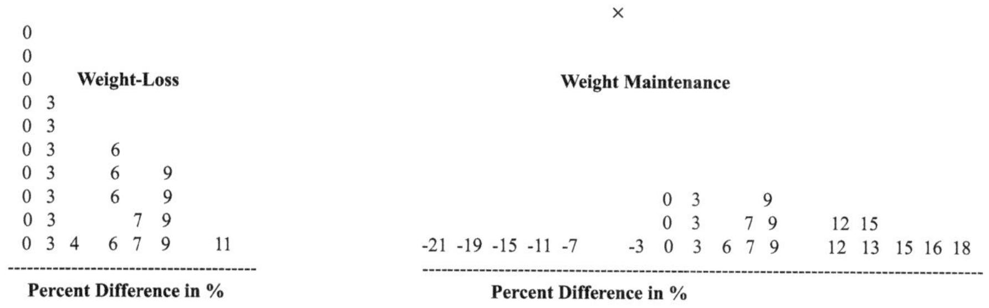

Fig. 5.11 Distributions of percent difference (P = 100×[B − E]/B)%

Table 5.3 Descriptive statistics of baseline and end-of-camp BMI values and pair indices

	Group I				Group II			
	Mean	Median	SD	Range	Mean	Median	SD	Range
Baseline	31.2	32.0	2.4	26 to 34	31.2	32.0	2.4	26 to 34
End-of-camp	30.0	30.0	2.0	26 to 34	30.0	30.0	2.0	26 to 34
Pair difference	1.2	1.0	1.2	0 to 4	1.2	2.0	3.3	−6 to 6
Pair ratio	0.96	0.97	0.04	0.88 to 1.00	0.97	0.94	0.11	0.82 to 1.21
Percent difference	4%	3%	4%	0.0 to 12%	3%	6%	11%	−21% to 18%

differences and not by the respective distributions of the baseline and end-of-camp values. Figures 5.9, 5.10, and 5.11 show that the distributions of the three pair indices differ distinctly between the two groups.

The distributions of the pair indices show the following at the end of the camp:

- Weight loss group: The BMI value of not any camper increased; those of 16 (64%) declined 9 (36%) remained unchanged.
- Weight maintenance group: The BMI values of 6 (24%) campers elevated, 3 (12%) stayed the same, and 16 (64%) declined.

- *Synoptic Descriptions of Pair Indices*

Table 5.3 shows the means, medians, standard deviations, and ranges of the three pair indices. It shows that the mean of the pair differences equals the difference between the baseline and end-of-camp means. Pair difference is the only pair index with this convenient property.

Example 5.2.2

One outcome of Cooper and Others (2014) (Example 5.1.5) is change in systolic blood pressure. The article reported:

> Systolic blood pressure declined in both the medical therapy-only group (by 15.6 ±25.8 mmHg) and the stent group (by 16.6±21.2 mmHg).

Medical-therapy-only group:	[----------------0-------▲------------------------]8			
(15.6∓2×25.8)	-36.0	15.6	67.2	
Medial-therapy -plus-stent group:	[-------------0---------▲----------------------]			
(16.6∓2×21.2	- 28.8	16.6	59.0	

Fig. 5.12 Speculated 95% observations regions for before–after treatment changes in systolic blood pressure

The values 15.6 ± 25.8 mm Hg and 16.6 ± 21.2 mm Hg denote the means and standard deviations of pair differences. The before-and-after systolic blood pressures of a subject constitute an observation-pair. A pair difference was computed from the observation-pair of each subject by subtracting after-treatment pressure from before-treatment pressure. It is a measure of change in systolic blood pressure; a positive pair difference indicates a decline. The means are positive and suggest that the means of systolic blood pressures of both groups declined. The standard deviations (25.8 mm Hg and 21.2 mm Hg) are large and submit that the distributions of the changes in both groups varied widely and included declines as well as elevations. However, the numbers and sizes of declines and elevations are unknown.

As more comprehensive descriptions of the distributions of changes are not available, the means and standard deviations of before and the after treatment systolic pressures were used to determine 95% observation-regions speculated by the Gaussian model, which are displayed schematically in Fig. 5.12. The speculated observation-regions are wide and conjecture that the distributions of changes in the two treatment groups are quite comparable. They vary in similar wide ranges and are skewed to right. Both include declines as well as elevations. It is astute to note that the assertion that systolic blood pressure declined in the treatment groups alluded to declines in means and not changes in individual subjects.

It is more prolific to describe distributions of the two sets of changes in detail and use percentages of clinically relevant declines to assess the effect of being in the two treatment groups.

Example 5.2.3

Leonardi and Others (2012) presented the results of a study that randomly assigned 142 patients with chronic moderate-to-severe plaque psoriasis to receive subcutaneous injection of 10, 25, or 150 mg of ixekizumab or placebo at 0, 2, 4, 8.12, and 16 weeks. The primary outcome of the study was the proportion of patients with reductions in the psoriasis area and severity index (PASI) by at least 75% at 12 weeks of follow-up. The following is one account of the primary outcome of the study:

> At 12 weeks, a reduction in the PASI score by at least 75% (the primary outcome) or 90% occurred in significantly more patients in the 25-mg, 75-mg, and 150-mg ixekizumab groups (P<0.001 for each vs. placebo) (Table 2 and Fig. 2).

The PASI scores of a subject at baseline and at 12 weeks constitute a pair. The primary outcome: a reduction in the PASI score by at least 75% is a percent difference. The difference between the baseline and week 12 PASI scores of a subject is expressed as a percentage of the baseline score. Table 2 shows that the percentages of subjects whose reductions in the PASI score at 12 weeks were at least 75% of their baseline scores are 8% among the subjects assigned to receive placebo and 29%, 77%, 83%, and 82% among subjects assigned to receive 10 mg, 25 mg, 75 mg, and 150 mg of ixekizumab, respectively. The percentages are descriptions of changes in individual subjects in the treatment groups. They unveil that, at 12 weeks, a reduction in the PSA score by at least 75% occurred more frequently in the ixekizumab groups than in the placebo group. It is the highest in 150 mg group. $P < 0.001$ suggested that the distinctions between the placebo group and the 25 mg, 75 mg, and 150 mg groups may be declared statistically significant.

5.3 Intelligent Reading and Informative Reporting

Accounts of revelations of paired quantitative data sets are often substantiated by descriptions of respective distributions of the data sets. The descriptions yield limited useful information regarding observation-pairs and may be used to make useful deductions only when the two data sets differ markedly. To read accounts of revelations of paired quantitative data sets intelligently, it is constructive to consider the following:

1. Revelations of paired quantitative data sets are shown by observation pairs and manifested by distributions of pair indices that characterize the observation pairs. The respective distributions of the two data sets yield limited information.
2. How a group of subjects changed after treatment is shown by their observation pairs and manifested by the distribution of a pair index. Changes in the means and medians of before- and after-treatment observations yield limited information regarding the changes in individual subjects.
3. *P*-values of distinctions between two paired quantitative data sets are usually the results of testing the statistical null hypotheses that insinuate the means of pair differences are coincidences. Small *P*-values suggest that the means of pair differences are probably not coincidental. They do not certify that all or most pair differences are positive or negative. It is productive to learn the percentage of germane observation pairs.

To report informatively, it is helpful to consider the following comments:

1. Do not simply declare that the distinction between two paired data sets is or is not "significant". Use a comprehensive description of the distribution of a pair index to describe the revelation of the data sets. Articulate the manifestation of the distribution of the pair index.
2. If sets of observations are obtained from a group of subjects before and after a treatment, use the distribution of a pair index to depict how the observations of the subjects changed. Percentage of relevant changes is often informative synoptic descriptions of the changes.

Table 5.4 Hemoglobin levels (g/dl) 12 months before and 3 months after eculizumab treatment[a]

Patient No.	1	2	3	4	5	6	7	8	9	10	11
12 months before treatment	10.3	8.3	10.1	9.3	11.9	9.8	12.8	9.5	10.7	8.5	8.5
3 months after treatment	10.0	8.8	10.7	9.4	10.6	10.6	13.5	9.8	11.4	8.8	10.0
Pair-difference (A – B)[†]	-0.3	0.5	0.6	0.1	-1.3	0.8	0.7	0.8	0.7	0.3	1.5

[a]Subjects who did not require transfusion during treatment

3. Percentages of clinically relevant observation-pairs are often informative synoptic descriptions of revelations of paired quantitative data sets.

Example 5.3.1

Hillmen and Others (2004) (Example 1.1.3) uses the following stylish statement to depict the effect of the study (infusion of 300 mg of eculizumab every week for four weeks, followed by a 900 mg dose one week later and 900 mg every week through 12 weeks):

> Hemoglobin levels did not increase significantly during the treatment period, although hemoglobin values in six patients stabilized without transfusion (Table 1).

It is unclear how the hemoglobin levels changed during treatment. To read intelligently, it is crucial to determine whether all changes are small. It was noticed that 12 months before and 3 months after eculizumab hemoglobin levels are shown in Table 1 of the article (Table 1.3). They were used to compute the pair differences shown in Table 5.4. The pair differences show that the changes in hemoglobin levels of nine subjects were small increases and those of two were small decreases. The changes in hemoglobin levels of the six subjects who did not require transfusion were small increases.

To report informatively, it is more forthright to cite the numbers of small increases and small decreases and note that the changes of the six subjects who did not require transfusion were all small increases.

Example 5.3.2

One finding of Zheng and Others (2018) (Example 4.3.4) was related as follows:

> Changes in spasticity from baseline to month 12 as measured on the Modified Ashworth Scale significantly favored the surgery group at all joints (elbow extension, P<0.001; forearm rotation, P=0.003; wrist extension, P=0.005; thumb extension, P=0.02, and extension of fingers two through five, P =0.008) (Table 2).

To read intelligently, it is important to note that the *P*-values suggest only that the distinctions between the means of changes of the two treatment group would be unlikely if chance were the explanation. The distinctions in means of changes may be declared statistically significant. The changes in means favored the surgery

```
        Surgery Group                          Control Group
|-2 -2                                   |
|-1 -1 -1 -1 -1 -1 -1 -1                 |-1
| 0  0  0  0  0                          | 0 0 0 0 0 0 0 0 0 0 0 0 0 0 0 0
                                         | 1
```

Fig. 5.13 Pair differences of baseline and 12 months after treatment scores of spasticity of elbow extension

group. However, it is unknown how the changes in the individual subjects differed between the treatment groups.

To read intelligently, it is productive to ascertain how the scores changed in the two treatment groups. Table 2 presents descriptions of distributions of changes. For instance, it uses −2 (2), −1 (11), 0 (5), and −1 (1), 0 (16), 1 (10) to depict the changes in the score on the Modified Ashworth Scale assessing spasticity of elbow extension in the surgery group and the control group, respectively. These are values of changes and numbers of changes equaling the values and descriptions of distributions of changes.

Scores on the Modified Ashworth Scale measuring spasticity range from 0 to 5, with higher scores indicating more severe spasticity. The scores of a subject at baseline and month 12 constitute a pair. The changes are pair differences computed as the month-12 scores minus the baseline scores. Negative values indicate improvements, and positive values indicate deteriorations. Figure 5.13 displays the changes graphically.

Figure 5.13 shows clearly that the changes of as many as 13 (72%) of the 18 subjects in the surgery group were improvements by one or two points on the Modified Ashworth Scale. In the control group, on the other hand, the score of only one subject (6%) improved (1 point), the scores of 16 (89%) did not change, and that of one worsened by 1 point.

It is more informative to use the percentages of improvements to depict the distinction between the two groups as compared with using *P*-values to corroborate the assertion that changes in spasticity favored significantly the surgery group. For instance, the percentages of subjects whose elbow extension improved (72% vs. 6%) accentuate forcefully how the surgery group and the control group differed.

Example 5.3.3

Acker and Others (2018) (Example 1.2.5) used the Minnesota Living with Heart Failure questionnaire to assess heart failure symptoms. Scores of the questionnaire range from 0 to 105, with higher scores indicating worse heart failure symptoms. The article reported:

> As measured on the Minnesota Living with Heart Failure questionnaire, there was a reduction from baseline in heart-failure symptoms of 46.9% in the repair group and 61.2% in the replacement group.

```
                                    Repair Group
Baseline              [----0------------------▲-----------------------]
(46.1∓2×27.2)       -8.1                    46.1                    100.5

Year-1            [----------0------------▲---------------------]
(24.5∓2×23.1)   -21.7                   24.5                   70.7

                                    Replacement Group
Baseline               [--0---------------------▲-----------------------]
(50.2∓2×27.4)        -4.6                      50.2                     105.0

Year-1            [----------0--------▲---------------]
(19.6∓2×19.4)    -19.2              19.6            58.4
```

Fig. 5.14 Speculated 95% observation-regions for the Minnesota living with heart failure questionnaire scores

To read intelligently, it is essential to determine what the percentages are and what they unveil. Three possibilities are:

1. Percent reduction in means: difference between mean of baseline scores and mean of month-12 scores expressed as a percentage of mean of baseline scores.
2. Mean of percent changes – the mean of the differences between the pair of baseline and 12-month scores of each subject expressed as percentages of the subject's baseline scores.
3. Percentage of subjects whose scores were reduced.

Table 1 uses 46.1 ± 27.2 and 50.2 ± 27.4 to denote the means and standard deviations of the baseline scores of the repair group and the replacement group, respectively; Table 3 uses 24.5 ± 23.1 and 19.6 ± 19.4 to denote the mean and standard deviation of the two groups at 1 year. The means yield that percentage of change in means is (46.1 − 24.5)/46.1 = 46.9% and (50.0 − 19.6)/50.0 = 60.8%. This suggests that 46.9% and 61.2% are probably percent reductions in the means of the two treatment groups. If so, they are not descriptions of the changes of individual subjects in the two groups.

Some clues regarding the changes of individual subjects from baseline may be reaped by using the means and standard deviations to determine 95% observation-regions speculated by the Gaussian model. The regions are displayed schematically in Fig. 5.14. They conjecture that the distributions of baseline and year-1 scores of each group overlapped extensively. In each group, there were probably both increases and decreases. The speculated 95% observation-regions also suggest that changes in the two groups were comparable. They also speculate the following:

1. The distributions of the baseline and post-treatment scores of the subjects in the repair group overlapped extensively. There were both declines and elevations. Probably the scores of the subjects whose baseline scores were above 70 declined.

Fig. 5.15 Speculated 95% observation-regions for the changes in PPT scores from baseline to year one

Diet-Exercise Group $(5.4\mp2\times2.4)$	[----------▲----------] 0.6 5.4 10.2
Diet Group $(3.4\mp2\times2.4)$	[--0------▲--------] -1.4 3.4 8.2
Exercise Group $(4.0\mp2\times2.5)$	[-0-------▲--------] -1.0 4.0 9.0

2. The distribution of the baseline and post-treatment scores of the subjects in the replacement group overlapped extensively. There are probably a few subjects whose baseline scores were above 58. The scores of these subjects declined.

The assertion that there was a reduction from baseline in heart failure symptoms of 46.9% in the repair group and 61.2% in the replacement group is an oversimplification and misleading. To report informatively, it is productive to depict the distributions of the changes in the two treatment groups. Percentages of relevant increases would be informative synoptic descriptions of the changes in the treatment groups and the distinction between the two groups.

Example 5.3.4

A study evaluated the effects of diet and exercise in adults who were 65 years of age or older and obese. Subjects were randomly assigned to a control group, a diet group, an exercise group, or a diet and exercise group. The primary outcome was a change in score on the modified physical performance test (PPT), a scale that ranges from 0 to 36 with higher scores indicating better physical status. The following is one account of the changes in physical performance presented by Villareal and Other (2011):

> The mean (±SD) on the Physical Performance Test (the primary outcome) increased more in the diet-exercise group than in the diet group or the exercise group; an increase of 5.4±2.4 points in the diet-exercise group (a 21% change from baseline) compared with increases of 3.4±2.4 points in the diet group (a 12% change) and 4.0±2.5 points in the exercise group (a 15% change) (Table 2 and Fig. 2).

To read intelligently, it is productive to note that the values 5.4 ± 2.4, 3.4 ± 2.4, and 4.0 ± 2.5 denote the means and standard deviations of changes in the physical performance test (PPT) scores at one year. Table 2 shows that the mean PPT scores at baseline are 28.0, 28.6, and 27.1 in the diet–exercise group, the diet group, and the exercise group, respectively. They yield $5.4/28.0 = 19\%$, $3.4/28.6 = 12\%$, and $4.1/27.1 = 15\%$. These results suggest that 21%, 12%, and 15% are the percentages of changes in means. They are not descriptions of changes of individual subjects.

The standard deviations are not small relative to the means. They suggest that there were probably both decreases and increases in each group. This is ratified by observation-regions speculated by the Gaussian model shown in Fig. 5.15. The regions speculate that the increases of some of the 28 subjects in the diet–exercise group are probably all increases, and that the changes of a few of the subjects in the diet group and a few of the subjects in the exercise group were small decreases. However, the sizes of the small increases in the diet–exercise group and the percentages of declines in the diet group and the exercise group are unknown.

It is more informative to depict the distributions of changes comprehensively and use percentages of relevant changes to depict the distinction among the four groups.

Review Questions

1. Do the means and standard deviations or medians and ranges of measurements obtained from a group of subjects before and after a treatment unveil how the measurements of the subjects changed individually?
2. Do distributions of measurements obtained from a group of subjects before and after a treatment unveil how the measurements of the subjects changed individually?
3. Is an assertion that the mean of a groups of subjects increased significantly after treatment an affirmation that observations of all or most subjects increased?
4. When observations obtained from a group of subjects before and after a treatment are analyzed to assess treatment effect, what are unveiled by the before-and-after treatment observation-pairs that are not unveiled by the set of before and the set of after treatment observations?
5. What is indicated by a graph that uses lines to connect pairs of observations of subjects before and after a treatment that is not indicated by comprehensive displays of the respective distributions of the before-and-after treatment data sets?
6. What is indicated by the mean and standard deviation of the pair differences of paired quantitative data sets that is not indicated by the means and standard deviations of the respective distributions of the data sets?
7. What is indicated by the median and range of the pair differences of paired quantitative data sets that is not indicated by the medians and ranges of the two data sets?
8. Does the mean of pair ratios of two paired quantitative data sets equal the ratio of the means the data sets?
9. Does the median of pair ratios of two paired quantitative data sets equal the ratio of the means the data sets?
10. How does difference between means of before and after treatment observations relate to mean of differences of before and after observations? How does percent change in means relate to mean of percent changes?
11. How does difference between medians of before and after treatment observation relate to median of differences between before and after treatment observations?
12. Is $P < 0.001$ a suggestion that all observations after treatment are increases or decreases?

Exercise

5.E.1. Review the before-and-after treatment ratings of pain shown in Table 1.13 and compute pair differences. Discuss the relative advantages of using each of the following to depict the effect of the pain reliever.

(a) Means and standard deviations of the set of before treatment and the set of after treatment ratings
(b) Medians and ranges of the before treatment and the after treatment ratings
(c) Graphical displays of the respective distributions of the before treatment and the after treatment ratings
(d) Mean and standard deviation of pair differences
(e) Median and range of pair differences
(f) A graphical display of the distribution of pair differences

5.E.2. Hillmen and Others (2004) (Example 5.1.1) stated: *Similarly, the numbers of reticulocytes remained relatively constant during eculizumab treatment.* Review Table 1.3 and determine values of a pair index to characterize the changes in reticulocytes counts of the subjects. Elaborate the relative advantage of using each of the following to depict how the reticulocyte counts remained relatively constant during eculizumab treatment.

(a) Means and standard deviations of the 12 months before treatment and the 3 months after treatment reticulocyte numbers
(b) Medians and ranges of the 12 months before treatment and the 3 months after treatment reticulocyte numbers
(c) Graphical displays of the distributions of the 12 months before and the 3 months after treatment numbers of reticulocytes
(d) Mean and standard deviation of pairwise differences.
(e) Median and range of the pair differences.
(f) Graphical display the distribution of the pair differences.

5.E.3. Review Figure 3B and Figure 4B of Russell and Others (2014) (Figs 2.16 and 5.3).

(a) Elaborate the suggestion of Figure 4B and discuss whether it unveiled how the mean glucose levels of the adolescents changed individually.
(b) Elaborate the suggestions of Figure 3B and discuss whether it unveiled how the mean glucose levels of the adolescents changed individually.

5.E.4. Hsu and Others (2004) (Example 5.1.4) reported that maximum capacity increased significantly in both treatment groups. This was corroborated by means and standard deviations of before ablation and after ablation measures of capacity and P-values.

(a) Elaborate the suggestions of the means and standard deviations of the set of before ablation and the set of after ablation measures of maximum capacity and P-value of the subjects with congestive heart failure

(123 ± 44, 144 ± 55 W, and $P < 0.00$) with respect to changes in the subjects.

(b) Elaborate the suggestions of the means and standard deviations of the set of before ablation and the set of after ablation measures of maximum capacity and the P-value of the group of controls (145 ± 44, 158 ± 52 W, and $P < 0.001$) with respect to changes in the controls.

5.E.5. Zheng and Others (2018) (Example 5.3.2) used $P = 0.003$ to corroborate the assertion that changes in spasticity of forearm rotation from baseline to month 12 as measured on the Modified Ashworth Scale significantly favored the surgery group. Table 2 used −2 (3), −1 (10), and 0 (5) and −1 (3), 0 (14), and 1 (1) to depict the distributions of the changes in the surgery and control groups, respectively.

(a) Elaborate what $P = 0.003$ suggests, particularly whether it is an assertion that all changes in the surgery group were more favorable improvements as compared with changes in the control group.

(b) Suggest a narrative of the distinction in changes in spasticity between the two groups.

References

Acker, M. A., et al. (2018). Mitral-valve repair vs. replacement for severe ischemic-artery stenosis. *The New England Journal of Medicine, 370*(1), 23–32.

Alexander, E. K., et al. (2004). Timing and magnitude of increases in levothyroxine requirements during pregnancy in women with hypothyroidism. *The New England Journal of Medicine, 351* (3), 241–249.

Cooper, C. J., et al. (2014). Stenting and medical therapy for atherosclerotic renal-artery stenosis. *The New England Journal of Medicine, 370*(1), 13–22.

Hillmen, P., et al. (2004). Effect of Eculizumab on hemolysis and transfusion requirements in patients with paroxysmal nocturnal hemoglobinuria. *The New England Journal of Medicine, 350*(6), 552–559.

Hsu, L.-F., et al. (2004). Catheter ablation for atrial fibrillation. *The New England Journal of Medicine, 351*(23), 2373–2383.

Leonardi, C., et al. (2012). Anti-interleukin-17 monoclonal antibody ixekizumab in chronic plaque psoriasis. *The New England Journal of Medicine, 366*(13), 1190–1199.

Lockley, S. W., et al. (2004). Effect of reducing interns' weekly work hours on sleep and attentional failure. *The New England Journal of Medicine, 351*(18), 1829–1837.

Russell, S. J., et al. (2014). Inpatient glycemic control with a bionic pancreas in type 1 diabetes. *The New England Journal of Medicine, 371*(4), 313–325.

Villareal, D. T., et al. (2011). Weight loss, exercise, or both and physical function in obese older adults. *The New England Journal of Medicine, 364*(13), 1218–1229.

Zheng, M.-X., et al. (2018). Trial of contralateral seventh cervical nerve transfer for spastic arm paralysis. *The New England Journal of Medicine, 378*(1), 22–34.

Chapter 6
Unpaired Qualitative Data Sets

Observations pertaining to occurrences of events are important in medical research. They are qualitative and are analyzed to assess the likelihoods of events. This chapter demonstrates that revelations of a set of qualitative observations are clearly manifested by percentages of observations belonging to categories that comprise the distribution of the data set. Revelation of unpaired qualitative data sets is clearly manifested by the respective distributions of the data sets.

When observations pertaining to the occurrence of events are analyzed, times to occurrence are readily available. Assessments of likelihoods of event based on times to occurrence are routinely used to supplement or in place of percentages of events. The use of such assessments is also examined in this chapter.

Section 6.1 previews examples of descriptions of revelations of unpaired qualitative data sets. Indications of percentages are probed in Sect. 6.2. Person-time incidence rates and Kaplan–Meier estimates are often presented as assessments of likelihood of events in addition to or in place of percentages. Suggestions of these assessments are explained in Sect. 6.3. Section 6.4 probes suggestions of measures of distinction. Section 6.5 presents examples of the evolution of likelihood during follow-up. Effects of traits on likelihoods of events in treatment groups and distinctions in likelihoods between treatment groups are often evaluated by subgroup analysis. Examples of subgroup analysis are reviewed in Sect. 6.6. Section 6.7 presents examples of intelligent reading and informative reporting.

6.1 Examples

This section uses examples to demonstrate how revelations of unpaired qualitative data sets are related in medical articles.

P. C. Chang, *Data Analysis of Medical Studies*,
https://doi.org/10.1007/978-3-031-49984-5_6

Example 6.1.1

Combes and Others (2018) reported the results of a study that randomly assigned 124 subjects with severe acute respiratory disease syndrome (ARDS) to receive immediate venovenous extracorporeal membrane oxygenation (ECMO) and 125 to receive control treatment (continued conventional mechanical ventilation). The following is a description of the primary end point of the study, mortality at 60 days:

> At 60 days, 44 patients (35%) in the ECMO group and 57 (46%) in the control group had died (relative risk, 0.76; 95% confidence interval [CI], 0.55 to 1.04, P=0.09) (Table 2). The hazard ratio for death within 60 days after randomization in the ECMO group, as compared with the control group, was 0.70 (95% CI, 0.47 to 1.04; P=0.07) (Fig. 2).

The article stated: *Randomization was stratified according to center and the period of ventilation before randomization (<72 hours* vs. *≥72 hours).* Randomization was performed by a randomized block design; the two groups of subjects and their data sets are unpaired although matched. Whether a subject died is a dichotomous observation. The two sets of dichotomous observations are unpaired. The percentages: 35% and 46% are synoptic descriptions of the distributions of two unpaired dichotomous data sets.

The percentages are assessments of the risk of death during the first 60 days of follow-up among subjects assigned to the two treatment groups. The relative risk 0.76 is a ratio of the cumulative incidence rates, 35 % /46% = 0.76. This suggests that the risk of death during the first 60 days of follow-up among the 124 subjects in the ECMO group was lower than and 7.6-tenth of that among the 125 subjects in the control group.

$P = 0.09$ is an improvised estimate of the probability that, if the study were replicated a score of times and chance were the only explanation, relative risks of replicates of the study diverge from 1.0 as much as or more than 0.76 would be 0.09. The 95% confidence interval [0.55 to 1.04] is an improvised estimate of the region that would include 95% of the relative risks of replicates of the study and chance were the only explanation of the difference among replicates. $P = 0.09$ is not smaller than the customary criterion (≤0.05), and the 95% confidence interval does not exclude 1.0. They both suggest that the relative risk of 0.76 should not be declared statistically significant and that the concern that it might be incidental should not be dismissed.

Boundaries of the 95% confidence interval [0.55 to 1.04] are 72% and 136% of the relative risk 0.76. They suggest that if the study were replicated a score of times, there might be relative risks as small as 76% and as large as 136% of the reported relative risk. The reproducibility of the reported relative risk is deemed inadequate.

Both $P = 0.09$ and the 95% confidence interval suggest that it is astute to limit the relative risk of 0.76 to the subjects of the study and not to make inference.

The hazard ratio 0.70 is a result of a statistical procedure known as the Cox proportional hazards regression analysis determined from the times to death during the first 60 days of follow-up. It is used as an assessment of the distinction in risks of death in 60 days between the two treatment groups and an insinuation that the risk of death during the first 60 days of follow-up of the subjects in the ECMO group was lower than and approximately 7.0-tenth of the risk of the subjects in the control group.

$P = 0.07$ is an improvised estimate of the probability that, if the study were replicated a score of times and chance were the only explanation, hazard ratios of the replicates diverge from 1.0 as much as or more than 0.70 would be 0.07. The 95% confidence interval [0.47 to 1.04] is an improvised estimate of the region that would include 95% of the hazard ratios of replicates of the study and chance were the only explanation of the difference among replicates. $P = 0.07$ is not smaller than the customary criterion (≤0.05), and the 95% confidence interval does not exclude 1.0. They both suggest that the hazard ratio 0.70 should not be declared statistically significant.

The boundaries of the 95% confidence interval [0.47 to 1.04] are 67% and 149% of the hazard ratio 0.70. This suggests that if the study replicated a score of times, there might be hazard ratios as small as 67% and as large as 149% of the reported hazard ratio. The reproducibility of the reported hazard ratio is inadequate.

The *P*-values and 95% confidence intervals suggest that it is astute to limit the ratio of the cumulative incidence rates (0.76) and the hazard ratio 0.70 to the subjects of the study and not to make inferences.

Figure 2 (Fig. 6.1) depicts estimates of the probability of survival in periods of increasing length (10–60 days). The heights of points on the curves signify the values of the estimates. Labels marked along a vertical line specify a scale for gauging values of estimates signified by heights of points. Lengths of follow-up

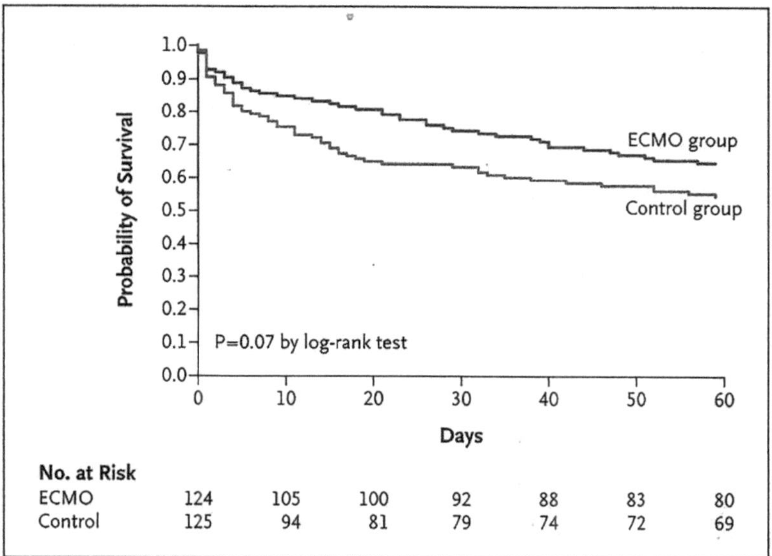

Figure 2. Kaplan–Meier Survival Estimates in the Intention-to-Treat Population during the First 60 Days of the Trial.

Fig. 6.1 Figure 2 of Combes and Others (2018)

periods are marked along a horizontal line in number of days. The two lines are the vertical and horizontal axes of the figure. The estimates are Kaplan–Meier estimates of the probability of survival, and the curves are Kaplan–Meier curves. The two curves suggest that the probability of survival declined steadily in the two treatment groups when the follow-up period lengthened and that the probability of survival in the ECMO group was consistently higher than that in the control group.

The article stated: "*Primary analyses were conducted according to the intention-to-treat principle and did not use a stratified test statistics.*" Figure 1 suggests that computation of the cumulative incidence rates used data of 3 of the 124 subjects assigned to the ECMO group who did not receive the treatment and 35 of the 125 assigned to the control group who received rescue ECMO. The cumulative incidence rates, their ratio, and the hazard ratio are not indisputable assessments of the effects of the treatments but are credible assessments of being assigned to the treatment groups. More credible assessments of treatment effects may be determined by using data of the 121 subjects who received only ECMO, 90 subjects who received conventional mechanical ventilation only, and 35 subjects who received conventional mechanical ventilation and rescue ECMO.

Example 6.1.2

The results of the Stabilization of Atherosclerotic Plague by Initiation of Darapladib (STABILITY) trial are reported in an article by the STABILITY Investigators (2014). This study randomly assigned subjects with stable chronic coronary heart disease to receive either a once-daily oral dose of darapladib or a matching placebo. Subjects were instructed to return for clinic visits 1, 3, and 6 months after randomization and thereafter every 6 months during the study. The primary end point was time to cardiovascular death, myocardial infarction, or urgent coronary revascularization. The following is a description of the risks of the primary end point:

> The primary end point occurred in 769 of 7924 patients (9.7%) in the darapladib group and in 819 of 7904 patients (10.4%) in the placebo group (hazard ratio in the darapladib group, 0.94; 95% CI, 0.85 to 1.03; P = 0.20) (Table 2 and Fig. 2).

The two groups of subjects were the results of random assignments. They and their data sets are unpaired. The occurrence of the primary outcome is a dichotomous observation. The percentages 9.7% and 10.4% are synoptic descriptions of the distributions of two unpaired dichotomous data sets and manifestations of the revelation of the data sets.

The percentages 9.7% and 10.4% are average incidence rates and assessments of risks of the primary end point during follow-up. Their ratio 9.7%/10.4% = 0.93 suggests that the risk of the primary end point of the darapladib group was slightly lower than and approximately 9.3-tenth of that of the placebo group during follow-up.

The hazard ratio 0.94 is a suggestion that the risk of the primary end point of the darapladib group is lower than and about 9.4-tenth of the risk of the placebo group. It was determined by the Cox proportional hazards regression analysis using times to event. It is an assessment of the relative difference in the risks of the primary end point between the two treatment groups and insinuates that the risk of the primary end point of the darapladib group is slightly lower than and approximately 9.4-tenth of the risk of the placebo group during follow-up.

$P = 0.20$ is an improvised estimate of the probability that hazard ratios of replicates of the study diverge from the null value 1.0 as much as or more than 0.94 if chance were the only explanation of the difference among replicates of the study. It is not smaller than 0.05 and suggests that the hazard ratio may not be declared statistically significant. The 95% confidence interval [0.85 to 1.03] does not exclude 1.0; it also suggests that the hazard ratio may not be declared statistically significant.

Boundaries of the 95% confidence interval [0.85 to 1.03] are 90% and 110% of the hazard ratio 0.94. They suggest that if the study replicated a score of times, hazard ratios of most replicates of the study would be relatively close to the hazard ratio 0.94. The hazard ratio is adequately reproducible.

Although the hazard ratio 0.94 should not be declared statistically significant, its reproducibility is adequate. It may be inferred to appropriate individuals.

The suggestion of the hazard ratio 0.94 that the risks of the primary end during follow-up are close between the two treatment groups is confirmed by Fig. 2 (Fig. 6.2). The figure displays Kaplan–Meier estimates of the probability of the primary end point in the two treatment groups in periods of increasing length since randomization. It shows that the estimates of probability of the primary end point in the two groups were close whether it was a few months or more than 36 months since randomization.

The average incidence rates, hazard ratios, and Kaplan–Meier curves are the results of the intention-to-treat analysis. Figure 1 of the article suggests that their

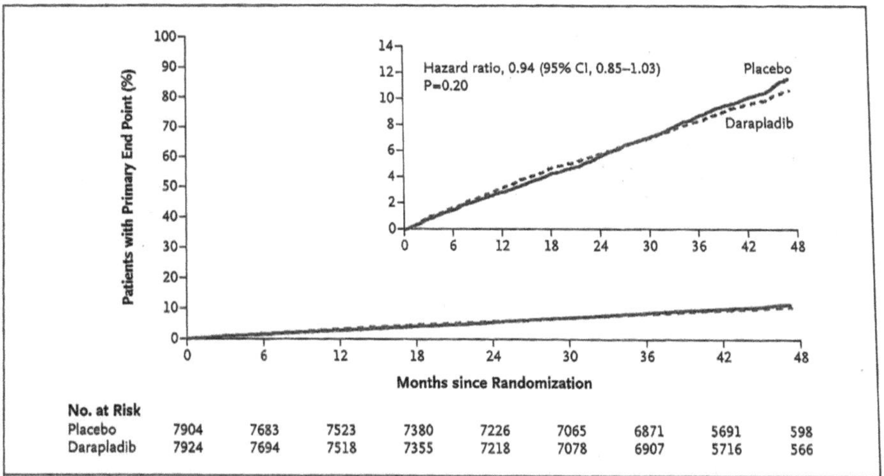

Figure 2. Kaplan–Meier Curves for the Primary End Point of Death from Cardiovascular Causes, Myocardial Infarction, or Stroke.
The inset shows the same data on an enlarged y axis.

Fig. 6.2 Figure 2 of the STATBILITY Investigators (2014)

determinations used data of many subjects with protocol violations such as not receiving or discontinuing assigned treatment or withdrawing from the study. They are not indisputable assessments of the effects of the treatments but credible assessments of being assigned to the treatment groups.

Example 6.1.3

The results of a study that randomly assigned 230 children who had tympanostomy tube otorrhea to receive antibiotic-glucocorticoid eardrops, oral antibiotics, and observation are presented by van Dongen and Others (2014). The study stratified subjects into blocks of size 6 according to age (<4 years vs. ≥4 years) and randomly assigned the children in each block to treatment groups. The block size is larger than the number of treatments. The three groups of children are unpaired although matched; their data sets we are analyzed as unpaired.

The primary outcome was treatment failure, defined as the presence of otorrhea in one or both ears 2 weeks after study group assignment. Observations pertaining to the occurrence of the primary outcome are dichotomous; the three sets of observations are unpaired dichotomous data sets. An account of the revelations of the three unpaired dichotomous data sets was related by van Dongen and Others (2014) as follows:

> At week 2, 5% of children treated with eardrops had otorrhea, as with 44% of those who received oral antibiotics (risk difference, −39 percentage points, 95% CI, −51 to −26; number needed to treat, 3) and 55% of those who were assigned to initial observation (risk difference, −49 percentage points; 95% CI, −62 to −37, number needed to treat, 2) (Table 2).

The percentages: 5%, 44%, and 55% are synoptic descriptions of three unpaired dichotomous data sets. They are assessments of risk of treatment failure during the first 2 weeks of follow-up. They unveiled that 5% of the subjects in the eardrops group, 44% of those in the oral antibiotics group, and 55% of those in the initial observation group had treatment failure. The risk differences −39 and −49 percentage points are measures of distinction in risks. They suggest that the risk of treatment failure in the eardrops group was 39 percentage points lower than that in the oral antibiotic group and 49 percentage points lower than that in the initial observation group.

The numbers needed to treat (three and two) are alternate expressions of the differences in the rates. They suggest that, to prevent one more treatment failure, three more children would be needed in the eardrops group instead of the oral antibiotic group, and two more would be needed in the eardrops group instead of the oral antibiotic group.

CI stands for confidence interval. Boundaries of the 95% confidence interval of the risk difference −39 percentage points: [−51 to −26] are 131% and 67% of the risk difference. Boundaries of the 95% confidence interval of the risk difference −49 percentage points: [−62 to −37] are 126% and 76% of the risk difference. They suggest that if the study replicated a score of times, there would be risk differences differing from the reported risk difference rather substantially. The reproducibility of the risk differences is inadequate. It is astute to limit them to the subjects of the study and consider them preliminary signals only.

Example 6.1.4

Gaudino and Others (2018) presented the results of an analysis of the combined data of six randomized controlled trials comparing radial artery grafts and saphenous vein grafts. The primary outcome was a composite of death, myocardial infarction, or repeat revascularization. The following is a description of the risks of the composite outcome:

> The incidence of the composite outcome of death, myocardial infarction, or repeat revascularization was significantly lower in the radial artery group than in the saphenous-vein group (25 vs. 39 events per 1000 patient-years; hazard ratio, 0.67; 95% confidence interval [CI], 0.49 to 0.90; P = 0.01) (Fig. 1 A).

The numbers 25 and 39 events per 1000 patient-years are person-year incidence rates and measures of risk of the composite outcome during follow-up. They suggest that there would be 25 events of the composite outcome in the radial artery group and 39 in the saphenous vein group if 1000 subjects were followed for one year.

The hazard ratio 0.67 is a result of the statistical procedure known as the Cox proportional hazard regression analysis. It is used as an insinuation that the risk of the composite outcome in the radial artery group was 6.7-tenth of the risk in the saphenous vein group. The hazard ratio 0.67 is close to the ratio of the person-year incidence rates 25/39 = 0.64, which suggests that if 100 subjects were followed for 10 years, the number of events of the composite outcome in the radial artery group is lower than and 6.4-tenth of the risk of the saphenous vein group.

The 95% confidence interval excludes the null value of hazard ratio 1.0, and $P = 0.01$ meets the customary criterion ≤0.05. They suggest that the hazard ratio 0.67 may be declared statistically significant; the concern that the ratio might be coincidental may be dismissed.

The 95% confidence interval [0.49 to 0.90] is wide relative to the hazard ratio 0.67. Its boundaries suggest that if the study replicated a score of times, there might be hazard ratios as small as or smaller than 49% and as large as or larger than 134% of the reported hazard ratio. The reproducibility of the hazard ratio 0.67 is inadequate. Although the hazard ratio 0.67 may be declared statistically significant, it is astute to limit it to the subjects of the study and use it as a preliminary signal only.

Example 6.1.5

Albers and Others (2018) (Example 3.1.7) use percentages of subjects who were deemed functionally independent to depict the severity of disability on the 90th day of follow-up. Functional independence was defined as a score on the modified Rankin scale of 0 to 2. Whether a subject is functionally independent is a dichotomous observation. The percentages of subjects who were functionally independent (45% and 17%) are informative synoptic descriptions of the two sets of dichotomous observations.

The two groups of subjects were the results of a randomized block design. They are unpaired. The two sets of observations pertaining to functional independence are unpaired dichotomous data sets. Their revelations are informatively unveiled by the two percentages.

Albers and Ohers (2018) used the risk ratio 2.67 to assess the degree of distinction between the two sets of dichotomous observations. 95% CI, 1.60 to 4.48, and P<0.001 were presented.

The risk ratio 2.67 is the ratio of the two percentages computed directly from the numbers of subjects whose scores were 0 to 2 in the two treatment groups (41 of 92 and 15 of 90). It suggests that the likelihood of being functionally independent in the endovascular therapy group was approximately 2.67 times that in the medical therapy group.

The 95% confidence interval of the risk ratio [1.60 to 4.48] excludes the null value of 1.0, and P<0.001 is below the customary criterion ≤ 0.05. They suggest that the ratio may be declared statistically significant; the concern that the ratio is a chance coincidence may be dismissed.

The 95% confidence interval [1.60 to 4.48] yields more information than just confirming the indication of $P < 0.001$ that the risk ratio may be declared statistically significant. It is wide; its boundaries suggest that if the study replicated a score of times, there might be risk ratios as small as or smaller than 60% and larger than 168% of the reported risk ratio. The reproducibility of the risk ratio 2.67 is deemed inadequate. Although the risk ratio may be declared statistically significant, its reproducibility is inadequate. It is astute to limit it to the subjects of the study and use it as a preliminary signal.

6.2 Incidence and Prevalence Rates

Percentages and proportions are expressions of the same quantity. The revelations of a set of qualitative observations are informatively manifested by percentages (proportions) of observations belonging to categories. The percentages (proportions) constitute the distribution of the data set. When two sets of qualitative observations are unpaired, their revelations are informatively manifested by their respective distributions.

- *Average and Cumulative Incidence Rates*

If observations of a data set pertain to occurrence of an event when a group of subjects are followed, revelation of the data set is cogently manifested by the percentage of subjects in whom the event occurred. The denominator of the percentage is the number of subjects in the group; it was determined by study design. The numerator is the number of subjects in whom the event occurred; it is an outcome of the study. It is rational to use the percentage as an assessment of the probability of event occurrence. It is called an average incidence rate if its numerator is the number of subjects in whom the event occurred during follow-up and a cumulative incidence rate if its numerator is the number of subjects in whom the event occurred in a period of fixed length during follow-up.

Average incidence rate

$$= \frac{\text{Number of events occurred during the course of follow-up}}{\text{Number of subjects followed}} \times 100\% \qquad (6.2.1)$$

Cumulative incidence rate

$$= \frac{\text{Number of events occurred in a period of given length during follow-up}}{\text{Number of subjects followed during the period of length}} \times 100\% \qquad (6.2.2)$$

When indication of an average incidence rate is ascertained, it is important to consider the length of follow-up. It may differ substantially from the cumulative incidence rates of short or extended periods.

- Remark

Using average and cumulative incidence rates as assessments of likelihood has its ground in the important mathematical distribution known as binomial distribution. A binomial distribution postulates how the probability that the number of successes in a series of mathematically independent trials relates to the number of trials and the probability of success of a single trial. The trials are deemed mathematically independent if the outcome of any one trial is not affected by the outcome of any other trial. The probability of success of individual trials is identical among all trials.

Average and cumulative incidence rates are computed by using numbers of subjects in whom events occurred as numerators and numbers of subjects in treatment groups as denominators. The numbers of subjects in the treatment groups are determined by study design; they are analogous to the number of trials of binomial distribution. The number of events is an outcome of the study; they are analogous to the number of successes of binomial distributions. It is rational to use the rates as estimates of the probability of event occurrence. An average incidence rate is a judicious assessment of the probability of an event during the entire period of follow-up, and a cumulative incidence rate is a judicious assessment of the probability of an event during a fixed length of time during follow-up.

- *Prevalence Rates*

If observations of a data set pertain to the presence of a condition at the time of the study or in the past, revelation of the data set is informatively unveiled by the percentage of YES observations in the data set. The denominator of the percentage is the number of subjects in the group; it was determined by study design. The numerator is the number of subjects who had the condition at the time of the study or in the past; it is an outcome of the study. The percentage is an assessment of the commonness of the condition; it is a prevalence rate.

$$\text{Prevalence rate} = \frac{\text{Number of subjects with a condition currently or in the past}}{\text{Number of subjects}} \times 100\% \quad (6.2.3)$$

- *Odds*

The likelihood and commonness of an event are sometimes assessed by odds. When one category of a set of qualitative observations is designated the YES category, the odds of YES among the observations equals:

$$\text{Odds of YES} = \frac{\text{Percent of Yes Observations}}{\text{Percent of NO Observations}} = \frac{\text{Number of YES Observations}}{\text{Number of NO Observations}} \quad (6.2.4)$$

- *Contingency Table for Unpaired Qualitative Data Sets*

Revelations of unpaired qualitative data sets are informatively paraded by a table displaying percentages and numbers of observations of data sets belonging to categories. The table is known as a contingency table, a two-way contingency table, or a two-way table. It is particularly useful when the number of categories or number of data sets is larger than two. Contingency tables depicting unpaired qualitative data sets are sometimes dubbed unpaired data two-way tables to be distinguished from paired data two-way tables that exhibit methodically revelations of paired qualitative data sets (Chap. 7).

The same format is followed in this book to present contingency tables. Headings of rows designate data sets, and headings of columns indicate categories. Each row displays percentages and numbers of observations of a data set belonging to categories that comprise the distribution of a data set. The rightmost cell of a row exhibits the summation of the percentages and numbers of the row. The summation of the numbers in a row is the total number of observations in a data set; the summation of the percentages in a row is 100% or within rounding error.

The percentages displayed in a row present a comprehensive description of the distribution of a data set. They are row percentages computed by using the number in the rightmost cell of each row to divide the numbers displayed in the row.

Example 6.2.1

Combes and Others (2018) (Example 6.1.1) used 35% and 46% to depict the risk of death in 60 days. The percentages are synoptic descriptions of two unpaired dichotomous data sets. Table 6.1 is a contingency table that presents comprehensive delineations of the distributions of the two dichotomous data sets. It shows that the denominators of the percentages are the numbers of subjects in the treatment groups, which were determined by study design, and that the numerators of the percentages are the numbers of deaths in 60 days, which are outcomes of the study. It is rational

Table 6.1 Percentages (numbers) of subjects died in 60 days

	Died in 60 days		
	YES	NO	TOTAL
	% (#)	% (#)	% (#)
Treatment			
ECMO	35% (44)	65% (80)	100% (124)
Control	46% (57)	54% (68)	100% (125)

Table 6.2 Percentages (numbers) of subjects in whom the primary end point occurred

	Primary end point		
	YES	NO	TOTAL
	% (#)	% (#)	% (#)
Treatment			
Darapladib	9.7% (769)	90.3% (7155)	100% (7924)
Placebo	10.4% (819)	89.6% (7085)	100% (7904)

to consider the denominators numbers of trials and the numerators numbers of success of binomial distributions. The percentages are functional assessments of risks of death in 60 days. They are cumulative incidence rates.

Example 6.2.2
The article by the STABILITY Investigators (2014) used the percentages: 7.9% and 10.4% to assess the risk of the primary end point of the study in the darapladib group and the placebo group during follow-up. The percentages are synoptic descriptions of two unpaired dichotomous data sets. Table 6.2 is a contingency table that presents comprehensive delineations of the two dichotomous data sets. It shows that the denominators of the percentages are the numbers of subjects in the treatment groups, which were determined by study design, and that the numerators are number of occurrence of the primary end point, which are outcomes of the study. It is rational to consider the denominators numbers of trials and numerators numbers of success binomial distributions. The percentages are functional estimates of probabilities of success and assessments of risks of the primary end point. They are average incidence rates.

Example 6.2.3
The article by van Dongen and Others (2014) (Example 6.1.3) uses cumulative incidence rates of 5%, 44%, and 55% to assess the risk of treatment failure (with otorrhea in one or both ears) 2 weeks after enrollment. These percentages are synoptic descriptions of three unpaired dichotomous data sets. Table 6.3 is a contingency table that presents comprehensive delineations of the three distributions.

The numbers of subjects in the treatment groups 76, 77, and 75 were determined by study design. It is rational to consider them numbers of trials of binomial distributions. It is judicious to use the percentages as assessments of probabilities of treatment failure.

Table 6.3 Percentages and numbers of treatment failure

	Treatment failure		
	YES	NO	TOTAL
	% (#)	% (#)	% (#)
Treatment			
Ear drops	5% (4)	95% (72)	100% (76)
Oral antibiotic	44% (34)	56% (43)	100% (77)
Observation	55% (41)	45% (34)	100% (75)

6.3 Person-Time Incidence Rate and Kaplan–Meier Estimate of Probability

Subjects of clinical trials are followed to monitor occurrence of events. Times to occurrence of event are readily available in addition to observations pertaining to occurrence of event. Person-time incidence rates and Kaplan–Meier estimates of probability are assessments of the likelihood of events that utilize not only data pertaining to the occurrence of events but also time to event. They are often reported in place of or together with incidence rates.

The lengths of time subjects are followed to monitor occurrence of event are called follow-up times. The onset of follow-up of a subject may be enrollment in the study, allocation to treatment groups, initiation or completion of treatments, or occurrence of some condition. The end of follow-up may be the occurrence of an event, scheduled termination of follow-up, disqualification, or loss to follow-up.

The follow-up time of a subject is dubbed a time-to-event if follow-up of the subject ended when the event of interest occurred. It is called a censored follow-up time if the subject was known to be event-free when follow-up ended according to the study protocol or the subject was lost to follow-up. The time-to-event of the subject is unknown.

6.3.1 Person-Time Incidence Rate

Like the average incidence rate, the person-time incidence rate is an assessment of the likelihood of event occurrence during follow-up. The person-time incidence rate is the ratio of the number of events relative to the sum of follow-up times. It is computed as follows:

$$\text{Person-time incidence rate} = \frac{\text{Number of subjects in whom event occurred during follow-up}}{\text{Sum of follow-up times of all subjects followed}} \quad (6.3.1)$$

Person-time incidence rates may be expressed as numbers of events per number of days, months, or years.

Example 6.3.1.1
The study reported by DeBaun and Others (2014) (Example 1.1.4) randomly assigned 99 subjects to the transfusion group and 97 to the observation group. The primary end point of the study was recurrence of infarct or hemorrhage. A narrative of the likelihood of the primary end point is presented in the article as follows:

> In an intention-to-treat analysis, the incidence rate of infarct recurrence was 2.0 per 100 person-years at risk in the transfusion group and 4.8 per 100 person-years at risk in the observation group, with an incidence rate ratio of 0.41 (95% confidence interval [CI], 0.12 to 0.99; P=0.04).

The values 2.0 and 4.8 per 100 person-years are person-time incidence rates. They suggest that if 100 subjects were followed for one year, the primary end point would occur in two of the subjects in the transfusion group and five of the subjects in the observation group.

The article reported: *In the transfusion group, 99 participants accumulated 304 patient-years (median, 3.0 years per patient); in the observation group, 97 participants accumulated 289 patient-years (median, 3.0 per patient).* The primary end point was observed in 6 subjects in the transfusion group and 14 in the observation group. These numbers and the accumulated patient-years yield:

$$\begin{aligned}&\text{Person} - \text{time incidence rate of the primary endpoint in the transfusion group}\\&= \frac{\text{Number of participants in the transfusion group in whom primary end point was documented}}{\text{Sum of follow} - \text{up times of all participants in the transfusion group}}\\&= \frac{6}{304} = 0.0197\\&= 2.0 \text{ per } 100 \text{ person} - \text{years.}\end{aligned}$$

$$\begin{aligned}&\text{Person} - \text{time incidence rate of the primary end point in the observation group}\\&= \frac{\text{Number of participants in the observation group in whom primary end point was documented}}{\text{Sum of follow} - \text{up times of all participants in the observation group}}\\&= \frac{14}{289} = 0.0484\\&= 4.8 \text{ per } 100 \text{ person} - \text{years.}\end{aligned}$$

The incidence rate ratio 0.41 is a ratio of the two person-year incidence rates (2.0/4.8 = 0.417). This suggests that the risk of infarct recurrence in the transfusion group was much lower than and approximately 4.1-tenth of the risk in the observation group.

The 95% confidence interval [0.12 to 0.99] excludes 1.0, and $P = 0.04$ is smaller than 0.05. They suggest that the rate ratio of 0.41 may be declared statistically significant, and the concern that it is coincidental may be dismissed.

The 95% confidence interval is wide relative to the incidence rate ratio. Its boundaries suggest that if the study replicated a score of times, there would be replicates yielding incidence ratios as small as 29% and as large as 241% of the reported incidence ratio 0.41. Although the incidence rate ratio may be declared "significant," its reproducibility is inadequate. It is astute to limit it to the subjects of the study and use it as a preliminary signal.

The person-year incidence rates are the results of intention-to-treat analysis that used data from all subjects assigned to the treatment groups. Figure 1 of the article shows that of the 99 subjects assigned to the transfusion group, 15 crossed over to the observation group, and 2 were lost to follow-up or withdrew. Of the 97 patients assigned to the observation group, 6 crossed over to the transfusion group, and 9 were lost to follow-up. Follow-up times of these subjects were included in the denominators of person-time incidence rates. The rates are not indisputable assessments of effects of the treatments on risks of the primary end point but more credible assessments of effects of being assigned to the treatment groups.

Example 6.3.1.2 Gaudino (378, 22)

Gaudino and Others (2018) (Example 6.1.4) used 25 and 39 events per 1000 patient-years to assess risks of the composite outcome of death, myocardial infarction, or repeat revascularization of the radial artery and the saphenous vein groups. These are person-time incidence rates. They suggest that there would be 25 events of the composite outcome in the radial artery group and 39 in the saphenous vein group if 1000 subjects were followed for one year.

6.3.2 *Kaplan–Meier Estimate of Probability*

Like cumulative incidence rats, Kaplan–Meier estimate is an estimate of likelihood of event in a period of fixed length. Like the person-time incidence rate, its computation uses follow-up times. It differs from the person-time incidence rate in that a person-time incidence rates is computed from the number of events and sums of follow-up times directly; a Kaplan–Meier estimate of probability is computed by using a fundamental law of probability that uses times-to-event and censored follow-up time differently.

Example 6.3.2.1 van Driel (378, 3)

An article by van Driel and Others (2018) presented the results of a study comparing interval cytoreductive surgery with and without hyperthermic intraperitoneal chemotherapy (HIPEC). Subjects of the study consisted of patients who had newly diagnosed stage II epithelial ovarian, fallopian tube, or peritoneal cancer. The primary end point was recurrence-free survival. The article stated:

> The probability of recurrence-free survival at 3 years was 8% in the surgery group (95% CI, 4 to 16) and 17% in the surgery-plus HIPEC group (95% CI, 11 to 26).

The percentages 8% and 17% are Kaplan–Meier estimates of probability. They suggest that the probability of being a recurrence-free survivor for 3 years is 8%

among the 123 subjects of the surgery group and 17% among the 121 subjects of the surgery plus HIPEC group.

The 95% confidence intervals [4% to 16%] and [11% to 26%] are wide relative to the estimates. The boundaries of [4% to 16%] are 50% and 200% of 8%. The boundaries of [11% to 26%] are 65% and 153% of 17%. They suggest that the reproducibility of the estimates of probability is inadequate. It is prudent to limit the estimates to the subjects of the study and use them as a preprimary signal only.

This is a rare case. The hazard ratio and the ratio of Kaplan–Meier estimate of probability disagree noticeably. The hazard ratio 0.66 suggests that the risk of the event of disease recurrence or death of the surgery plus HIPEC group is substantially lower than and only 6.6-tenth of the risk of the surgery-only group. Ratio of the Kaplan–Meier estimates of probability: $0.81/0.89 = 0.91$ suggests that the risk in the surgery plus HIPEC group is only slightly lower than and about 9.1-tenth of the risk in the surgery-only group.

Example 6.3.2.2 Kadish (350, 21)

The results of a study evaluating the effect of prophylactic implantation of a cardioverter-defibrillator (ICD) in preventing sudden death were reported by Kadish and Others (2004). The study randomly assigned 458 patients with nonischemic dilated cardiomyopathy, a left ventricular ejection fraction of less than 36%, and premature ventricular complexes or nonsustained ventricular tachycardia to receive standard medical therapy (229) or standard medical therapy plus a single-chamber ICD (229). The following is a narrative of outcome:

> On the basis of Kaplan–Meier curves, the rate of death from any cause at one year was 6.2 percent in the standard therapy group and 2.6 percent in the ICD group. At two years, it was 14.1 percent in the standard therapy group and 7.9 percent in the ICD group.

The percentages are Kaplan–Meier estimates of the probability of death from any cause. They suggest that of the 229 subjects assigned to receive the standard therapy, the estimated probability of death in 1 year was 6.2%, and the estimated probability of death in 2 years was 14.1%. Among the 229 subjects assigned to receive the ICD, the estimated probability of death in 1 year was 2.6%, and the estimated probability of death in 2 years was 7.9%.

The article stated that all analyses were conducted according to the intention-to-treat principle. Of the 229 subjects assigned to the ICD group, two declined implantation of the device, one had the device explanted, and one had the device deactivated. Of the 229 subjects assigned to the standard therapy group, 23 received ICDs. There were also other complications and deviations from the study protocol. Thus, the Kaplan–Meier estimates are not indisputable assessments of the effects of treatments on the risk of death but assessments of the effects of being assigned to the treatment groups.

6.4 Distinction Measures

Distinction in likelihoods of event between treatment groups is often assessed by ratio or difference of incidence rates or Kaplan–Meier estimates of probability. The hazard ratio is a trendy measure of distinction in the risks of events.

6.4.1 Rate Difference and Rate Ratio

Revelations of a dichotomous data set are informative unveiled by its percentage of YES observations. The difference and ratio of the percentages of YES of unpaired dichotomous data sets are informative measures of the degree of distinction between the data sets. Difference and ratio of incidence rates and Kaplan–Meier estimates of probability are useful assessments of distinction in likelihoods of event; difference and ratio of prevalence rates are useful assessments of distinction in commonness of event. The differences and ratios are dubbed rate differences and rate ratios.

When rates of treatment group 1 and treatment group 2 are written as rate *(1)* and rate *(2)*, the difference and ratio of the rates are computed as:

$$\text{RD} = \text{Rate-Difference} = \text{Rate}(1)\text{–}\text{Rate}(2) \qquad (6.4.1.1)$$

$$\text{RR} = \text{Rate-Ratio} = \frac{\text{Rate}(1)}{\text{Rate}(2)} \qquad (6.4.1.2)$$

A rate difference > 0 and a rate ratio >1.0 unveil that rate (1) is higher than rate (2); a rate difference < 0 and a rate ratio < 1.0 unveil that rate (1) is lower than rate (2). The null value of the rate difference is 0 and that of the rate ratio is 1.0. They unveiled that two rates are equal. The extent to which the rate difference and rate ratio deviate from their null values are quantitative measures of the degree of distinction.

It is important to consider magnitudes of rates when indication of rate difference and rate ratio are appraised. If rate (1) and rate (2) are small, their difference is small, but their ratio may noticeably deviate from 1.0. If rate (1) and rate (2) are large, their difference may be not small, but their ratio may be close to 1.0. For instance, if rate (1) = 2% and rate (2) = 1%, their difference is 1% and suggest that the rates are close, but their ratio is 2 and suggests that rate (1) is twofold of rate (2). If rate (1) = 88% and rate (2) = 98%, their difference equals −10%, and their ratio equals 0.90. The rate difference reveals that rate (1) is as much as 10 percentage points lower than rate (2); the two rates differ noticeably. The rate ratio suggests that rate (1) is 90 percent of rate (2); the two rates are relatively close.

- *NNT*

NNT is an alternative expression of differences in incidence rates. When incidence rates of treatment 1 and treatment 2 are written as rate (1) and rate (2), NNT is computed as:

$$\mathrm{NNT} = \frac{100}{\mathrm{Rate}(1)\text{–}\mathrm{Rate}(2)}, \text{ if Rate}(1) \text{ and Rate}(2) \text{ are percentages.} \quad (6.4.1.3)$$

$$\mathrm{NNT} = \frac{1}{\mathrm{Rate}(1)\text{–}\mathrm{Rate}(2)}, \text{ if Rate}(1) \text{ and Rate}(2) \text{ are proportions.} \quad (6.4.1.4)$$

If rate (1) and rate (2) are credible assessments of treatment effects, NNT is the number of subjects needed to treat by treatment 1 instead of treatment 2 to prevent one event. If rate (1) and rate (2) are credible assessments of the risks of being assigned to treatments, NNT is the number of subjects needed to assign to receive treatment 1 instead of treatment 2 to prevent one event.

Example 6.4.1.1

The article by van Dongen and Others (2014) (Example 6.1.3) used cumulative incidence rates (5%, 44%, and 55%) to assess risks of treatment failure (presence of otorrhea in one or both ears) 2 weeks after study group assignment. Differences of the cumulative incidence rates: −39 and −49 percentage points were used to assess the degree of distinctions in risks of the primary outcome between treatment groups. They are rate differences. The rate difference −39 percentage points unveiled that the cumulative incidence rate of the eardrops group is 39 percentage points lower than that of the oral antibiotics group. The rate difference −49 unveils that the cumulative incidence rate of the eardrops group is 49 percentage points lower than that of the observation group.

Distinctions in the risk of treatment failure were also measured by two numbers, 3 and 2, which were referred to as the "*number needed to treat.*" The number 3 is the result of rounding 100/(5% – 44%) = 2.56 to its nearest positive integer. It suggests that three subjects are needed in the eardrop group instead of the oral antibiotic group to prevent one more treatment failure. The number 2 is the result of 100/(5% –55%) = 2. The percentages are the results of intention-to-treat analysis; their computations used data from subjects with protocol violations. They are not indisputable assessments of the effects of the treatments but more credible assessments of the effects of being assigned to the treatment groups. The numbers 3 and 2 are the numbers need to assign. The number 3 suggests that three subjects are needed in the eardrops group instead of the oral antibiotic group to prevent one more treatment failure. The number 2 suggests that two subjects are needed in the eardrops group instead of the observation group to prevent one more treatment failure.

Distinctions in risks may also be assessed by rate ratios. The ratio 5%/44% = 0.11 indicates that the risk of treatment failure among the subjects of the eardrops group was decidedly lower than and just slightly over 1-tenth of the risk of the subjects in the oral antibiotics group. The ratio 5%/55% = 0.09 indicates that the risk of treatment failure of the eardrops group was decidedly lower than and less than 1-tenth of the risk of the observation group.

Example 6.4.1.2

DeBaun and Others (2014) (Example 6.3.1.1) uses person-time incidence rates to assess risks of infarct recurrence (2.0 and 4.8 per 100 person-years) in the transfusion and observation groups. It uses a ratio of person-time incidence rates of 0.41 to assess the distinction in risks between the two treatment groups. It is a rate ratio and suggests that the risk in the transfusion group is lower than and approximately 4.1-tenth of the risk in the observation group.

The article also states the following:

> The prevalence of the primary end point was 6% (6 of 99 participants) in the transfusion group and 14% (14 of 97 participants) in the observation group (Table 2).

and

> The absolute risk reduction was 8 percentage points, the relative risk reduction was 58%, and the number needed to treat was 13.

The absolute risk reduction (8 percentage points) is a rate difference (6–14% = −8%). The risk of the primary end point of the transfusion group is 8 percentage points lower than the risk of the observation group. The relative risk reduction (58%) is the rate difference relative to the rate of the observation group ([14–6%]/14% = 57%). The distinction in the risks of the primary end point between the treatment groups is approximately 58% of the risk in the observation group.

The number 13 is the result of rounding 100/(6–14%) = 12.5 to its nearest integer. The percentages 6% and 14% are the results of intention-to-treat analysis; they are not indisputable assessments of effects of the treatments (Example 6.3.1.1). The number 13 is the number of subjects needed to assign to the transfusion group instead of the observation group to prevent one incidence of the primary end point.

Ratios of the person-year incidence rates and average incidence rates (2.0/4.8 = 0.41 and 6%/14% = 0.43) are close. They submit a similar degree of difference in risks between the two treatment groups.

Example 6.4.1.3

Kadish and Others (2004) used Kaplan–Meier estimates of probability to assess risks of death from any cause in 1 and 2 years of follow-up (Example 6.3.2.2). The degree of distinction in the risks of death between treatment groups may be measured by rate difference or rate ratio. The Kaplan–Meier estimates are relatively small; their difference and ratio yield conflicting intimations.

The difference of the 1-year estimates 2.6–6.2% = −3.6%, and the ratio of the 1-year estimates 2.6%/6.2% = 0.42. The rate difference (−3.6%) indicates that the risk of death from any cause in 1 year in the ICD group was merely 3.6 percentage points lower than that in the standard therapy group; the rate ratio of 0.42 indicates that the risk of death from any cause in 1 year in the ICD group was much lower and less than half (4.2-tenth) of the risk in the standard therapy group.

The difference of the 2-year estimates 7.9 – 14.1% = −6.2% and the ratio of the 2-year estimates 7.9%/14.1% = 0.56.

The rate difference (−6.2%) submits that the risk of death from any cause in 2 years in the ICD group was just 6.2 percentage points lower than that in the standard therapy group; the rate ratio 0.56 submits that the risk of death from any cause in 2 years in the ICD group was much lower and close to half (5.6-tenth) of the risk in the standard therapy group.

Example 6.4.1.4

An article by van Gelder and Others (2002) presented the results of a study that compared the effects of rate control with rhythm control for the treatment of persistent atrial fibrillation. The study randomly assigned 522 subjects who had persistent atrial fibrillation after a previous electrical cardioversion to a rate–control group or a rhythm–control group. Subjects in the rate–control group received rate-slowing medication and oral anticoagulant drugs; those in the rhythm–control group underwent serial cardioversions and received antiarrhythmic and oral anticoagulant drugs. The two treatment groups and their data sets are unpaired.

The primary end point was the composite of death from cardiovascular causes, heart failure, thromboembolic complications, bleeding, implantation of a pacemaker, or severe adverse effects of antiarrhythmic drugs. The incidence of the primary end point was described as follows on one occasion:

> The primary end point occurred in 44 of the 256 patients in the rate-control group (17.2 percent) and in 60 of the 266 patients in the rhythm-control group (22.6 percent) (Table 2). The absolute difference of – 5.4 percent represents a trend in favor of rate control.

The percentages 17.2% and 22.6% are the average incidence rates and measures of risks of the primary end point during the course of follow-up. The absolute difference −5.4% is a rate difference (17.2–22.6% = −5.4%). It unveils that the risk of the primary end point of the rate–control group was 5.4 percentage points lower than the risk of the rhythm–control group.

The ratio of the average incidence rates: 17.2%/22.6% = 0.76 indicates that the risk of the primary end point in the rate–control group was 7.6-tenth of the risk in the rhythm–control group.

The article stated: *The incidence of the primary end point was calculated for all participants, irrespective of whether they actually received the assigned treatment (on the intention-to-treat principle).* The average incidence rates are not indisputable assessments of the effects of rate control and rhythm control but more credible assessments of the effects of being assigned to receive the treatments. The absolute difference of −5.4% and the rate ratio of 0.76 are credible assessments of the distinction in the effects of being assigned to treatment groups.

The intimations of the rate difference (−5.4%) and the rate ratio 0.76 differ noticeably. The rate difference seems small and suggests that the risk of the primary end point in the rate–control group is just 5.4 percentage points lower than the risk in the rhythm–control group. The rate ratio 0.76 suggests that the risk of the primary end point in the rate–control group is approximately 7.6-tenth of the risk in the rhythm–control group.

6.4.2 Hazard Ratio

Hazard ratio is a popular assessment of distinction in risks between treatment groups. It is a result of the Cox proportional hazards regression analysis that uses the Cox proportional hazards model to presume how time to event relates to treatment groups.

The Cox proportional hazards model is quite robust. Hazard ratios are usually close to ratios of measures of risks such as incidence rates and Kaplan–Meier estimates.

A limitation of Cox proportional hazards regression analysis is that it yields only hazard ratios as assessments of distinctions in risks between treatment groups but not assessments of risks in the treatment groups. The cox proportional model is technical and computation of hazard ratio is complicated and requires a computer.

Example 6.4.2.1

Combes and Others (2018) (Example 6.1.1) used cumulative incidence rates of 35% and 46% as assessments of risks of death in 60 days in the ECMO and the control groups. The distinction in the risks between the two treatment groups was measured by a relative risk 0.76. It is a ratio of the two cumulative incidence rates (35%/46% = 0.76) and suggests that the risk of death within 60 days in the ECMO group was lower than and approximately 7.6-tenth of the risk in the control group.

A hazard ratio 0.70 was also cited. Its suggestion was not commented on. It is a result of a regression analysis that used the Cox proportional hazards model to presume how time to death relates to treatment groups. Its computation used the follow-up times of the two groups of subjects.

The hazard ratio: 0.70 is relatively close to the ratio of the cumulative incidence rates (0.76). It suggests that the risk of death in 60 days among the 124 subjects of the ECMO group was approximately 7.0-tenth of the risk among the 125 subjects of the control group.

Example 6.4.2.2

The STABILITY Investigators (2014) (Example 6.1.2) used average incidence rates (9.7% and 10.4%) to assess the risk of the primary end point of the study. The rates suggest that the risks of the primary end point of both treatment groups were not high. Their ratio 9.7%/10.4% = 0.93 suggests that the risk in the darapladib group was slightly lower than and approximately 9.3-tenth of the risk of the control group.

A hazard ratio 0.94 was presented in parenthesis. Its suggestion was not noted. It is a result of a regression analysis that used the Cox proportional hazards model to presume how time to event relates to treatment groups. Its computation used the follow-up times of the two groups of subjects.

The hazard ratio: 0.94 is close to the ratio of average incidence rates (0.93) and suggests that the risk of the primary end point among the 7924 subjects of the darapladib group was slightly lower than the risk among the 7904 subjects of the control group.

Example 6.4.2.3

Gaudino and Others (2018) (Example 6.1.4) cited: "25 vs. *39 events per 1000-patient-years; hazard ratio, 0.67; 95% confidence interval [CI], 0.49 to 0.90; P = 0.01*" in parenthesis to corroborate the assertion that the incidence of the composite outcome was significantly lower in the radial artery group than in the saphenous vein group. The numbers are person-year incidence rates and assessments of risks of the composite outcome in the two treatment groups during follow-up. Their ratio 25/39 = 0.64 is a rate ratio and a measure of the distinction in risks between the two treatment groups. It suggests that if 100 subjects were followed for 10 years, the number of events in the radial artery group will be smaller than and approximately 6.4-tenth of the number in the saphenous vein group.

The hazard ratio 0.67 is a result of a regression analysis that used the cox proportional hazards model to presume how time to the occurrence of the composite outcome relates to treatment groups. Computation of the hazard ratio 0.67 use follow-up times of the two groups of subjects.

The hazard ratio: 0.67 is relatively close to the ratio of the person-year incidence rates (0.64). It suggests that the risk of the composite outcome among the 534 subjects in the radial artery group was 6.7-tenth of the risk among the 502 subjects in the saphenous vein group.

Table 3 shows that the average incidence rates of the primary outcome were 12.5% in the radial artery group and 18.7% in the saphenous vein group. Their ratio 12.5%/18.7% = 0.67 is a rate ratio. It suggests that the risk of the primary outcome during the course of follow-up in the radial artery group was approximately 6.7-tenths of the probability in the SV group.

The hazard ratio 0.67 is close to the ratio of person-year incidence rates (0.64) and equals the ratio of the average incidence rates.

The 95% confidence interval of the hazard ratio [0.49 to 0.90] excludes the null value of a ratio 1.0, and $P = 0.01$ is smaller than 0.05. They suggest that the hazard ratio may be declared statistically significant. The boundaries of the 95% confidence interval are 73% and 134% of the hazard ratio 0.67. They suggest that if the replicated a score of times, there would be hazard ratios as small as 73% and as large as 134% of the reported hazard ratio. The hazard ratio 0.67, although it may be declared statistically significant, is not adequately reproducible. It is astute to limit it to the subjects of the study and use it only as a preliminary signal.

Example 6.4.2.4

Recurrence-free survival was the primary outcome of the study reported by van Driel and Others (Example 6.3.2.1). The article reported:

> In the intention-to-treat analysis, 110 of the 123 patients (89%) in the surgery group and 99 of the 122 patients (81%) in the surgery-plus-HIPEC group had disease recurrence or death (hazard ratio, 0.66; 95% confidence interval [CI], 0.50 to 0.87; stratified P = 0.003) (Fig. 2A).

The percentages 81% and 89% are average incidence rates and assessments of the risk of having the event of disease recurrence or death during follow-up. They suggest that the risks of the primary outcome are high in both treatment groups. Their ratio 81%/89% = 0.91 suggests that the risk of the surgery plus HIPEC group was slightly lower than and approximately 9.1-tenth of the risk in the surgery only group.

The hazard ratio 0.66 is a result of the Cox proportional hazard regression analysis that used the Cox proportional hazard model to presume how time to event relates to treatment groups. It is presented here as an insinuation that the risk of the primary outcome during follow-up in the surgery plus HIPEC group was noticeably lower than and only 6.6-tenth of the risk in the surgery-only group.

The confidence interval of the hazard ratio excluded 1.0, and $P = 0.003$ meet the customary requirement of ≤ 0.05. They suggest that the hazard ratio may be declared statistically significant; the concern that the ratio might be coincidental may be dismissed.

The boundaries of the 95% confidence interval of the hazard ratio [0.50 to 0.87] conjecture that if the study replicated a score of times, the hazard ratios of close to 95% of the replicates would vary between 76% and 132% of the reported hazard ratio. Although the hazard ratio 0.66 may be declared statistically significant, its reproducibility is rather inadequate. It is astute to limit it to the subjects of the study and consider it a preliminary signal.

In this case, the ratio of the average incidence rates and the hazard ratio (0.91 vs. 0.66) differ considerably. This discrepancy is unusual but occurred throughout the article. The computations of the average incidence rates and their ratio are simple, and their indications are clear. The hazard ratios, on the other hand, were computed by an elaborate procedure and used the Cox proportional hazard model to presume how time to the event of disease recurrence or death relate to treatment groups. It is possible that the proportional hazard condition of the model is not realistic.

The average incidence rates and hazard ratios are the results of the intention-to-treat analysis. Their computations used data from 4 of the 122 subjects assigned to the surgery plus HIPEC group who did not receive the assigned treatment and 1 of the 123 subjects assigned to the surgery-alone group who did not receive the assigned treatment. They are not indisputable assessments of treatment effects but more credible assessments of effects of being in the treatment groups.

6.4.3 Odds Ratio

The distinction between two unpaired qualitative data sets is sometimes measured by the ratio of the odds of YES in the data sets. The odds of YES in a dichotomous data set is the quotient of percentages of YES and NO observations. When one category of a qualitative data set is designated the YES category, the odds of YES equals:

$$\text{Odds of YES} = \frac{\text{Percent of YES}}{\text{Percent of NO}} = \frac{\text{Number of YES}}{\text{Number of NO}} \tag{6.4.3.1}$$

The odds ratio is often written as OR. When two unpaired qualitative data sets are designated data set 1 and data set 2, the odds ratio equals:

$$\text{OR} = \frac{\text{Odds of YES in Data Set 1}}{\text{Odds of YES in Data Set 2}} \tag{6.4.3.2}$$

It is the odds ratio for unpaired qualitative data sets and an assessment of the distinction in odds of YES between the two sets.

- *Odds Ratio and Rate Ratio*

One property of the odds ratio is that it differs from its corresponding rate ratio negligibly if the percentage of YES is small. The discrepancy becomes noticeable when the percentage is 10% or larger and is further amplified when the percentage is larger. This is demonstrated by Table 6.4.

- *Exposure Odds Ratio of Case–Control Study*

The odds ratio is particularly useful when data are the results of case–control studies. A case–control study enrolls patients with a disease as its cases and individuals free of the disease as its controls. Exposures to one or more risk factors for the disease are ascertained. Its purpose is to gain some insight into the association of the risk of the disease with exposure to risk factors. However, case–control studies yield only assessments of the prevalence of exposure to risk factors among diseased cases and disease-free controls. They do not yield assessments of the risk of disease.

Data from case–control studies yield percentages of cases and controls who were exposed to risk factors. The denominators of the percentages are the numbers of cases and controls that are determined by study design. The numerators of the percentages are the numbers of cases and controls who were exposed to risk factors. They are manifestations of the association of the risk of the disease with risk factors. The percentages are assessments of the prevalence of exposure to the risk factors among the cases and controls. They are not assessments of risks of disease.

When data are obtained from a case–control study, the percentages of cases and controls who were exposed to a risk factor are called exposure odds and are computed as:

$$\text{Exposure odds among Cases} = \frac{\text{Percent of Exposed Cases}}{\text{Percent of Unexposed Cases}} = \frac{\text{Number of Exposed Case}}{\text{Number of Unexposed Case}},$$

and

$$\text{Exposure odds among Controls} = \frac{\text{Percent of Exposed Controls}}{\text{Percent of Unexposed Controls}} = \frac{\text{Number of Exposed Controls}}{\text{Number of Unexposed Controls}} \tag{6.4.3.3}$$

The ratio of the exposure odds among cases relative to the exposure odds among controls is called an exposure odds ratio. It is computed as:

Table 6.4 Ratio of odds and ratio of percentages (set 1 relative to set 2)

	Percentages of YES											
Data set 1	2%	4%	6%	8%	10%	20%	40%	1%	3%	5%	10%	20%
Data set 2	1%	2%	3%	4%	5%	10%	20%	2%	6%	10%	20%	40%
Rate ratio	2.000	2.000	2.000	2.000	2.000	2.000	2.000	0.500	0.500	0.500	0.500	0.500
Odds ratio	2.020	2.042	2.064	2.087	2.111	2.250	2.667	0.495	0.485	0.474	0.444	0.375

$$\text{Exposure odds ratio} = \frac{\text{Exposure Odds among Cases}}{\text{Exposure Odds among Controls}} \tag{6.4.3.4}$$

The exposure odds ratio is used as an auxiliary estimate of the risk ratio of interest, the ratio of a measure of risk of the disease among exposed subjects relative to that among unexposed subjects. This use of the exposure odds ratio is supported by the notion that the exposure odds ratio would be close to the risk ratio of interest, the ratio of the percentage of cases of the disease among individuals who were exposed to the risk factor trait relative to that among those who were not exposed to the risk factor, if the disease was rare. It is also sanctioned by the contention that the exposure odds ratio is an operative estimate of the risk ratio of interest as long as the study is meticulously designed and executed so that enrollments of the cases and the controls were not related to their exposure histories.

Example 6.4.3.1

To investigate whether α_{2C}Del322-325 and β_1-Arg389 receptor variants would predispose individuals to risk of heart failure, Small and Others (2002) enrolled 159 cases of heart failure and 189 controls (individuals who were apparently healthy did not have a history or symptoms of cardiovascular diseases and had not been taking any medication for extended periods). The cases and controls were compared with respect to genotype assessments of α_{2C}Del322-325 and β_1-Arg389 receptor variants. Data of black and white subjects were analyzed separately. The following is a description of the data of black subjects:

> Indeed, 52.6 percent of the black patients with heart failure were homozygous for the α_{2C} polymorphism compared with only 16.6 percent of the black controls. The unadjusted odds ratio for heart failure among participants who were homozygous for α_{2C}Del322-325 compared with participants who were not was 5.54 (95 percent confidence interval, 2.68 to 11.45: $P<0.001$).

The cases and controls were identified separately. The group of black cases and the group of black controls are unpaired. Whether a subject is homozygous for α_{2C}Del322-325 is a dichotomous observation. The percentages: 52.6% and 16.6% are descriptions of two unpaired dichotomous data sets.

The denominators of the percentages: 78 and 84 are the number of black cases and black controls. They were determined by study design. It is judicious to consider them mathematical constants and assessments of prevalence of homozygosity for α_{2C}Del322-325. The odds ratio 5.54 is the ratio of the odds of homozygosity for α_{2C}Del322-325 among the black cases (52.6%/47.4%) and the odds among the black controls (16.6%/83.4%). The odds are functions of the prevalence rates; their ratio 5.54 suggests that the odds of homozygosity for α_{2C}Del322-325 among the 78 black cases was 5.54 times the odds among the 84 black controls. It is not an assessment of distinction in risks of heart failure.

The odds ratio 5.54 is an exposure odds ratio. It is used as an auxiliary estimate of the risk ratio—ratio of an assessment of the risk of heart failure among black individuals who are homozygous for α_{2C}Del322-325 relative to that among the black individuals who are not and an insinuation that the risk of heart failure among black individuals who are homozygous for α_{2C}Del322-325 is about 5.54 times that among black individuals who are not.

The 95% confidence interval of the odds ratio: [*2.68 to 11.45*] excludes 1.0 and P<0.001 is smaller than 0.05. They suggest that the odds ratio may be declared statistically significant, and the concern that it is incidental may be dismissed. However, the confidence interval is wide. Its boundaries suggest that if the study replicated a score times, there would be odds ratios as small as 48% and as large as 207% of the reported odds ratio. The reproducibility of the odds ratio 5.54 is inadequate. Although it could be declared statistically significant, it is astute to limit it to the subjects of the study and consider it a preliminary clue only.

Example 6.4.3.2

This example uses a fake modification of the study of Small and Others (2002) to demonstrate that fractions of diseased cases of case–control studies are not valid assessments of risk of the disease among subjects who were and were not exposed to risk factors. They, to a considerable extent, are the results of the numbers of cases and controls of the study.

Table 6.5 is a two-way contingency table that displays the percentages and numbers of black cases and controls of Small and Others (2002) who are homozygous for α_{2C}Del322-355. The numbers of subjects who were and were not homozygous for α_{2C}Del322-355 were 41 + 14 = 55 and 37 = 70 = 107, respectively. The fractions of heart failure cases are 41/55 = 0.75 among the 55 subjects who are homozygous for α_{2C}Del322-355 and 37/107 = 0.35 among the 107 subjects who are not. Their ratio is 0.75/0.35 = 2.17.

The denominators of the fractions of heart failure cases are the results of the association of heart failure with homozygosity for α_{2C}Del322-355, and the numerators of the fractions are part of the study design. The fractions, to a considerable extent, are affected by the numbers of cases and controls included in the study. They are not valid assessments of risks of heart failure.

Table 6.6 displays the data of the fake modification of the study of Small and Others (2002). The study enrolled the same number of black cases of heart failure but ten times the number of black controls (840). The percentages of cases and controls who are and are not homozygous for α_{2C}Del322-325 (52.6% and 47.4%,

Table 6.5 Percentages and numbers of black cases and controls homozygous for α_{2C}Del322-325

	Homozygous for α_{2C}Del322-325		
	YES	NO	SUM
Cases	52.6% (41)	47.4% (37)	100% (78)
Controls	16.7% (14)	83.3% (70)	100% (84)

Table 6.6 Data of a fictitious modification of the study reported by Small and Others (2002)

	Homozygous for α_{2C}Del322-325		
	YES	NO	SUM
Black cases	52.6% (41)	47.4% (37)	100% (78)
Black controls	16.6% (140)	83.3% (700)	99% (840)

respectively) are identical to those of the data of Small and Others (2002). The exposure odds ratio is also the same *(5.54)*. The faked study shows the same manifestation of the association of the risk of heart failure and homozygosity for α_{2C}Del322-325 as the study of Small and Others (2002) but unmistakably distinct fractions of heart failure cases among subjects who are and are not homozygous for α_{2C}Del322-325.

Data from the faked study show that a total of 181 subjects are homozygous for α_{2C}Del322-355, and a total of 737 are not. The fraction of heart failure cases is $41/181 = 0.23$ among the 181 subjects who are homozygous for α_{2C}Del322-325 and $37/737 = 0.05$ among the 737 who are not. Their ratio $0.23/0.05 = 4.60$. The fractions of heart failure cases among the subjects who are and are not homozygous for α_{2C}Del322-325 (0.23 and 0.05) and their ratio 4.60 differ distinctly from those of the data of Small and Others (2002) (0.75 and 0.35, respectively, and 2.14), although the association between risk of heart failure and homozygosity for α_{2C}Del322-355 demonstrated by the data of the two studies are identical. One reason for the discrepancy between the fractions of heart failure cases of the two studies is that the number controls of the study reported by Small and Others (2002) is close to the number of cases (78 and 84), but the number of controls of the fake study is more than ten times the number of cases (840 vs. 78).

Example 6.4.3.3

Weaver (347, 14): Odds ratio of clinical trial

The results of a study evaluating the effect of hyperbaric oxygen therapy on the risk of cognitive sequelae in subjects with symptomatic carbon monoxide poisoning were reported by Weaver and Others (2002). The study randomly assigned 152 eligible subjects to receive either hyperbaric oxygen therapy or normobaric oxygen therapy. Randomization was performed by using a randomized block design. The two treatment groups and their data sets are unpaired although matched.

The following is a description of the primary end point—incidence of cognitive sequelae six weeks after randomization to treatment groups:

> By the time the results of interim analysis became available, 152 patients had been enrolled. For all 152 patients in the intention-to-treat population, cognitive sequelae at six weeks were less frequent in the hyperbaric-oxygen group (25.0 percent) than in the normobaric-oxygen group (46.1 percent; unadjusted odds ratio, 0.39 [95 percent confidence interval, 0.20 to 0.78]; P=0.007) (Table 2).

The percentages 25.0% and 46.1% are percentages of subjects having cognitive sequelae at six weeks in the two treatment groups. Their denominators are numbers of subjects assigned to treatment groups that are part of study design. It is rational to consider them mathematical constants. The percentages are cumulative incidence rates and assessments of the risks of cognitive sequelae at six weeks. Their ratio $25.0/46.1\% = 0.54$ submits that the risk of cognitive sequelae at six weeks of the hyperbaric oxygen group was lower than and 5.4-tenth of the risk of the normobaric oxygen group.

The unadjusted odds ratio 0.39 suggests that the odds of having cognitive sequelae at six weeks in the hyperbaric oxygen group: (25.0 % /(100.0 % −

25.0%) is lower than and approximately 3.9-tenth of the odds in the normobaric oxygen group: 44.1%/(100% −46.1%).

The 95% confidence interval of the odds ratio: [0.20 to 0.78] excludes the null value (1.0), and $P = 0.007$ is smaller than 0.05. They suggested that the odds ratio could be declared statistically significant. It is all right to dismiss the concern that the odds ratio is coincidental.

The boundaries of the 95% confidence interval [0.20 to 0.78] are 51% and 200% of the reported odds ratio and suggest that the reproducibility of the odds ratio 0.39 is inadequate. Although the odds ratio could be declared statistically significant, it is astute to limit it to the subjects of the study and use it as a preliminary clue only.

The study is a randomized trial. The percentages: 25.0% and 46.1% are cumulative incidence rates and established assessments of likelihoods. Their ratio 0.54 is an established assessment of distinction in likelihoods. The odds are not established assessments of likelihood; the odds ratio is not an established assessment of distinction in likelihoods. The odds ratio (0.39) differs from the ratio of cumulative incidence rates (0.54) considerably. It is astute to use the odds ratio with care.

6.5 Progression of Likelihood

Average and person-time incidence rates are assessments of likelihoods of events during follow-up. Cumulative incidence rates and Kaplan–Meier estimates are assessments of likelihoods in periods of fixed length. They do not unveil how likelihood progressed when the length of follow-up increased. Their difference and ratio do not unveil how distinction in likelihoods progressed during the course follow-up. Similarly, hazard ratios are assessments of distinction in risk of events during follow-up or in periods of given length. They do not unveil how distinction in risks progressed during the course of follow-up. One way to show how likelihoods and distinction in likelihoods progressed during the course of follow-up is to show how cumulative incidence rates or Kaplan–Meier estimates of probability progressed in periods of increasing length. The estimates and rates may be displayed by a graph or a table.

Example 6.5.1

Combes and Others (2018) (Example 6.1.1) used cumulative incidence rates of 35% and 46% to depict the risks of death in 60 days in the ECMO group and the control group. The cumulative incidence rates are assessments of risk of death in 60 days; they did not unveil how the risks progressed when length of follow-up increased.

Figure 2 of Combes and Others (2018) (Fig. 6.1) was cited in parenthesis as part of the narrative that cited the cumulative incidence rates of death at 60 days. It yielded much valuable information even though its indications were not noted.

The figure exhibits Kaplan–Meier estimates of the probability of survival in periods of increasing length. The heights of points on the curves signify the values of the estimates of probability of death. Labels marked along a vertical line specify a scale that gauges values of estimates signified by heights of points on the curves. The lengths of the periods are marked along a horizontal line in increments of 10 days. The two lines are the vertical and horizontal axes of the figure.

The red curve suggested that the risk of death in the ECMO group increased gradually to approximately 0.35 at 60 days of follow-up. The blue curve suggests that the risk of death in the control group increased gradually at a quicker rate when follow-up lengthened to 20 days and then at a slower rate to approximately 0.46 at 60 days of follow-up.

The two curves showed that the risk of death was consistently lower in the ECMO group than in the control group. The distinction became more notable when follow-up was longer than 10 days.

Example 6.5.2

The article by van Driel and Others (2018) (Example 6.3.2.1) used Kaplan–Meier estimates of probability to assess likelihoods of recurrence-free survival at 3 years in the surgery group and the surgery plus HIPEC group (8% and 17%). Figure 2 (Fig. 6.3) uses Kaplan–Meier curves to show how the likelihood of recurrence-free survival fell in periods of increasing length. The heights of points on the curves signify the values of the estimates of the probability of recurrence-free survival. Labels marked along a vertical line specify a scale that can be used to gauge values of estimates signified by heights of points on the curves. The lengths of the periods are marked along a horizontal line in increments of 10 years. The two lines are the vertical and horizontal axes of the figure.

The red curve suggests that the probability of recurrence-free survival of the surgery plus HIPEC group declined quickly to approximately 0.17 when follow-up was three years and then slowly to approximately 0.10 when follow-up was 5 years. The blue curve suggests that the probability of recurrence-free survival of the surgery-only group declined at a quicker rate to approximately 0.08 when follow-up was three years and then slowly to approximately 0.05 when follow-up was 5 years.

The probability of recurrence-free survival in the surgery plus HIPEC group was consistently higher than that in the surgery-only group; the distinction was more notable between one and three and half years of follow-up.

Example 6.5.3

Gaudino and Others (2018) (Example 6.1.4) used person-time incidence rates to assess risks of the composite primary outcome of the radial artery and saphenous vein groups (25 and 39 events per 1000 patient-years). The rates are synoptic assessments of risks during follow-up; they do not unveil how the risks progressed during follow-up.

Figure 1A (Fig. 6.4) displays graphically the cumulative incidence rates of the composite primary outcome of the two treatment groups in periods of increasing length. The blue curve suggests that the rate of the composite primary outcome of the saphenous vein group increased steadily to close to 25% at 9 years of follow-up. The red curve suggests that the risk of the composite primary outcome of the radial artery group was slightly lower than the risk of the saphenous vein group in short and extended periods of follow-up. It reached 20% after approximately 9 years of follow-

Fig. 6.3 Figure 2 of van Driel and Others (2018)

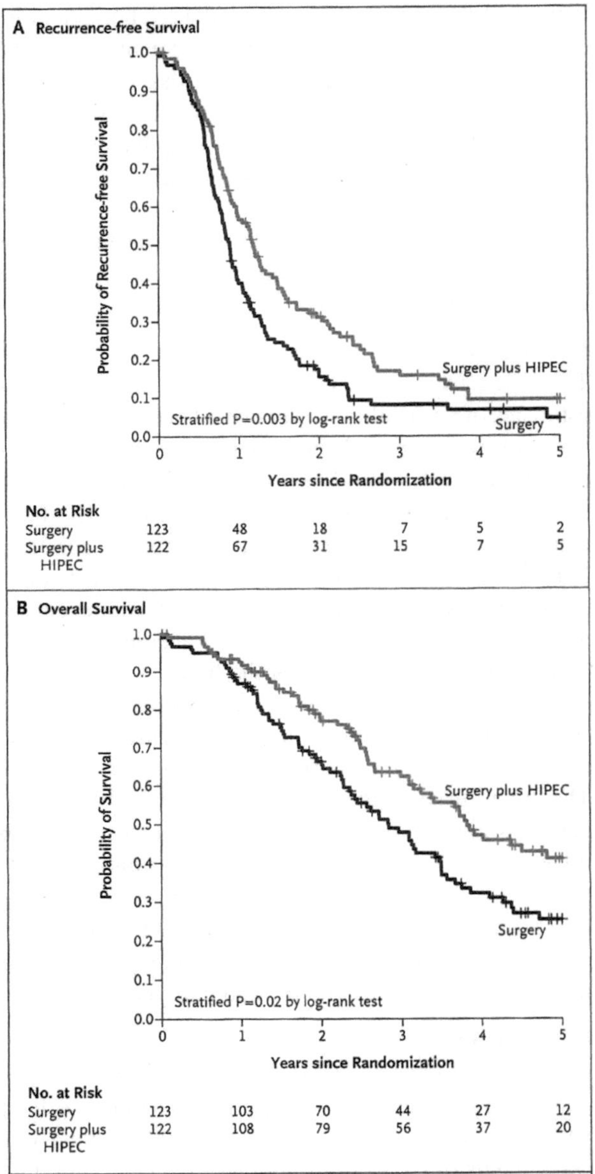

Figure 2. Kaplan–Meier Estimates of Recurrence-free Survival and Overall Survival.
Panel A shows Kaplan–Meier estimates of recurrence-free survival among patients in the intention-to-treat population. Events of disease recurrence or death were observed in 110 patients (89%) in the surgery group and in 99 patients (81%) in the surgery-plus-HIPEC group. Panel B shows Kaplan–Meier estimates of overall survival among patients in the intention-to-treat population. A total of 76 patients (62%) in the surgery group and 61 (50%) patients in the surgery-plus-HIPEC group died.

Fig. 6.4 Figure 1 of Gaudino and Others (2018)

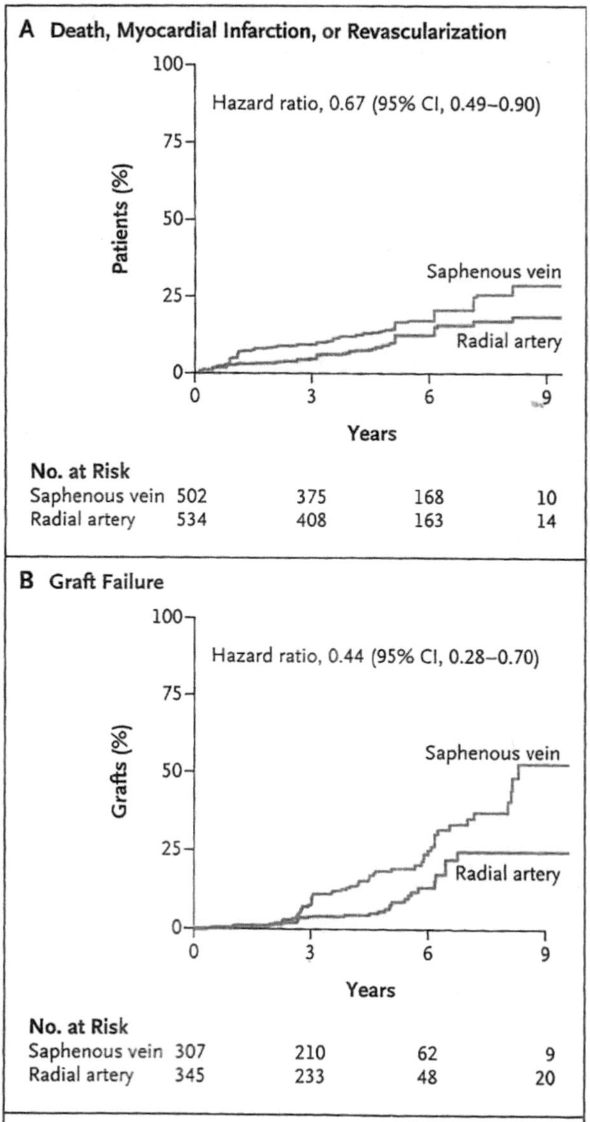

Figure 1. Cumulative Incidence of the Primary Composite Outcome of Death, Myocardial Infarction, or Repeat Revascularization and of Graft Failure in the Intention-to-Treat Analysis.

up. The risk of death, myocardial infarction, or revascularization was consistently lower in the radial artery group than in the saphenous vein group when the length of follow-up increased from 1–9 years.

6.6 Subgroup Analysis

Incidence rates (average, cumulative, or person-time) and Kaplan–Meier estimates of probability are useful assessments of likelihood of events. Ratios and differences of incidence rates and Kaplan–Meier estimate and hazard ratios are assessments of distinction in likelihood between treatment groups. They are determined from observations pertaining to the occurrence of events. Traits of subjects that might affect likelihoods and their distinctions are not involved. It is unknown how the likelihoods and their distinctions were affected by traits such as sex, age, and health conditions.

6.6.1 Subgroup Analysis

A productive way to evaluate how likelihoods of events in treatment groups and their distinctions are affected by a trait is to evaluate the likelihoods in subgroups of subjects specified by attributes of the trait. This is known as a subgroup analysis.

When there are two or more traits of interest, the effect of each trait is appraised by evaluating likelihoods in subgroups of subjects specified by attributes of each trait. The joint effect of traits may be appraised in two ways. One is to evaluate risks in subgroups of subjects specified by combinations of the attributes of the traits; another is to use attributes of the traits to determine an index and evaluate risks in subgroups specified by the index.

- *Subgroup and overall measures of likelihood*

The results of subgroup analyses are informatively depicted by measures of likelihoods and measures of distinctions in likelihoods computed by using data from subjects in subgroups. For clarity, these are dubbed subgroup measures. Measures computed by using data from all subjects are dubbed overall measures.

Overall measures and subgroup measures are closely related. Overall incidence rates (average and cumulative) are weighted average of the subgroup rates when numbers of subjects in subgroups are used as weights. Overall person-time incidence rates are weighted average of the subgroup rates when sums of follow-up times of subjects in subgroups are used as weights. Overall distinction measures are close to weighted averages of the subgroup distinction measures when numbers of subjects in subgroups are used as weights.

Example 6.6.1.1

One feature of van Gelder and Others (2002) (Example 6.4.1.4) is that it presented the results of a subgroup analysis. It stated:

> Table 3 shows the incidence of the primary end point according to sex and blood pressure status. Among women and patients with hypertension, the incidence of the primary end point was higher with rhythm control than with rate control.

Table 3 (Table 6.7) shows average incidence rates of the primary end point in subgroups of male and female subjects and subgroups of normotensive and hypertensive subjects. The table reveals the following with respect to the effect of blood pressure status:

- Risks of the primary end point in treatment groups
  1. The average incidence rate of the rate–control group in the subgroup of normotensive subjects was close to that in the subgroup of hypertensive subjects (17.1% and 17.3%).
  2. The average incidence rate of the rhythm–control group was markedly lower in the subgroup of normotensive subjects than in the subgroup of hypertensive subjects (12.5% vs. 30.8%).

- Distinction in risks of the primary end point between the treatment groups.
  1. In the subgroup of normotensive subjects, the average incidence rate of the rate–control group was 4.6 percentage points higher than that of the rhythm–control group (17.1% vs. 12.5%).
  2. In the subgroup of hypertensive subjects, in contrast, the average incidence rate of the rate–control group was 13.5 percentage points lower than that of the rhythm–control group (17.3% vs. 30.8%).

The disparities between the subgroups of normotensive and hypertensive subjects suggest that it is important to consider blood pressure status when risk of the primary end point of the two treatment groups and their distinction are evaluated.

Remark: It is of interest to note that the overall average incidence rates equal the weighted averages of the average incidence rates of the subgroup average incidence rates using numbers of normotensive and hypertensive subjects as weights. Indeed,

Rate control: $(146 \times 17.1\% + 110 \times 17.3\%)/(146 + 110) = (25 + 19)/(146 + 110) = 44/256 = 17.2\%$

Rhythm control: $(120 \times 12.5\% + 146 \times 30.8\%)/(169 + 97) = (15 + 45)/(126 + 146) = 60/266 = 22.6\%$

Table 6.7 Table 3 of van Gelder and Others (2002)

TABLE 3. INCIDENCE OF THE PRIMARY END POINT ACCORDING TO SEX AND BLOOD-PRESSURE STATUS.

GROUP	RATE CONTROL	RHYTHM CONTROL	ABSOLUTE DIFFERENCE (90% CI)*
	no./total no. (%)		
All patients	44/256 (17.2)	60/266 (22.6)	−5.4 (−11.0 to 0.4)
Men	34/161 (21.1)	29/169 (17.2)	3.9 (−3.2 to 11.1)
Women	10/95 (10.5)	31/97 (32.0)	−21.5 (−30.8 to −12.1)
Normotensive patients	25/146 (17.1)	15/120 (12.5)	4.6 (−2.5 to 11.8)
Hypertensive patients	19/110 (17.3)	45/146 (30.8)	−13.5 (−22.2 to −4.9)

*CI denotes confidence interval.

Example 6.6.1.2

One feature of the article by van Driel and Others (2018) (Example 6.3.2.1) is that it reported the results of subgroup analyses. It stated:

> Subgroup analyses of recurrence-free survival (Fig. 3) and overall survival (Fig. S2 in the Supplementary Appendix) showed that the effect of HIPEC was consistent across the prespecified stratification factors and post hoc subgroups.

To read intelligently, it is constructive to review Fig. 3 (Fig. 6.5) which displays hazard ratios assessing in subgroups specified by five variables. The hazard ratios of all subgroups were below 1.0 and suggested that the risk of disease recurrence or death in the surgery plus HIPEC group was lower than the risk in the surgery-only group across the subgroups specified by the five variables.

The hazard ratios of the subgroup of subjects who did and did not have previous surgery were 0.47 and 0.71, respectively. They suggest that the distinction in the risks between the two treatment groups was more substantial in the subgroup of subjects who had previous surgery than that in the subgroup of subjects who did not have previous surgery. Previous surgery is a crucial factor when the distinction in the risks of disease recurrence or death between the two treatment groups is evaluated.

The hazard ratios are relatively close between subgroups specified by the other factors. Little is lost if factors such as age, histologic type, number of involved regions, and laparoscopy before surgery are ignored when the distinction in the risks of the event of disease recurrence or death between the two treatment groups is evaluated.

The 99% confidence intervals of all hazard ratios included 1.0 and suggested that the hazard ratios could not be declared statistically significant; the concern that they were coincidental could not be dismissed. The intervals are wide and suggest that the reproducibility of the hazard ratios is low. It is astute to limit them to the subjects of the study and consider them preliminary indications only.

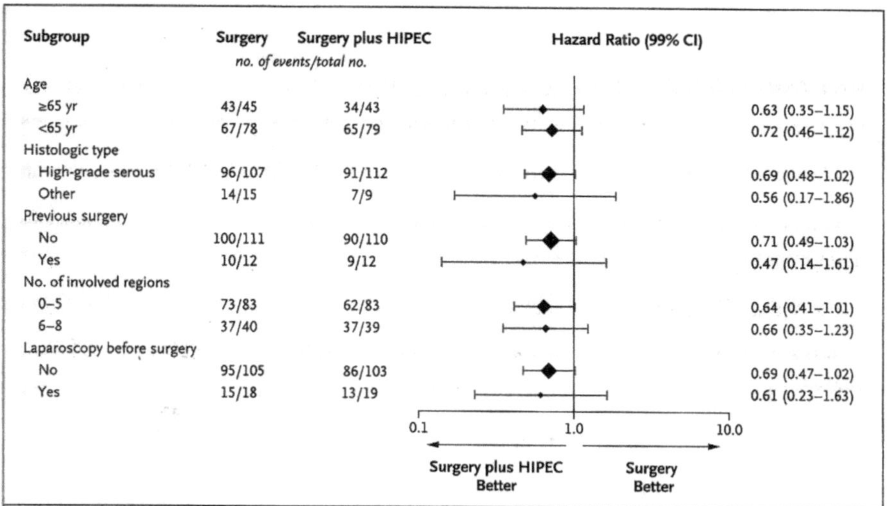

Figure 3. Prespecified Subgroup Analyses of Recurrence-free Survival.
Histologic data were missing (i.e., no tumor sample was available for review) for one patient in each group. Histologic type was determined on the basis of centrally reviewed pathological assessment. Previous surgery and the number of involved regions in the abdominal cavity were used as stratification factors at randomization. All the patients had received neoadjuvant chemotherapy. The size of each diamond is proportional to the amount of data available.

Fig. 6.5 Figure 3 of van Driel and Others (2018)

Example 6.6.1.3

Goldenberg and Others (2014) presented the results of a study that used data from the multicenter automatic defibrillator implantation trial with cardiac resynchronization therapy (MADIT-CRT) to evaluate the effects of cardiac resynchronization with defibrillator (CRT-D) and implantable cardioverter defibrillator (ICD) on long-term survival. One feature of the article is that it presented descriptions of risks of death from any cause of two levels of subgroup analysis. Assessments of risks in subgroups of subjects with and without left bundle branch block were described in separate sections. Each section presented descriptions of assessments of risks in subdivisions of the subgroup.

Subgroups of subjects with and without a left bundle branch block.

Table 2 of the article (Table 6.8) showed that the hazard ratios are 0.63 and 1.31 in the subgroups of subjects with and without left bundle branch block, respectively. The hazard ratio 0.63 suggests that the risk of death from any cause in the CRT-D group was lower than and approximately 6.3-tenth of the risk in the ICD-only group among the subgroup of subjects with left bundle branch block. The hazard ratio 1.31 suggests that the risk of death from any cause in the CRT-D group was not lower but higher than and approximately 1.31 times the risk in the ICD-only group among the subgroup of subjects without left bundle branch block. It is important to evaluate the

Table 6.8 Table 2 of Goldenberg and Others (2014)

Table **2.** Hazard Ratios for End Points with CRT-D versus ICD Alone, According to the Presence or Absence of Left Bundle Branch Block

End Point	No. of Events	No. of Patients	Left Bundle Branch Block		Non-Left Bundle Branch Block		
			Hazard Ratio (95% CI)	*P* Value	Hazard Ratio (95% CI)	*P* Value	*P* Value for Interaction[a]
Death from any cause							
Unadjusted analysis	292	1818	0.63 (0.47–0.84)	0.002	1.31 (0.87–1.96)	0.19	0.004
Adjusted analysis[b]	267	1681	0.59 (0.43–0.80)	<0.001	1.57 (1.03–2.39)	0.04	<0.001
Nonfatal heart-failure event							
Unadjusted analysis	442	1818	0.42 (0.33–0.52)	<0.001	1.10 (0.79–1.53)	0.59	<0.001
Adjusted analysis[b]	405	1681	0.38 (0.30–0.48)	<0.001	1.13 (0.80–1.60)	0.48	<0.001
Nonfatal heart-failure event or death							
Unadjusted analysis	577	1818	0.50 (0.41–0.61)	<0.001	1.21 (0.90–1.63)	0.21	<0.001
Adjusted analysis[b]	530	1681	0.45 (0.37–0.56)	<0.001	1.27 (0.94–1.73)	0.12	<0.001

[a]The P value for interaction represents the likelihood that the difference between the treatment effect on patients with left bundle branch block and the treatment effect on those without left bundle branch block occurred by chance alone

[b]Models were adjusted for the following covariates: age at enrollment, serum creatinine level of 1.4 mg per deciliter (120 μmol per liter) or more, smoking status at enrollment, presence or absence of diabetes mellitus, cause of cardiomyopathy (ischemic vs. nonischemic), left ventricular end-systolic volume at baseline indexed by body-surface area, QRS duration at baseline (≥150 msec vs. <150 msec), and NYHA class III or IV more than 3 months before enrollment (yes vs. no). Covariates were identified from a best-subset regression analysis

distinction in the risks of death from any cause between the two treatment groups among the subjects with and without left bundle branch block separately.

In the section **CRT-D IN PATIENTS WITH LEFT BUNDLE BRANCH BLOCK**, the article stated:

> Kaplan–Meier estimates of death from any cause during the period from enrollment through 7 years of follow-up in the two treatment groups are shown in Figure 1A. The curves diverge at 1 year and continue to have separate paths thereafter, with significantly lower mortality among patients randomly assigned to CRT-D therapy than among patients randomly assigned to ICD therapy alone (P = 0.002, by the log-rank test without adjustment). Thus, at 7 years of follow-up, the cumulative rate of death from any cause among patients with left bundle branch block was 29% in the ICD-only group, compared with 18% in the CRT-D group. The survival difference corresponded to nine patients who would need to be treated with CRT-D to save one life within 7 years.

In the section **CRT-D IN PATIENTS WITHOUT LEFT BUNDLE BRANCH BLOCK**, the article stated:

> Among patients without left bundle branch block, Kaplan–Meier survival analysis did not show a significant difference between the two treatment groups in the cumulative probability of death from any cause during the period from enrollment through 7 years of follow-up (P = 0.21 by the log-rank test without adjustment) (Fig. 2B).

Figure 2A (Fig. 6.6) shows that in the subgroup of subjects with left bundle branch block, the Kaplan–Meier estimate of the probability of death from any cause in the CRT-D group increased at a slower rate and was consistently lower in short and extended periods of follow-up than the estimate of the ICD-only group. Figure 2B shows that, in the subgroup of subjects without left bundle branch block, the Kaplan–Meier estimate of the probability of death from any cause in the CRT-D group, on the other hand, increased at a faster rate and was consistently higher than the estimate of the ICD-only group until the length of follow-up extended to 5 years. The estimates in the two treatment groups were close in periods of 6 years or longer.

The contrasting indications of the subgroups of subjects with and without left bundle branch block, suggests that it is important to consider the presence of left bundle branch block when the risk of death from any cause, is evaluated.

Subdivisions of the subgroup of subjects with left bundle branch block

Risks of death from any cause of the subgroup of subjects with left bundle branch block were further evaluated by using seven traits to divide subjects into subdivisions. The following is a description of the risks of death from any cause in the subdivisions specified by the seven traits:

> The effects of CRT-D therapy on mortality among patients with left bundle branch block in seven prespecified subgroups are shown in Figure 3. The survival benefit with CRT-D was consistent in each subgroup analyzed, including patients with ischemic cardiomyopathy and those with nonischemic cardiomyopathy, men and women, and patients with a longer QRS period (≥150 msec) and those with a shorter QRS period (<150 msec); there were no significant treatment-by-subgroup interactions.

Figure 3 (Fig. 6.6) shows that among subjects with left bundle branch block, hazard ratios were all under 1.0 in the subdivisions of subjects specified by each of seven traits. They suggest that among the of subjects with left bundle branch block, the risk of death from any cause in the CRT-D group was lower than that in the ICD group in subdivisions specified by each of the seven traits.

Hazard ratios of subdivisions specified by some traits were not close. Among the subjects with left bundle branch block, the hazard ratios of the male and female subdivisions were 0.69 and 0.48, respectively, and those of the subdivisions of subjects with smaller and larger left ventricular end-systolic volume (LVESV) ($\leq$ 170 ml and $>$ 170 ml) were 0.56 and 0.71, respectively. It is astute to pay some attention to these traits of the subjects when the distinction in the risks of death from any cause between the two treatment groups among subjects with left bundle branch block is evaluated.

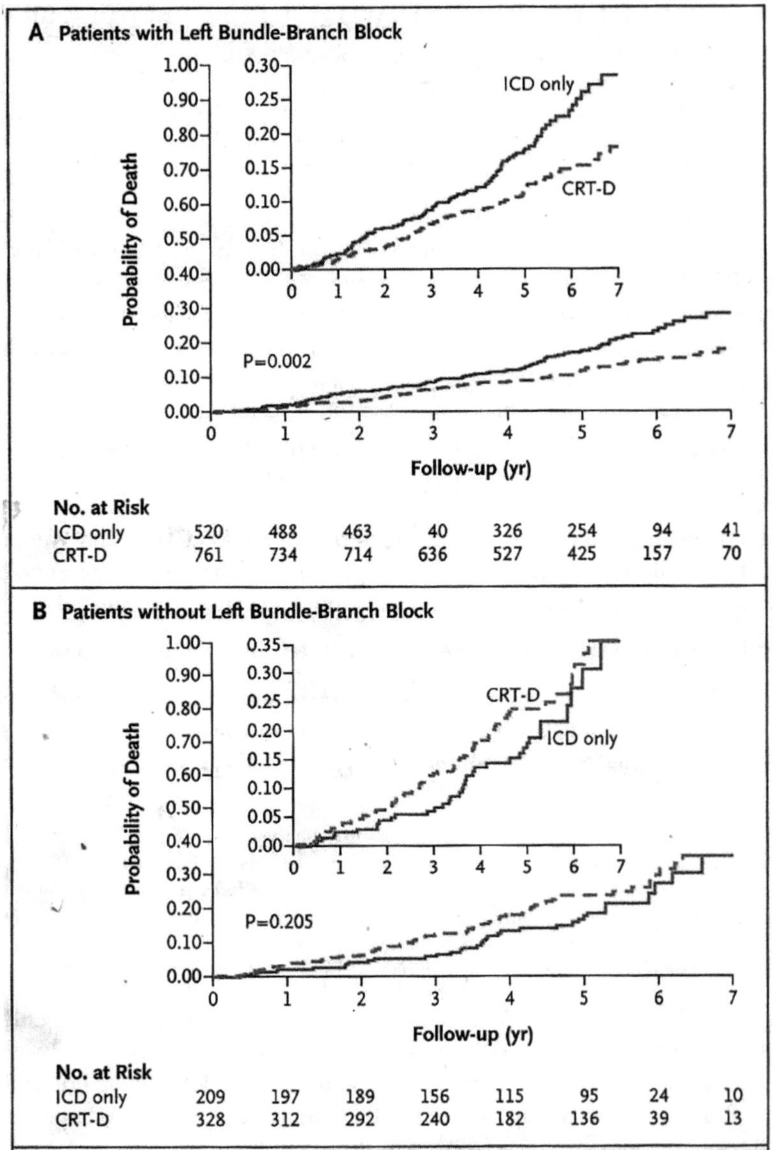

Figure 2. Kaplan–Meier Estimates of the Cumulative Probability of Death from Any Cause among Patients with and Those without Left Bundle-Branch Block.

CRT-D denotes cardiac-resynchronization therapy with defibrillator, and ICD implantable cardioverter–defibrillator. The insets show the same data on an enlarged y axis.

Fig. 6.6 Figure 2 of Goldenberg and Others (2014)

Subgroups of subjects with and without left bundle branch block

The following is a description of the risks of death in subdivisions of the subgroup of subjects without left bundle branch block:

> The lack of a survival benefit associated with CRT-D in patients without left bundle branch block was consistent among those with a longer QRS duration (≥ 150 msec) or a shorter QRS duration (< 150 msec) and among patients with QRS morphologic findings showing right bundle branch block or intraventricular conduction delay (Fig. S4 in the Supplementary Appendix).

As Fig. S4 of the Supplementary Appendix is not readily available, it is unknown how the CRT-D group was associated with a lack of survival benefit in subjects without left bundle branch block. Table 2 shows that the hazard ratio of the subgroup of subjects without left bundle branch block was 1.31 and suggested that the risk of death from any cause of the CRT-D group was higher than and approximately 1.31 times the risk of the ICD-only group among subjects without left bundle branch block. Probably, the hazard ratios of all subdivisions of the subgroup of subjects without left bundle branch block specified by each of the eight adjusting variables were higher than 1.0 or relatively close to the hazard ratio of the subjects without left bundle branch block (1.57).

Intention-to-treat

Goldenberg and Others (2014) stated: *All analyses in the present study were carried out on an intention-to-treat basis (i.e., according to the original treatment assignment, regardless of in-trial or posttrial crossovers). During long-term follow-up, 171 of the 1818 patients (9%) crossed over from ICD therapy alone to CRT-D therapy, and 92 (5%) crossed over from CRT-D to ICD therapy alone.* Assessments of the risks of death and other outcomes included data from subjects who crossed over from one therapy to the other. They are not indisputable assessments of the effects of treatments but more credible appraisals of the effects of being assigned to the treatment groups (Fig. 6.7).

6.6.2 Adjusted Measures of Likelihood and Distinction in Likelihoods

The measures of likelihood and distinction in likelihoods discussed in the previous sections are crude. Their computations used only observations pertaining to occurrence of event or follow-up time and number of subjects. Factors that might affect the likelihoods, such as sex, age, and physical conditions, are not involved. They are oversimplifications if likelihoods or distinction in likelihoods differ considerably between subgroups of subjects specified by some factors. They are referred to as crude measures for clarity sometimes. Generally, measures of likelihood such as incidence rates (cumulative, average, or person-time) and Kaplan–Meier estimate of probability and measures of distinction in likelihoods such as rate difference, rate ratio, and hazard ratio are crude unless otherwise indicated.

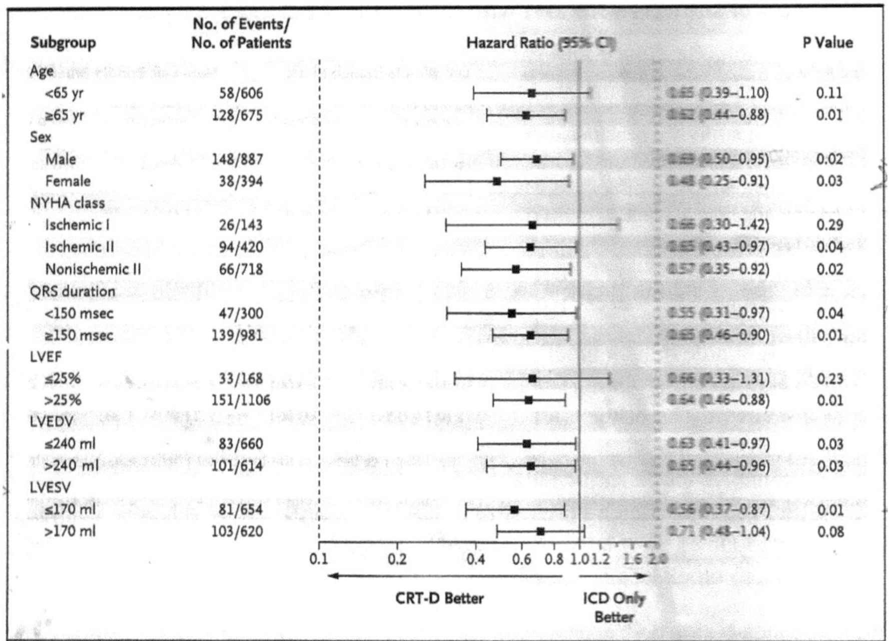

Figure 3. Risk of Death from Any Cause, According to Treatment Group, in Subgroups of Patients with Left Bundle-Branch Block.

Findings are based on univariate Cox proportional-hazards regression models and an interaction-term analysis. LVEDV denotes left ventricular end-diastolic volume, LVEF left ventricular ejection fraction, LVESV left ventricular end-systolic volume, and NYHA New York Heart Association.

Fig. 6.7 Figure 3 of Goldenberg and Others (2014)

Measures of likelihoods and distinctions in likelihoods may be determined by using observations of some variables in addition to observations pertaining to occurrence of event or time to follow-up time. These measures are called adjusting measures; the additional variables are called their adjusting variables. Adjusted measures are often reported in addition to or in place of crude measures.

Adjusted measure are usually close to their corresponding crude measures. Like crude measures, adjusted measures are oversimplifications if crude measures of the subgroups specified by one or more adjusting variables differ noticeably. Adjusted measures are useful only if the measures of the subgroups specified by each adjusting variable are close. When adjusted measures are cited, it is important to demonstrate that they are not oversimplifications.

For instance, an incidence rate adjusted for sex is determined by suing observations pertaining to sex in addition to observations pertaining to the occurrence of events and the number of observations. Sex is its adjusting variable. It is usually close to the crude incidence rate. It and the crude incidence rate are oversimplifications if the crude incidence rates of the female and male subjects differ substantially. It is a useful measure of likelihood only if the incidence rates of the subgroups of female and male subjects are close.

A hazard ratio adjusted for age is determined by using ages in addition to follow-up times and group membership.

Age is its adjusting variable. It and the crude hazard ratio are oversimplifications if the crude hazard ratios of younger and older subjects differ substantially. It is a useful measure of distinction in risks only if the hazard ratios of the subgroups of female and male subjects are close.

Removal, Control, or Concealment?

Adjusted measures are sometimes alluded to as measures with the effects of adjusting variables "removed" or "controlled." They are special types of averages of the subgroup measures of the subgroups specified by their adjusting variables. The effects of the adjusting variables on the measures are concealed, not removed or controlled.

The effects of the adjusting variables of adjusted measures are informatively demonstrated by the subgroup measures of the subgroups specified by the adjusting variables. If the subgroup measures of the subgroups specified by one or more adjusting variables differ considerably, the effects of the variables are concealed. The adjusted measure is an oversimplification and misleading when it is applied to the subgroups. This is often the case.

Adjusted measures of likelihood and distinction in likelihoods are useful only if the subgroup measures in the subgroups specified by each adjusting variable are close. This is rarely the case.

Example 6.6.2.1

The article by van Gelder and Others (2002) (Example 6.3.2.1) used the absolute difference −5.4 percentage points to assess distinction in risks of the primary end point between the rate–control and the rhythm–control groups (17.2% and 22.6). The absolute difference is a crude rate difference. Its computation used only observations of occurrence of the primary end point and numbers of subjects in treatment groups. Table 3 (Table 6.7) shows that the subgroup absolute differences of the normotensive and hypertensive subjects differed markedly (4.6 vs. −13.5 percentage points). The absolute difference of –5.4 percentage points is an oversimplification. It is misleading when it is applied to the normotensive and the hypertensive subjects.

The article also used rate differences adjusted for hypertension to assess the distinction. It stated:

> The noninferiority of rate control compared with rhythm control was confirmed in an ancillary analysis with statistical adjustment for the unbalanced distribution of patients with hypertension between the two groups; the adjusted absolute difference was –4.2 percent, and the corresponding 90 percent confidence interval was −10.0 to 1.5 percent.

The statistical adjustment referred to a regression analysis that used a model to presume that the subgroup differences of the normotensive and hypertensive subjects are identical. The adjusted absolute difference of −4.2% is a result of this presumption and an average of the subgroup absolute differences of the subgroups. It is close to the crude absolute difference (−5.4%). Like the crude absolute difference, it is between the differences of the subgroups of hypertensive and the normotensive subjects (4.6% and −13.5%). It is misleading when it is applied to the normotensive and the hypertensive subjects.

The effect of hypertension on the distinction in risks of the primary end point between the two treatment groups is demonstrated by the disparity of the absolute difference between the subgroups of hypertensive and normotensive subjects (4.6% and −13.5%). It was not removed or controlled but was concealed by the adjusted absolute difference (−4.2%).

Example 6.6.2.2
Table 2 of Goldenberg and Others (2014) (Table 6.8) shows crude and adjusted hazard ratios of subgroups of subjects with and without left bundle branch block. A footnote of the table indicates that the adjusted hazard ratios were determined by the Cox proportional hazard model using as many as eight adjusting variables. The model presumed that the hazard ratios are identical among subdivisions specified by each adjusting variable.

The adjusted hazard ratios are relatively close to their corresponding unadjusted crude hazard odds ratios. For instance, the crude and adjusted hazard ratios for death from any cause of the subjects with left bundle branch block are 0.63 and 0.59, respectively. The crude and adjusted hazard ratios for death from any cause of the subjects without left bundle branch block are 1.31 and 1.51, respectively.

Figure 3 (Fig. 6.6) shows that the hazard ratios of the subdivisions of the subgroup of subjects with left bundle branch block specified by age (0.65 and 0.62), NYHA class (0.66, 0.65, and 0.57), QRS duration (0.55 and 0.65), LVEF (0.66 and 0.64), and LVEDV (0.63 and 0.5) are close to the unadjusted crude and the adjusted hazard ratios of the subgroup (0.63 and 0.59). They suggest that the distinctions in the risks of death from any cause between the subjects of the two treatment groups were not related to these variables.

However, the hazard ratios of the subdivisions of male and female subjects (0.69 vs. 0.48) and those of the subdivisions of subjects whose left ventricular end-systolic volumes (LVESV) at baseline were ≤170 ml and > 170 ml (0.56 vs. 0.71) differed noticeably. The crude and adjusted hazard ratios of the subgroup of subjects with left bundle branch block (0.63 and 0.59) are rather misleading when they are applied to the subdivisions specified by sex and LVEDV.

The adjusted hazard ratios are relatively close to their corresponding unadjusted crude ratios. Little is lost if they are not displayed.

6.6.3 *P-Value for Interaction*

P-values for interactions are sometimes cited. A *P*-value for interaction is a result of testing the statistical significance of the disparity of a measure of distinction in likelihoods between two subgroups specified by a variable. A small *P*-value suggests that the disparity in the measures of distinction between two subgroups may be declared statistically significant. It does not unveil how the measures of distinction differ. To read intelligently, it is productive to look for measures of distinction in subgroups. To report informatively, it is more enlightening to present the measures of distinction in subgroups.

Example 6.6.3.1

Gaudino and Others (2018) (Example 6.1.4) devoted a section to depict the results of subgroup analyses. The following is one narrative of the results of using seven variables to divide subjects into subgroups.

> The interaction term analysis (Fig. 2) showed a greater benefit with regard to major adverse cardiac events in association with radial-artery grafts than with saphenous-vein grafts in patients younger than 75 years of age (P = 0.008), in women (P = 0.01) and, nominally, in patients without renal insufficiency (P = 0.02). Diabetes (P = 0.35), a left ventricular ejection fraction of less than 35% (P = 0.37), and previous myocardial infarction (P = 0.45) did not modify the treatment effect. The radial-artery-craft target vessel did not significantly influence the treatment effect (P = 0.42).

The interaction term analysis referred to that Cox proportion hazards regression analysis that included in its regression function products of the variable indicating treatment group and variables indicating traits. The products are interaction terms. The its coefficient of an interaction term represents the magnitudes of disparity in the hazard ratios between subgroups specified by attributes of the traits. A small *P*-value ($\leq$0.05) suggests that the disparity in the hazard ratios between subgroups specified by the attributes of a trait would be particularly unlikely if chance were the explanation. It does not unveil how the hazard ratios differ between subgroups.

For instance, $P = 0.008$ suggests that the disparity in the hazard ratios between the subgroups of younger and older subjects would be particularly unlikely if chance were the explanation. It does not unveil how the hazard ratios of the younger and older subjects differed. $P = 0.35$ suggests that the disparity in the hazard ratios between the subgroups of subjects with and without diabetes would not be particularly unlikely if chance were the explanation. It does not unveil how close the hazard ratio of the two subgroups were.

Figure 2 (Fig. 6.8) exhibits hazard ratios for the primary composite outcome of subgroups specified by seven variables and *P*-values for interaction. The hazard ratios of the subgroups unveil. The figure unveils the following, for instance:

- The hazard ratios of the subgroups of younger and older subjects (younger and older than 75 years of age) were 0.6 and 1.00, respectively. The hazard ratio 0.6 suggests that the risk of the primary composite outcome of the radial artery group was substantially lower than and only 6-tenth of the risk of the saphenous vein group among the subjects of the younger subgroup (younger than 75 years); the hazard ratio 1.0 suggests that the risk of the radial therapy group was the same as that of the saphenous vein group among the subjects of the older subgroup (at least 75 years of age). The *P*-value for interaction (0.008) suggests only that the disparity between the subgroup hazard ratios (0.61vs. 1.00) would be particularly unlikely if chance were the explanation.

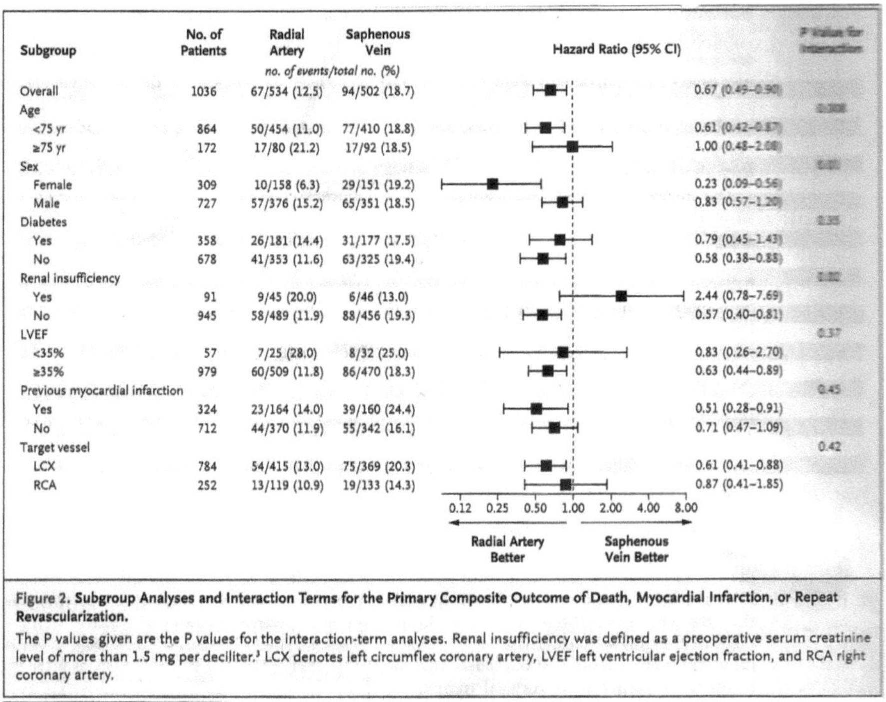

Fig. 6.8 Figure 2 of Gaudino and Others (2018)

- The hazard ratios of the female and male subgroups were 0.23 and 0.83, respectively. The hazard ratio 0.23 suggests that the risk of the primary composite outcome of the radial artery group was markedly lower than and only 2.3-tenth of the risk of the saphenous vein group among the female subjects. The hazard ratio 0.83 suggests that the risk of the primary composite outcome of the radial artery group was slightly lower than and approximately 8.3-tenth of the risk of the saphenous vein group among the female subjects. The *P*-value for interaction (0.01) suggests only that the disparity between the subgroup hazard ratios (0.23 vs. 0.83) would be unlikely if chance were the explanation.
- The hazard ratios of the subgroups of subjects with and without renal insufficiency were 2.44 and 0.57, respectively. The hazard ratio 2.44 suggests that the risk of the primary composite outcome of the radial artery group was markedly higher than and 2.44 times that of the saphenous vein group among subjects with renal insufficiency. The hazard ratio 0.57 suggests that the risk of the primary composite outcome of the radial artery group was lower than and approximately 5.7-tenth of the risk of the saphenous vein group among the subjects without renal insufficiency. The *P*-value for interaction (0.02) suggests only that the disparity between the subgroup hazard ratios (92.44 vs. 0.57) would be particularly unlikely if chance were the explanation.

The disparities in hazard ratios between subgroups specified by some variables are rather noticeable, although their *P*-values for interaction are not lower than 0.05. For example:

- The hazard ratios of the subgroups of subjects with and without diabetes differed noticeably (0.79 vs. 0.58). They suggested that the distinction in risks of the primary composite outcome between the radial artery group and the saphenous vein group was more noticeable in the subgroup of subjects with diabetes than in the subgroup of subjects without diabetes. The *P*-value for interaction: 0.35 is not below 0.35. It is not considered a suggestion of particularly unlikely result if chance were the explanation.
- The hazard ratio of the subgroups of subjects whose left ventricular ejection fractions were <35% differ noticeably (0.83 vs. 0.63). They suggested that the distinction in risks of the primary composite outcome between the radial artery group and the saphenous vein group was more noticeable in the subgroup of subjects whose left ventricular ejection fractions were <35% compared with the distinction in the subgroup of subjects whose left ventricular ejection fractions were ≥35%. The *P*-value for interaction: 0.37 is not below 0.05. It is not considered a suggestion of particularly unlikely result if chance were the explanation.
- The hazard ratio of the subgroups of subjects whose target vessels were denotes left circumflex coronary artery (LCX) and right coronary artery (RCA) differed noticeably (0.61 vs. 0.87). They suggested that the distinction in risks of the primary composite outcome between the radial artery group and the saphenous vein group was more noticeable in the subgroup of subjects whose target vessels were LCX than in the subgroup of subjects whose target vessels were RCA. The *P*-value for interaction: 0.42 is not below 0.05. It is considered a suggestion of particularly unlikely result if chance were the explanation.

The hazard ratios of the subgroups are more informative than the *P*-values for interaction.

Example 6.6.3.2

Goldenberg and Others (2014) (Example 6.6.1.3) stated:

> The differential effect of CRT-D on outcomes according to QRS morphologic findings was significant for all end points (P<0.05 for interaction of treatment with QRS morphologic, in unadjusted and adjusted analyses) (Table 2).

This is a statistical result. It is important to know how the differential effect of CRT-D on outcomes according to QRS morphologic findings was assessed and what the *P*-value for interaction suggested.

The STATISTICAL ANALYSIS section stated:

> The benefit of CRT-D therapy compared with ICD therapy alone among patients with left bundle branch block and those without left bundle branch block was assessed by including a

> term for interaction between treatment and presence or absence of left bundle branch block in the multivariate Cox models.

A footnote of Table 2 states:

> The P-value for interaction represents the likelihood that the difference between the treatment effect on patients with left bundle branch and the treatment effect on those without left bundle branch block occurred by chance alone.

The differential effect of CRT-D on outcomes was measured by hazard ratios assessing distinction in risks of end points between the CRT-D group and the ICD group. A small *P*-value for interaction suggests that the disparity between the hazard ratios of the subgroups with and without left bundle branch block would be unlikely if chance were the only explanation. The disparity could be declared statistically significant. It did not unveil how the hazard ratios of the subgroups of subjects differed.

How the differential effect of CRT-D on outcome varied according to QRS morphologic findings was plainly indicated by the hazard ratios of the subgroups of subjects with and without left bundle branch block shown in Table 2. The unadjusted (crude) hazard ratios for death from any cause of the subgroups of subjects with and without left bundle branch block differed markedly (0.63 vs. 1.31). The adjusted hazard ratios of the two subgroups are 0.59 and 1.57, respectively.

It is more productive to note the subgroup hazard ratios and stress their contradictory indications than using *P*-values for interaction to depict the differential effect on outcomes according to QRS morphologic findings.

Example 6.6.3.3

Combes and Other (2018) (Example 6.1.1) reported:

> Subgroup analyses showed no significant interaction of 60-day mortality with baseline characteristics, ARDS severity, or randomization at ECMO centers versus non-ECMO centers (Fig. S9 in the supplementary Appendix).

The subgroup analyses referred to the Cox regression analysis that included in its regression function the products of the variable indicating treatment group and the variables indicating baseline characteristics, ARDS severity, and randomization at ECMO centers. The disparity of the hazard ratios between the subgroups specified by each of the variables was not declared statistically significant. It is unknown how the hazard ratio differed between the subgroups specified by each of these variables. It is astute to review Fig. S9 in the Supplementary Appendix to find assessments of 60-day mortality in subgroups specified by these factors.

To report informatively, it is more revealing and more effective to show measures of risk in treatment groups and measures of distinction in risks between treatment groups by subgroups specified by each of these factors. It then would be clear how the risks of the treatment groups and the distinctions in the risks between the treatment groups were related to these factors.

6.7 Intelligent Reading and Informative Reporting

A few more examples of intelligent reading and informative reporting are reviewed in this section. The following suggestions are presented here as references.

Intelligent Reading

1. Ascertain whether revelations of data are the results of intention-to-treat analysis, per-protocol analysis, or some variations of the two approaches. Ascertain whether measures of effects are credible assessments of effects of being assigned to treatment groups or effects of treatments. If there is not sufficient information, assume that they are measures of the effects of being assigned to treatment groups.
2. Scrutinize the clinical implications of "significant" and "not significant" data revelations. Keep in mind that the expression "significant" is routinely used in the sense of statistical significance and means only that it is all right to dismiss the concern that data revelations are incidental.
3. Small *P*-values suggest only that revelations of data would be unlikely if chance were the only explanation and that it is alright to dismiss the concern that the revelations are incidental. "Significant" revelations are not necessarily clinically important, and statistically not significant distinctions are not necessarily trivial.
4. Identify the statistics portraying revelations of data whether the revelations are or are not declared "significant." Probe their suggestions. Keep in mind that the reproducibility of statistically significant revelations of data may be inadequate.
5. Whether a revelation of data is or is not declared statistically significant, use its 95% confidence interval to appraise its reproducibility.
6. When the likelihood of an event is assessed by an average or person-time incidence rate, it is important to note the length of the follow-up period.
7. If a distinction in likelihoods is depicted by a difference or ratio of measures of likelihoods, ascertain the indication of the difference or ratio in light of the magnitudes of measures of likelihoods.
8. If the degree of distinction is appraised by an adjusted distinction measure, looked for the measures of the subgroups specified by its adjusting variables. An adjusted distinction measure is an oversimplification if the measures of the subgroups specified by its one of its adjusting variables vary substantially. It would be a convenient single measure of distinction applicable to subgroups of subjects defined by its adjusting variables only if the measures of the subgroups are comparable. This occurs occasionally.
9. If a distinction in risks between treatment groups is depicted by a hazard ratio, ascertain its indication in light of measures of the risks of the treatment groups.
10. Read with care assertions that distinction measures stayed unchanged by adjustment. Adjusted measures are usually close to their corresponding unadjusted crude measures. The result that a measure stayed unchanged by adjustment is not an affirmation that the measure was not affected by the adjusting variables. This may occur when the measures of the subgroups specified by one or more adjusting variables differed substantially.

11. A P-value for interaction is a result of testing the statistical significance of the disparity of a measure of distinction between subgroups specified by a variable. It does not unveil how and how much measures of distinction varied between subgroups. Look for the distinction measures in the subgroups.
12. Use results of subgroup analysis to probe indications of results of multivariate analysis such as adjusted measures and P-values for interaction.
13. The term "relative risk" may be used to refer to ratios of various measures of distinction in risks. Find out whether a relative risk is a ratio of average incidence rates, cumulative incidence rates, person-time incidence rates, Kaplan–Meier estimates of probability, or odds ratio. To report informatively, it is important to make it clear that a relative risk is a ratio of which measures of risk.

Informative Reporting

To report informatively, it is essential to be plain and easy to understand. Clarity is more important than sophistication. Avoid the use of ambiguous technical terms. Articulate clinical implications of results of statistical analysis plainly. The following suggestions are presented here as references.

1. Indicate clearly whether revelations of data are assessments of effects of being assigned to treatment groups or effects of treatments. Describe characteristics and numbers of subjects whose data were included or excluded.
2. Do not simply report statistical results. Articulate their suggestions clearly.
3. Do not simply state whether a distinction between treatment groups is or is not significant. Depict how the treatment groups differed.
4. When measures of distinction are cited to depict distinction in likelihoods between treatment groups, cite also measures of likelihoods of treatment groups. Articulate what the measures suggest.
5. Do not simply present 95% confidence interval or P-values. Identify the involved statistics and elaborate their suggestions.
6. Do not simply cite graphical displays. Elaborate their suggestions.
7. When evolutions of likelihoods of event are depicted graphically, exhibit values of measures of likelihood and measures of distinction at selected points in time. Articulate suggestions of the graph.
8. Use results of subgroup analyses to depict effects of variable on likelihoods and distinctions in likelihoods. The effects are informatively unveiled by measures of likelihoods and measures of distinction in subgroups specified by the variables.
9. Present results of corresponding subgroup analyses to substantial results of regression analyses such as adjusted measures of likelihood and adjusted measures of distinction and P-values for interaction.
10. Report adjusted measures such as adjusted incidence rates and adjusted hazard ratios only if measures of subgroups specified by each adjusting variable are close.

11. Do not simply cite *P*-values of interactions or stating interaction is or is not statistically significant. Use measures of distinctions in likelihoods in subgroups to depict how the subgroup differed.
12. Indicate clearly whether a relative risk is a ratio of average incidence rates, cumulative incidence rates, person-time incidence rates, Kaplan–Meier estimates of probability, or odds.

Example 6.7.1

One feature of Molina and Others (2014) (Example 2.2.1) is that it reported the results of intention-to-treat analysis as well as per-protocol analysis. It stated:

> Figure 2 (Fig. 2.4) shows that the percentages of treatment failures in the two analyses differed, particularly the percentages of treatment failure in the benznidazole group (38.4% vs. 5.9%). To read intelligently, it is critical to determine how the percentages of treatment failure were computed and what they intimated.

and

> The intention-to-treat analysis included all patients who underwent randomization. Patients who were lost to follow-up, those who dropped out owing to adverse events, and those who had positive results on a rt-PCR assay at any time after completion of treatment were considered to have treatment failure. The per-protocol analysis included patients who completed treatment and follow-up (patients lost to follow-up were excluded unless rt-PCR testing after treatment was positive).

Figure 1 of the article shows that the following subjects were excluded from the per-protocol analysis:

1. In the benznidazole group, five patients withdrew due to adverse events, and four were lost to follow-up.
2. In the high-dose posaconazole group, one withdrew owing to pregnancy.
3. In the low-dose posaconazole group, three patients did not receive the assigned drug, and three were lost to follow-up.

The article also reported:

> From the end of the treatment period to the end of the follow-up period, consistent negative rt-PCR results were documented in 16 patients in the benznidazole group, 2 in the low-dose group, and 5 in the high-dose group.

These numbers are shown in Table 6.9 for convenience.

Table 6.9 suggests that the percentages of treatment failure of the intention-to-treat analysis were computed from data of the 26 subjects assigned to each treatment group as follows:

1. Benznidazole group (38.4% = 10/26). Its numerator (10) included 1 subject who had one or more positive RT-PCR assays, 5 who withdrew due to adverse events, and 4 who were lost to follow-up.
2. High-dose posaconazole group (80.7% = 21/26). Its numerator (21) included 20 subjects who had one or more positive RT-PCR assays and 1 who became pregnant.

Table 6.9 Numbers of subjects used in analyses

Treatment group	Benznidazole	High-dose posaconazole	Low-dose posaconazole
Subjects assigned	26	26	26
Consistent negative RT-PCR assay	16	5	2
One or more positive RT-PCR assay	1	20	18
Adverse events	5	0	0
Did not receive assigned treatment	0	0	3
Became pregnant	0	1	0
Lost to follow-up	4	0	3
Received assigned treatment fully and completed follow-up	17	25	20

3. Low-dose posaconazole group (92.3% = 24/26). Its numerator (24) included 18 subjects who had one or more positive RT-PCR assays, 3 who did not receive assigned treatment, and 3 who were lost to follow-up.

The percentages of treatment failure of the per-protocol analysis were computed as follows:

1. Benznidazole group (1/17 = 5.9%). Its numerator (1) is the number of subjects who had one or more positive RT-PCR assays (1), and its denominator is the number of subjects who received benznidazole fully and completed follow-up (17). Data from five patients withdrew due to adverse events, and four patients lost to follow-up were excluded.
2. High-dose posaconazole group (20/25 = 80.0%). Its numerator is the number of subjects who had one or more positive RT-PCR assays (20), and its denominator is the number of subjects who received only high-dose posaconazole and did not become pregnant (25). Data from one subject who became pregnant were excluded.
3. Low-dose posaconazole group (18/20 = 90.0%). Its numerator is the number of subjects who had one or more positive RT-PCR assays (18), and its denominator is the number of subjects who received low-dose posaconazole and completed follow-up (25). Data from the three patients who did not receive the assigned treatment and the three patients who were lost to follow-up were excluded.

The two analyses defined treatment failure differently. The intention-to-treat analysis considered one or more positive RT-PCR assays, adverse events, not receiving assigned treatment, becoming pregnant, and being lost to follow-up all treatment failures. The per-protocol analysis considered only having positive RT-PCR as treatment failure. The percentages of the intention-to-treat analysis are percentages of subjects whose treatment failed among all subjects assigned to treatment groups. The percentages of the per-protocol analysis are percentages of subjects whose treatment failed among subjects who received assigned treatment fully and completed follow-up.

The percentages of treatment failure of the intention-to-treat analysis (panel A) and the per-protocol analysis (panel B) are flawed when they are used to assess treatment effects. The percentages of treatment failure of the intention-to-treat analysis have the flaw that lost to follow-up, drop out owing to adverse events, not receiving assigned treatment, and becoming pregnant are counted treatment failures in addition to positive result on a RT-PCR assay at any time after completions of treatment. The percentages of treatment failure of the per-protocol analysis have the flaw that dropping out owing to adverse event is overlooked. It is important to evaluate them with care.

One way to read intelligently and report informatively is to consider the results of a modified per-protocol analysis that include one or more positive RT-PCR assays and withdrawing due to adverse event as treatment failure and use data of subjects who received only assigned treatment and completed follow-up. The percentages of treatment failure are 6/22 = 27.3% in the benznidazole group, 20/25 = 80.0% in the high-dose posaconazole group, and 18/20 = 90.0% in the high-dose posaconazole group.

Example 6.7.2
One feature of Fig. 2 of Gaudino and Others (2018) (Fig. 6.8) is that it displayed not only hazard ratios for the primary composite outcome by subgroups but also average incidence rates of the primary composite outcome by subgroups. The rates are valuable supplements to the hazard ratios. They unveil how the risk of the primary composite outcome of the treatment groups is related to the variables. Their ratios are close to hazard ratios. The following are some examples.

- Age
  - The average incidence rate of the radial artery group of the subgroup of younger subjects (< 75 years of age) was substantially lower than that of the subgroup of older subjects (11.0% vs. 21.2%).
  - The incidence rates of the saphenous vein group of the subgroups of younger and older subjects were particularly similar (18.8% vs. 18.5%).
  - The ratio of the average incidence rates of the subgroup of younger subjects: 11.0%/18.8 = 0.59 is substantially lower than the ratio of the subgroup of older subjects: 21.2%/18.5 = 1.15. They are close to the hazard ratio of the subgroups (0.61 and 1.00).
- Sex
  - The average incidence rate of the radial artery group of the subgroup of female subjects was substantially lower than that of the subgroup of male subjects (6.3% vs. 15.2%).
  - The incidence rate of the saphenous vein group of the subgroup of female subjects was slightly higher than the rate of the subgroup of male subjects (19.2% vs. 18.5%).
  - Among the female subjects, the ratio of the incidence rates 6.3%/19.2% = 0.33 is in the same direction as but relatively higher than the hazard ratio 0.23.

Among the male subjects, the ratio of the incidence rates 15.2%/18.5% = 0.82 is close to the hazard ratio 0.83.

- Renal Insufficiency
  - The average incidence rate of the radial artery group of the subgroup of subjects with renal insufficiency was substantially higher than that of the subgroup of subjects without renal insufficiency (20.0% vs. 11.9%).
  - The average incidence rates of the saphenous vein group of the subgroups of subjects with renal insufficiency were lower than the rate of the subgroup of subjects without renal insufficiency (13.0% vs. 19.3%).
  - The ratio of the average incidence rates of the subgroup of subjects with renal insufficiency: 20.0%/13.0% = 1.54 is substantially higher than in the same direction as but substantially lower than the ratio of the subgroup of subjects without: 11.9%/19.3% = 0.62. Their suggestions agree with those of the hazard ratios of the subgroups (2.44 and 0.57).

The numbers of subjects in subgroups may be used to demonstrate that overall incidence rates are weighted averages of incidence rates of subgroups and that overall hazard ratios are close to weighted averages of hazard ratios of subgroups. For instance:

Age

- When the numbers of subjects of the radial artery group in the younger and older groups (454 and 80) are used as weights, the weighted average of the average incidence rates of the radial surgery group is 454×11.0% + 80×21.2%/(454 + 80) = 67/534 = 12.5%, which is the overall incidence rate of the radial artery group.
- When the numbers of subjects of the saphenous vein artery group in the younger and older subgroups (410 and 92) are used as weights, the weighted average of the average incidence rates of the saphenous vein group is 410×18.8% + 92×18.5%/(410 +92) = 94/502 = 18.7%, which is the overall average incidence rate of the saphenous vein group.

Sex

- When the numbers of subjects of the radial artery group in the subgroup of female and male subjects (158 and 376) are used as weights, the weighted average of the average incidence rates of the radial artery group is 158×6.3% + 376×15.2%/(158 + 376) = 67/534 = 12.5%, which is the average incidence rate of the radial artery group.
- When the numbers of subjects of the saphenous vein artery group in the subgroup of female and male subjects (151 and 351) are used as weights, the weighted average of the average incidence rates of the saphenous vein group is 151×19.2% + 351×18.5%/(151 + 351) = 94/502 = 18.7%, which is the average incidence rate of the saphenous vein group.

Age

When the numbers of subjects in the subgroups of younger and older subjects (454 + 410 = 955 and 80 + 92 = 172) are used as weights, the weighted average of the hazard ratios of the subgroups of younger and older subjects is 955×0.61 + 172×1.00)/(955 + 172) = 0.6695, which equals the overall hazard ratio 0.67.

Sex

When the numbers of subjects in the subgroups of female and male subjects (158 +151 = 309 and 376 +351 = 727) are used as weights, the weighted average of the hazard ratios, it is 309×0.23 + 727×0.83)/(376 + 727) = 0.65, which is close to the overall hazard ratio 0.67.

- *Overall hazard ratios are close to weighted averages of hazard ratios of subgroups using numbers of subjects in subgroups as weights.*

Example 6.7.3 Desjardins (379, 2)

A study enrolled 61 consecutive adult patients who had recurrent supratentorial WHO grade IV malignant glioma with measurable disease. Seven doses of convection-enhanced, intratumoral delivery of the recombinant nonpathogenic polio-rhinovirus chimera (PVSRIPO) were evaluated. One result is presented by Desjardins and Others (2018) as follows:

> However, overall survival among the patients who received PVSRIPO reached a plateau beginning at 24 months, with the overall survival rate being 21% (95% CI, 11 to 33) at 24 months and 36 months, whereas overall survival in the historical control group continued to decline, with overall survival rates of 14% (95% CI, 8 to 21) at 24 months and 4% (95% CI, 1 to 9) at 36 months (Fig. 1).

This account was effectively corroborated by Fig. 1 (Fig. 6.9), which displays percentages of subjects who survived in periods of increasing length graphically; values of the percentages are also exhibited. The figure shows the following:

- The percentage of survivors among the 61 patients in the PVSRIPO group declined quickly to 21% as the follow-up period lengthened to 20 months but remained unchanged when the follow-up period lengthened.
- The percentage of survivors among the 104 historical controls declined at a similar rate to 21% when the follow-up period lengthened to approximately 20 months and continued to decline to as low as 4% or lower when the follow-up period lengthened to 36 months or longer.

The values of the percentages of surviving subjects in periods of increasing length are valuable. Readers who are interested in assessing the progression of the percentages of survivor and their distinctions do not have to figure out approximate values of the percentages laboriously.

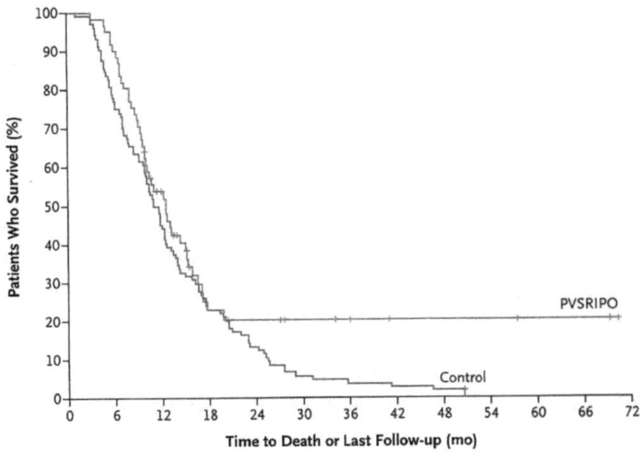

No. at Risk													
PVSRIPO	61	55	29	10	8	6	5	3	3	3	2	2	–
Control	104	80	47	24	14	6	4	3	2	–	–	–	–

Group	Total No. of Patients	No. of Deaths	Median Survival (95% CI)	Survival Rate (95% CI)						
				6 Mo	12 Mo	18 Mo	24 Mo	36 Mo	48 Mo	60 Mo
			mo				*percent*			
PVSRIPO	61	44	12.5 (9.9–15.2)	90 (79–96)	54 (40–65)	23 (12–35)	21 (11–33)	21 (11–33)	21 (11–33)	21 (11–33)
Control	104	103	11.3 (9.8–12.5)	77 (68–84)	45 (36–54)	23 (16–32)	14 (8–21)	4 (1–9)	2 (<1–6)	–

Figure 1. **Overall Survival among Patients Who Received PVSRIPO and Historical Controls.**
Tick marks indicate censored data. PVSRIPO denotes recombinant nonpathogenic polio–rhinovirus chimera.

Fig. 6.9 Figure 1 of Desjardins and Others (2018)

Example 6.7.4

The study reported by van Driel and Others (2018) (Example 6.4.2.4) is unusual in that the hazard ratio and ratio of average incidence rates of the event of disease recurrence or death differ noticeably (0.66 vs. 0.91). The results of subgroup analyses suggest that the hazard ratio and the ratio of average incidence rates of the event of disease recurrence or death in subgroups also differed noticeably.

Figure 3 (Fig. 6.5) shows graphically the hazard ratios of the subgroups of subjects specified by five factors. Numbers of subjects who had the event of disease recurrence or death in the treatment groups are shown by subgroup. The number may be used to compute average incidence rates in subgroups that are assessments of the risks of the event of the treatment groups in the subgroups. Table 6.10 shows the average incidence rates, their ratios, and hazard ratios in the subgroups. The subgroup average incidence rates unveil much valuable information including the following:

Table 6.10 Average incidence rates of disease recurrence or death of treatment groups and their ratios

	Surgery plus HIPEC	Surgery only	Rate ratio	Hazard ratio
Overall age	81% (99/122)	89% (110/123)	0.91	0.66
≥65 yrs	79% (34/43)	96% (43/45)	0.82	0.63
<65 yrs	82% (65/79)	86% (67/78)	0.95	0.72
Histologic type				
High-grade serious	81% (91/112)	90% (96/107)	0.90	0.69
Other	78% (7/9)	93% (14/15)	0.84	0.56
Previous surgery				
No	82% (90/110)	90% (100/111)	0.91	0.71
Yes	75% (9/12)	83% (10/12)	0.90	0.47
No. of involved regions				
0–5	75% (62/83)	88% (73/83)	0.85	0.64
6–8	95% (37/39)	93% (37/40)	1.02	0.66
Laparoscopy before surgery				
No	83% (86/103)	90% (95/105)	0.92	0.69
Yes	68% (13/19)	83% (15/18)	0.82	0.61

- Like the overall average incidence rates (0.81 and 0.89), the average incidence rates of the subgroups specified by the five variables are close to 1.0 and suggest that the risks of the event of disease recurrence or death of the treatment groups are high in subgroups specified by the variables. For instance, the average incidence rates of the surgery plus HIPEC group of the younger and older subgroups, 79% and 82%, are relatively close to 1.0. The average incidence rates of the surgery-only group of the younger and older subgroups, 96% and 86%, are also close to 1.0.
- Like the ratio of overall average incidence rates (0.91), the ratios of average incidence rates of the subgroups are relatively close to 1.0 and differ the hazard ratios substantially.

To read intelligently, it is important to note the substantial disparities between the hazard ratios and ratios of average incidence rates. To report informatively, it is critical to stress the substantial disparities between hazard ratios and ratios of average incidence rates.

The average incidence rates were directly computed from the numbers of events and numbers of subjects in the treatment groups. The indications of the rates and their ratios are clear. The hazard ratios, on the other hand, were computed by using a mathematical model and a sophistic computer algorithm. Its indication is not clear. Usefulness of hazard ratios is questionable if the Cox proportional hazard condition is not comparable with the data.

The Kaplan–Meier curves of Figure 2A of van Driel and Others (2018) (Fig. 6.3) suggests that the risk of the event of disease recurrence or death of the surgery plus HIPEC group was close to that of the surgery-only group when follow-up periods were shorter than 1 year or longer than 4 years but noticeably lower when periods of follow-up were between 1 and 4 years. The proportional hazards condition of the Cox proportional hazard model may be unreliable. The hazard ratios may not be valid assessments of the distinction in the risks of the event of disease recurrence or death between the two treatment groups during the course of follow-up.

Figure 2A suggests that the Kaplan–Meier estimates of the probability of the event of disease recurrence or death in the two treatment groups were close to the average incidence rates (0.81 and 0.89) when periods of follow-up were longer than 4 years. They confirm the indication of the ratio of average incidence rates that the risks in the two treatment groups were close.

To report informatively, it is constructive to stress indications of average or cumulative incidence rates and their ratios.

Example 6.7.5

The article by STABILITY Investigators (2014) (Example 6.1.2) stated:

> There were no significant effects of darapladib on any of the components of the primary end point (cardiovascular death, myocardial infarction, or stroke) or on all-cause mortality. The hazard ratio for the effect of darapladib on myocardial infarction was 0.89 (95% CI, 0.77 to 1.03; P=0.11).

The hazard ratio for myocardial infarction: 0.89 and (95% CI, 0.77 to 1.03: $P = 0.11$) are presented as an example to corroborate the assertion that there were no significant effects of darapladib on any of the components of the primary end point. The 95% confidence interval [0.77 to 1.03] includes the null value of hazard ratio 1.0, and $P = 0.11$ is not smaller than 0.05. They suggest that hazard ratio 0.89 would not be declared statistically significant.

To read intelligently, it is astute to note that the assertion that there were no significant effects of darapladib on any of the components of the primary end point meant only that the hazard ratios assessing the distinctions in the risks of the components of the primary end point between the two treatment groups were not declared statistically significant. It is not an assertion that the hazard ratios are not useful.

For instance, the hazard ratio 0.89 is relatively close to 1.0 and an insinuation that the risk of myocardial infarction of the darapladib group was only slightly lower than and approximately 8.9-tenth of the risk of the placebo group. The boundaries of the 95% confidence interval [0.77 to 1.03] are 87% and 116% of 0.89. They suggest that the hazard ratio is moderately reproducible. The revelation of the data that the risk of myocardial infarction in the darapladib group was slightly lower than that of the placebo group would be supported by many replicates of the study if the study were replicated a score of times.

It is more informative to present assessments of the risks of the components of the primary end point and assessments of the distinctions in the risks between treatment groups. These assessments would show clearly how close the risks of the components of the primary end point were between the treatment groups.

- *Subgroup Analysis*

The article also presented the results of a subgroup analysis. It stated:

> The treatment effect with respect to the primary end point was consistent in almost all prespecified subgroups. The only interactions below the P=0.10 levels were among smokers (P=0.04 for interaction) and white patients (P=0.08 for interaction) (Fig. S2 in the Supplementary Appendix)."

To read intelligently, it is critical to determine how the treatment effect was measured, what the characteristics of the subgroups were, and what $P = 0.04$ and $P = 0.08$ suggested.

Average incidence rates and hazard ratios were cited to assert that the risk of the primary end point in the darapladib group was slightly lower than that in the placebo group (Example 6.1.2). This suggests that treatment effects were assessed by average incidence rates and distinctions in risk are assessed by hazard ratios. Most likely, the assertion: "*The treatment effect with respect to the primary end point was consistent in almost all prespecified subgroups*" meant that the average incidence rates and hazard ratios of almost all subgroups confirmed that the risk of the primary end point in the darapladib group was lower than that in the placebo group.

The P-values for interaction $P = 0.04$ and $P = 0.08$ suggest that the disparity between the hazard ratios of the subgroups of smokers and nonsmokers and that between the subgroups of white and nonwhite subjects are smaller than 0.10. The P-values do not unveil how large the disparities were. They do not unveil whether the incidence rates of the subgroups were low or high, and whether the hazard ratios of the subgroups were close to or distant from 1.0.

It is more informative to present average incidence rates and hazard ratios of the subgroups. The incidence rates would unveil how the effects of the two treatments varied between subgroups specified by each variable; the hazard ratios would unveil how distinctions in risks varied between the treatment groups.

Example 6.7.6

Kadish and Others (2004) (Example 6.3.2.2) presented the results of two subgroup analyses in a section titled SUBGROUP ANALYSIS. It stated:

> Although the study was not powered to detect differences within subgroups, several prespecified analyses were performed regarding variables that could affect survival (Fig. 2). A Cox proportional hazards model was used to analyze differences in survival in predefined subgroups. Men had a relative risk of death from any cause of 0.49 (95 percent confidence interval, 0.27 to 0.90; P=0.018) after the implantation of an ICD. Patients with NYHA class III heart failure had a relative risk of death of 0.37 (95 percent confidence interval, 0.15 to 0.90; P=0.02) after receiving an ICD (Fig. 3).

The two values: 0.49 and 0.37 are hazard ratios. They suggest that the risks of death from any cause of the ICD group was substantially lower than the risk of the standard therapy group among subjects of the subgroup of male subjects and the subgroup of subjects with NYHA class III. It is unknown whether the hazard ratio of female subjects was close to 0.49 and whether the hazard ratios of the subjects whose NYHA classes are I, II, and III differed were close to 0.37.

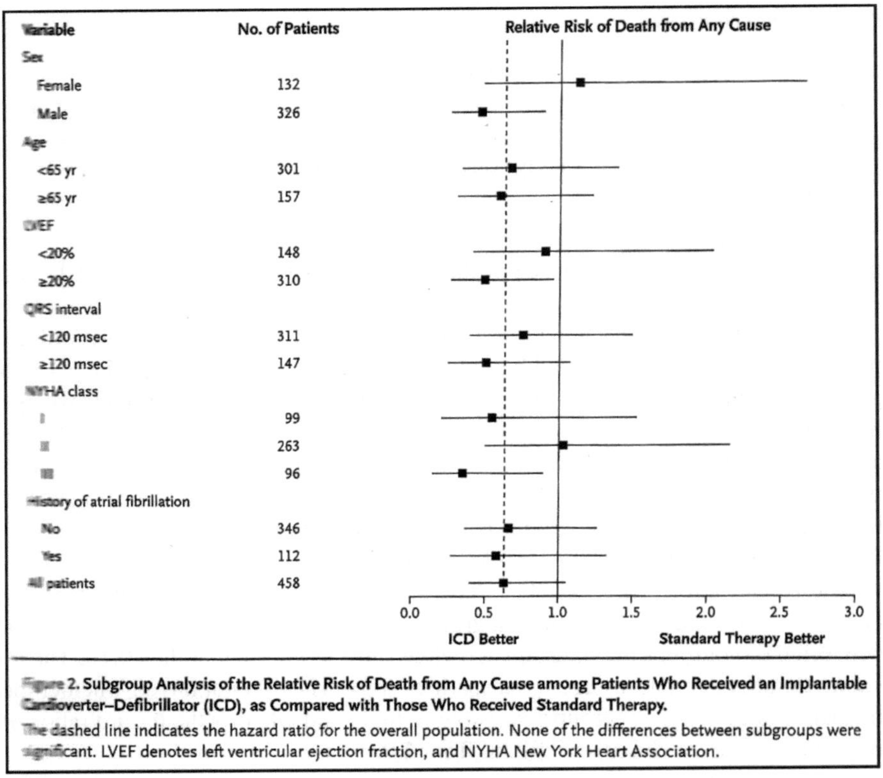

Fig. 6.10 Figure 2 of Kadish and Others (2004)

Figure 2 (Fig. 6.10) presents more information. It suggests, for instance, that the hazard ratios of the male and female subjects are approximately 0.49 and 1.20, respectively. The risk of death of the ICD group, compared with the risk of the standard therapy group, was much lower than and only 4.9-tenth among male subjects but slightly higher and approximately 1.2 times among female subjects. The hazard ratios of the subgroups of subjects whose NYHA classes were I, II, and III were approximately 0.50, 1.1, and 0.37, respectively. The risk of death in the ICD groups was lower among subjects whose NYHA classes were I or III but slightly higher among subjects whose NYHA classes were II.

The hazard ratios were relatively close between subgroups of subjects younger and older than 65 years of age and between subgroups of subjects with and without a history of atrial fibrillation. Little would be lost if these two variables were not considered when distinction in risks of death between the two treatment groups is appraised.

Figure 2 shows that 95% confidence intervals of subgroup hazard ratios are rather wide. The reproducibility of the hazard ratios of the subgroups is inadequate. It is astute to consider the hazard ratios of subgroups only preliminary clues.

To report informatively, it is productive to refer to Figure 2 and stress the suggestions of hazard ratios of subgroups. Articulate how distinctions in risks of death between treatment groups was affected by the variables.

Figure 2 shows the hazard ratios and 95% confidence intervals graphically and the numbers of subjects in the subgroups. The figure would be more informative if values of hazard ratios, boundaries of their 95% confidence intervals, and numbers of events are also shown. The numbers of events are particularly useful. They can be used to compute average incidence rates to assess risks of death from any cause in treatment groups by subgroups.

Example 6.7.7

Distinction in risks of death from any cause between the ICD group and standard therapy group was narrated as follows in Kadish and Others (2004) (Example 6.6.1.2) on one occasion:

> The unadjusted hazard ratio for death among patients who received ICD compared with those who received standard therapy was 0.65 (95 percent confidence interval, 0.40 to 1.06). The hazard ratio was unchanged (0.65) after adjustment for the period of heart failure.

It is unclear what the assertion that the hazard ratio was unchanged after adjustment for the period of heart failure suggested. Adjusted hazard ratios are usually close to their corresponding unadjusted crude hazard ratios. The adjusted hazard ratio 0.65 is an average of the hazard ratios of the subgroups of subjects whose durations of heart failure were short and long. It may be close to the unadjusted crude hazard ratios whether the hazard ratios of the subgroups of subjects whose durations of heart failure were short and long were close or differed substantially. That the hazard ratio was unchanged after adjustment is not a certification that the distinction in risks of death between the ICD group and the standard therapy group was not related to duration of heart failure.

It is more productive to present the measures of risk of death in the treatment groups and their distinction by subgroups of subjects whose durations of heart failure were short and long and articulate their suggestions.

Example 6.7.8

The following is a description of the association between heart failure and homozygosity for α_{2C}*Del322-325* in black subjects presented by Small and Others (2002) (Example 6.1.5):

> There was no evidence of significant confounding by age or sex, and the sex- and age-adjusted odds ratio for heart failure among participants who were homozygous for α_{2C}Del322-325 was 5.65 (95% confidence interval, 2.67 to 11.95; $P<0.001$).

It is unclear how the sex and age adjusted odds ratio for heart failure among participants who were homozygous for α_{2C}Del322-325 was 5.65 related to the asserting that there was no evidence of significant confounding by age or sex. The adjusted odds ratio of 5.65 is close to the unadjusted crude odds ratio of 5.54. However, this may occur even if the odds ratios of female and male subjects differed substantially and the odds ratios of younger and older subjects also differed substantially. It is more informative to show odds ratios of subgroups of female and male subjects and those of subgroups of younger and older subjects. The subgroup odds ratios indicate clearly how the association of heart failure with homozygosity for α_{2C}Del322-325 related to age and sex.

Review Questions

1. Why are the results of intention-to-treat analyses often disputable assessments of treatment effects and distinction in treatment effects?
2. What are suggested by *P*-values of measure of distinctions in risks of event between treatment groups?
3. Is statistical significance a certification of clinical importance?
4. Does statistical significance submit high reproducibility?
5. Is it possible that a statistically not significant finding adequately reproducible?
6. What do 95% confidence intervals suggest?
7. What does the 95% confidence interval of a revelation of data suggest that it is not suggested by the *P*-value of the revelation?
8. How do the indications of average incidence rate, cumulative incidence rate, person-time incidence rate, and Kaplan–Meier estimates of probability differ?
9. When hazard ratios are reported as assessments of distinctions in risks between treatment groups, why it is important to report some measures of risks in groups?
10. What are unveiled by Kaplan–Meier curves and graphical displays of cumulative incidence rates of periods of increasing length that are not unveiled by a single incidence rate?
11. How does a distinction measure adjusted for a variable relate to the distinction measures in subgroups specified by the variable?
12. Are adjusted distinction measures often oversimplifications and misleading?
13. What is suggested when a distinction measure is unchanged after adjustment for a variable?
14. What is suggested by a *P*-value for interaction?
15. Is the effect of the adjusting variable of an adjusted distinction measure removed, controlled, or concealed?
16. What is the most informative way to portray the effect of a variable on risks in treatment groups and their distinction?
17. Why are odds ratio used to assess distinction in risks of disease between subjects who were and were not exposed to a risk factor when data are obtained from case–control studies?
18. How are rate ratio and odds ratio related?

Exercise

6.E.1 Elaborate the suggestions of Figure 2B of van Driel and Others (2018) (Fig. 6.3).

6.E.2 Elaborate the suggestions of Figure 1B of Gaudino and Others (2018) (Fig. 6.4).

6.E.3 Review Figure 3 of van Driel and Others (2018) (Fig. 6.5).

(a) Elaborate the indications of the hazard ratios of the subgroups of subjects with and without previous surgery (0.71 and 0.47).
(b) Elaborate what the 99% confidence intervals of hazard ratios of the subgroups suggest.
(c) Use a table to display, by subgroups of subjects with and without previous surgery, numbers of events, numbers of total subjects in treatment groups, and average incidence rates.
(d) Elaborate the imitations of the average incidence rates of each treatment group of the subgroups of subjects with and without previous surgery.
(e) Elaborate the imitations of the ratio of average incidence rates of the treatment groups of the subgroups of subjects with and without previous surgery.
(f) Compute the crude overall average incidence rates of the two treatment groups and their ratio. Elaborate the suggestions for the overall rates and their ratio.
(g) Compare the suggestions of the hazard ratio and ratio of average incidence rates of the subgroups of subjects who did and did not have previous surgery.
(h) Suggest an approximate value of the hazard ratio adjusted for previous surgery and elaborate its suggestion.
(i) Discuss whether the adjusted hazard ratio is more useful than the crude hazard ratio 0.66.

6.E.4 Review Figure 2 of Gaudino and Others (2018) (Fig. 6.8).

(a) Elaborate the indications of the hazard ratios of the subgroups of subjects with and without renal insufficiency previous to surgery (2.44 and 0.57).
(b) Elaborate the suggestion of the 95% confidence intervals of hazard ratios of the subgroups.
(c) Use a table to display, by subgroups of subjects with and without renal insufficiency surgery, numbers of events, numbers of total subjects in treatment groups, and average incidence rates.
(d) Elaborate the imitations of the average incidence rates of each treatment group of the subgroups of subjects with and without renal insufficiency.
(e) Elaborate the imitations of the ratio of average incidence rates of the treatment groups of the subgroups of subjects with and without renal insufficiency.
(f) Compute the crude overall average incidence rates of the two treatment groups and their ratio. Elaborate the suggestions of the overall rates and their ratio.
(g) Compare the suggestions of the hazard ratio and ratio of average incidence rates of the subgroups of subjects who did and did not have renal insufficiency.
(h) Suggest an approximate value of the hazard ratio adjusted for renal insufficiency and elaborate its suggestion.
(i) Discuss whether the adjusted hazard ratio is more useful than the crude hazard ratio 0.67.

6.E.5 Review Table 2 of Goldenberg and Others (2014) (Table 6.8).

(a) Elaborate the suggestions of the hazard ratios for nonfatal cardiac event of the subgroups of subjects with and without left bundle branch block of the unadjusted analysis (0.42 and 1.10).
(b) Elaborate the suggestions of the 95% confidence intervals and *P*-values of the hazard ratios for nonfatal cardiac event of the subgroups of subjects with and without left bundle branch block of the unadjusted analysis.
(c) Elaborate the suggestion of the *P*-value for interaction for nonfatal heart failure event of the unadjusted analysis (<0.001).
(d) Elaborate the suggestions of the hazard ratios for nonfatal cardiac event of the subgroups of subjects with and without left bundle branch block of the adjusted analysis (0.38 and 1.13).
(e) Elaborate the suggestions of the 95% confidence intervals and *P*-values of the hazard ratios for nonfatal cardiac event of the subgroups of subjects with and without left bundle branch block of the adjusted analysis
(f) Elaborate the suggestion of the *P*-value for interaction for nonfatal heart failure event of the adjusted analysis (<0.001).

E.6 Review Figure 3 of Goldenberg and Others (2014) (Fig. 6.7).

(a) Elaborate the suggestions of the hazard ratios for death from any cause of the subdivisions of the subgroup of subjects with left bundle branch block whose LVESV levels were $\leq$ 170 ml and $>$ 170 ml.
(b) Elaborate the suggestions of the 95% confidence intervals and *P*-values of the hazard ratios.
(c) Suggest an approximate value of the hazard ratio for death from any cause adjusted for LVESV level and discuss whether it is more useful than the unadjusted crude hazard ratio 0.63.

6.E.7 Review Table 3 of van Gelder and Others (2002) (Table 6.7).

(a) Elaborate the suggestions of percentages of subjects who had the primary end point according to sex.
(b) Demonstrate how the percentages of all patients of each treatment group are related to the percentages of the subgroups.
(c) Demonstrate how the absolute difference of all patients is related to the absolute differences of the subgroups.
(d) Suggest a likely value for the absolute difference in average incidence rates adjusted for sex and discuss whether it is a realistic assessment of distinction in risks of the primary end point between the treatment groups applied to male and female subjects.

6.E.8 Review Figure 2 of Kadish and Others (2004) (Fig. 6.10).

(a) Elaborate what the figure unveiled with respect LVEF.
(b) Suggest a likely approximate value of the hazard ratio adjusted for LVEF and discuss how useful it is.

(c) If the adjusted hazard ratio is close to the unadjusted crude hazard ratio 0.65 and unveils that the hazard ratio did not changed after adjustment for LVEF, discuss why the closeness of the adjusted and unadjusted hazard ratios is or is not an indication that little is lost if LVEF is not considered when distinction in risks of the primary end point between the subjects in the two treatment groups is evaluated.

6.E.9 Table 2 of Small and Others (2002) shows that the number of subjects homozygous for α_{2C}-Del322-325 was 6 among 81 white cases of heart failure and 2 among 105 white controls.

(a) Use a two-way table to exhibit the percentages and numbers of white cases and white controls homozygous for α_{2C}-Del322-325. Discuss what the percentages indicate.
(b) Compute the exposure odds ratio of the white subjects—ratio of the odds of homozygosity for α_{2C}-Del322-325 among the white cases relative to the odds among the white controls. Explain what it insinuates.
(c) Compute the fractions of heart failure cases among the white subjects homozygous for α_{2C}-Del322-325 and those among the white subjects not homozygous for α_{2C}-Del322-325 and the ratio of the fractions.
(d) Explain why the fractions are or are not valid measures of risk of heart failure and their ratio is not a valid measure of the relative distinction in risks of heart failure between the two types of subjects.
(e) Use a two-way table to display the data if the study was repeated by enrolling the same number of white cases (81) but ten times the number of white controls (1050) and yielded the same percentages of cases and controls homozygous for α_{2C}-Del322-325 as well as the same exposure odds ratio.
(f) Use the data of the fictitious study to compute the fractions of heart failure cases among the subjects who were and those who were not homozygous for α_{2C}-Del322-325 and the ratio of the fractions.
(g) Compare the fractions and their ratio computed from the data of Small and Others (2002) and those from the data of the fictitiously repeated study. Discuss what the results suggest.

References

Albers, G. W., et al. (2018). Thrombectomy for stroke at 6 to 16 hours with selection by perfusion imaging. *The New England Journal of Medicine, 378*(8), 708–718.

Combes, A., et al. (2018). Extracorporeal membrane oxygenation for severe acute respiratory distress syndrome. *The New England Journal of Medicine, 378*(21), 1965–1975.

DeBaun, M. R., et al. (2014). Controlled trial of transfusions for silent cerebral infarcts in sickle cell anemia. *The New England Journal of Medicine, 371*(8), 699–710.

Desjardins, A., et al. (2018). Recurrent glioblastoma treated with recombinant poliovirus. *The New England Journal of Medicine, 379*(2), 150–161.

Gaudino, M., et al. (2018). Radial-artery or saphenous-vein grafts in coronary-artery pass surgery. *The New England Journal of Medicine, 378*(22), 2069–2077.

Goldenberg, I., et al. (2014). Survival with cardiac-resynchronization therapy in mild heart failure. *The New England Journal of Medicine, 370*(18), 1694–1701.
Kadish, A., et al. (2004). Prophylactic defibrillation implantation in patients with nonischemic dilated cardiomyopathy. *The New England Journal of Medicine, 350*(21), 2151–2158.
Molina, I., et al. (2014). Randomized trial of posaconazole and benznidazole for chronic chagas' disease. *The New England Journal of Medicine, 370*(20), 1899–1908.
Small, K. M., et al. (2002). Synergistic polymorphisms of β_1 and α_{2C}-adrenergic receptors and the risk of congestive heart failure. *The New England Journal of Medicine, 347*(15), 1135–1142.
The STABILITY Investigators. (2014). Darapladib for preventing ischemic events in stable coronary heart disease. *The New England Journal of Medicine, 370*(18), 1702–1711.
van Dongen, M. A., et al. (2014). A trial of treatment for acute otorrhea in children with tympanostomy tubes. *The New England Journal of Medicine, 371*(8), 723–733.
van Driel, W. J., et al. (2018). Hyperthermic intraperitoneal chemotherapy in ovarian cancer. *The New England Journal of Medicine, 378*(3), 230–240.
van Gelder, I. C., et al. (2002). A comparison of rate control and rhythm control in patients with recurrent persistent atrial fibrillation. *The New England Journal of Medicine, 347*(23), 1834–1840.
Weaver, L. K., et al. (2002). Hyperbaric oxygen for acute carbon monoxide poisoning. *The New England Journal of Medicine, 347*(14), 1057–1067.

Chapter 7
Paired Qualitative Data Sets

Chapter 5 demonstrates that revelations of paired quantitative data sets are plainly manifested by the distribution of an index of observation-pair and not by the respective distributions of the data sets. Similarly, revelations of paired qualitative data sets are plainly manifested by the distribution of the observation-pairs and not the respective distributions of the data sets.

When two sets of qualitative data are paired, the observations of the two data sets form observation-pairs; the categories to which the observations belong specify distinct types of observation-pairs. The percentages of observation-pairs belonging to the distinct types constitute the distribution of the observation-pairs. They unveil plainly the revelation of paired data sets. The percentages of observations of the data sets belonging to categories constitute the distributions of the observations of the data sets. They yield limited useful information.

One pivotal property of paired qualitative data sets is that the distribution of observation-pairs is exclusive to the data sets and yields precise descriptions of respective distributions of the data sets, but the converse is not true. There are several scenarios of the distribution of observation-pairs that yield the same respective distributions of the data sets. This pivotal property of paired qualitative data sets is frequently overlooked. Revelations of paired qualitative data sets are often depicted by description of the respective distributions of the data sets, although the statistical significance of revelations of paired qualitative data is routinely assessed by procedures for paired data sets.

This chapter uses examples to demonstrate the magnitude of using percentages of observation-pairs to depict revelations of paired qualitative data sets. Section 7.1 reviews examples. The importance of using the distribution of observation-pairs to attest revelations of paired qualitative data sets is demonstrated in Sect. 7.2. Synoptic descriptions of revelations of paired dichotomous data sets are examined in Sect. 7.3. Section 7.4 presents examples of intelligent reading and informative reporting.

P. C. Chang, *Data Analysis of Medical Studies*,
https://doi.org/10.1007/978-3-031-49984-5_7

7.1 Examples

This section uses examples to demonstrate the importance of using descriptions of distributions of observation-pairs to depict revelations of paired qualitative data.

Example 7.1.1
Pike and Smith (1972) noted in a letter to the editor that the estimated relative risk, 2.9, used by Vianna and Others (1971) to assess the risk of Hodgkin's disease in subjects who underwent tonsillectomy relative to the risk in subject who did not might be an underestimate. The study reported by Vianna and Others (1971) is a case–control study that assessed the association of Hodgkin's disease with tonsillectomy. It enrolled 109 patients with Hodgkin's disease as cases and 109 individuals free of Hodgkin's disease and other malignant or chronic illnesses as controls. Each control was identified by matching with a case with respect to age, sex, race, county of residence, and date of hospital admission. There is a one-to-one pairing of the cases and controls; the group of cases and the group of controls are paired. The set of observations of the cases and the set observations of the controls are paired.

Vianna and Others (1971) stated:

> Cases and controls differed significantly in their histories of prior tonsillectomy ($p < 0.01$) (see accompanying table). The estimated relative risk of developing Hodgkin's disease among those with a history of tonsillectomy was 2.9 times as great as those who had not been tonsillectomized.

Pike and Smith (1973) showed that the estimated relative risk, 2.9, was computed as $(0.66/0.34)/(0.40/0.60) = 2.9$. Here, 0.66 and 0.40 are the proportions of cases and controls who had a history of tonsillectomy, (0.66/0.34) is the odds of having a history of tonsillectomy among cases, and (0.40/0.60) the odds among controls. The estimated relative risk: 2.9 is an odds ratio for unpaired dichotomous data sets (Equation 6.4.3.2). Its computation did not take the pairings of the cases and the control into consideration.

As descriptions of case–control pairs were not available in Vianna and Others (1971), Pike and Smith (1973) used data from Johnson and Johnson (1972) to show that the estimated relative risk 2.9 may be an underestimate.

Johnson and Johnson (1972) reported the results of a case–control study similar to that of Vianna and Others (1971). The study evaluated tonsillectomy histories of 85 cases of Hodgkin's disease and their closely matched sibling controls. The control of each case was a sibling of the same sex and within five years of age. Whether a subject had a history of tonsillectomy is a dichotomous observation. There are four types of case–control pairs.

Johnson and Johnson (1972) reported that 41 of 85 Hodgkin's disease cases and 33 of the controls had a history of tonsillectomy. Matched controls of seven of the cases with intact tonsils had undergone tonsillectomy. Pike and Smith (1972) used these numbers to determine the numbers of the four types of case–control pairs and displayed the numbers in a table which shows:

1. Both cases and controls of 26 case–control pairs underwent tonsillectomy.
2. The cases of 15 case–control pairs underwent tonsillectomy, but the controls did not.
3. The cases of 7 case–control pairs did not undergo tonsillectomy, but the controls did.
4. Both cases and controls of 37 case–control pairs did not undergo tonsillectomy.

Pike and Smith (1973) suggested that the appropriate estimate of relative risk is 15/7 = 2.14. This is the odds ratio for paired dichotomous data sets (Eq. 7.3.1). It suggests that the risk of Hodgkin's disease among subjects with a history of tonsillectomy is higher than and approximately 2.14 times higher than the risk among subjects without a history of tonsillectomy.

The numbers of cases and controls with a history of tonsillectomy were 41 and 33, respectively. They yield that the odds ratio for unpaired dichotomous data sets equals (41/44)/(33/52) = 1.47. It is smaller than the odds ratio for paired dichotomous data sets (2.14) and an underestimate.

If the odds ratio for paired dichotomous data sets were computed from the data of Vianna and Others (1971), it would be greater than the estimated relative risk (2.9) used by Vianna and Others (1971) to assess the risk of developing Hodgkin's disease among those with a history of tonsillectomy relative to the risk among those without a history of tonsillectomy. The estimated relative risk (2.9) of Vianna and Other (1971) is an underestimate.

Example 7.1.2

Madhi and Others (2014) presented the results of a study evaluating the efficacy of a trivalent inactivated influenza vaccine (IIV3). One assessment of the effect of the vaccine in HIV-uninfected pregnant women was related as follows:

> A greater proportion of IIV3 recipients had seroprotective HAI titers after vaccination as compared with placebo recipients (Table 3).

Table 3 shows the numbers and percentages of subjects who had seroprotective HAI (hemagglutination inhibition) titers (≥1:40) before and after vaccination. The percentages and numbers of recipients with seroprotective HAI titers (≥1:40) were greater after vaccination. For instance, the percentage of the A/H3N2 strain of IIV3 recipients having seroprotective HAI titers increased 55.7 percentage points from 23.2% to 78.9%. The percentage of placebo recipients having a seroprotective HAI titer increased 2 percentage points from 25.0% to 27.0%. These are changes in the percentages of recipients who had seroprotective HAI titers; they are not percentages of recipients whose HAI titers changed from <1:40 to ≥140. The percentage of subjects whose HAI titers changed from ≥1:40 to <1:40 is unknown.

Example 7.1.3 Bullen (312, 21)

Bullen and Others (1985) presented the results of a study that evaluated the effect of strenuous exercise on hormonal conditions. Women with ovulation and luteal adequacy were randomly assigned to a weight loss or a weight maintenance group.

Table 7.1 Table 4 of Bullen and Others (1985)

Table 4 Effects of exercise Cycles I and II in the weight-loss group[a]

Abnormality	Exercise I ($N = 16$)	Exercise II ($n = 16$)	P Value
	No. of subjects (%)		
None	1 (16)	0(0)	NS
Clinical disorders			
Abnormal bleeding	3 (19)	6 (38)	NS
Delayed menses	1 (6)	12 (75)	<0.001
Hormonal disturbance			
Abnormal luteal function	10 (63)	2 (13)	<0.010
Loss of LH surge	5 (31)	12 (75)	<0.025

[a]NS denotes not significant. and LH luteinizing hormone

Hormonal conditions of the subjects were evaluated during two consecutive menstrual cycles. The following is a narrative of the results:

> The possible evolution of the disorders as training progressed was assessed by comparing their incidence in the first and second training periods (Tables 3 and 4). No differences in incidence were found between exercise cycles I and II within the weight-maintenance group. In the weight loss group, abnormal luteal function occurred significantly more often during exercise cycle I than exercise cycle II ($P < 0.01$). Delayed menses and loss of the surge in luteinizing hormone, on the other hand, predominated during exercise cycle II ($P < 0.001$ and $P < 0.025$, respectively).

Table 4 (Table 7.1) reveals that in the weight loss group, the percentage of subjects with abnormal luteal function was 63% during cycle I and 13% during cycle II. The percentage of subjects who lost luteinizing hormone surge was 31% during cycle I and 75% during cycle II. These percentages are descriptions of the conditions of the 16 subjects as a group during two consecutive menstrual cycles. They unveiled that in the weight loss group, the percentage of subjects with abnormal luteal function declined 50 percentage points from 63% during cycle I to 13% during cycle II; the percentage of subjects who lost luteinizing hormone surge increased 44 percentage points from 31% during cycle I to 75% during cycle II. They do not reveal how the conditions of the 16 subjects evolved. It is unknown the conditions of how many subjects changed from normal luteal function during cycle I to abnormal luteal function during cycle II and how many subjects changed from abnormal luteal function during cycle I to lost luteinizing hormone surge during cycle II. It is perplexing that the percentage of subjects with abnormal luteal function declined from 63% to 13%. Did the hormonal conditions of many subjects improve from abnormal luteal function to normal luteal function?

Example 7.1.4

Fawzi and Others (2004) presented the results of a study investigating the effects of vitamin supplements on the progression of HIV in pregnant women. A total of 1078 HIV-infected pregnant women were randomly assigned to one of the following four regimens:

1. Vitamin A alone: 30 mg of beta carotene plus 5000 IU of vitamin A
2. Multivitamins excluding vitamin A: 20 mg of vitamin B_1, 20 mg of vitamin B_2, 25 mg of vitamin B_6, 100 mg of niacin, 50 μg of vitamin B_{12}, 500 mg of vitamin C, 30 mg of vitamin E, and 0.8 mg of folic acid
3. Multivitamin plus vitamin A at the same doses as 1
4. Placebo

Table 7.2 Conditions at baseline and end of follow-up in the vitamin A–alone group

	WHO stage				Died	Stage IV or died	≥ Stage III	≥ Stage II increases
	1	2	3	4				
Baseline	77.8% (212)	19.6% (53)	2.6% (7)	–	–	–	–	–
End of follow-up				8.5% (23)	23.9% (65)	88.0% (79)	60.1% (165)	49.3%(134)

Subjects were followed by monthly visits. Revelations of the data of the primary outcome: progression to WHO stage IV or death from AIDS-related causes were narrated as follows on one occasion:

> A total of 299 of the 1078 women progressed to WHO stage 4 or died of AIDS-related causes: 67 of 271 women who received multivitamins (24.7 percent), 70 of 268 who received multivitamins plus vitamin A (26.1 percent), 79 of 272 who received vitamin A alone (29.0 percent), and 83 of 267 women who received placebo (31.1 percent) (Table 2).

The numbers and percentages are partial descriptions of changes in the four groups of subjects during the study. They yielded limited information regarding the disease progression of individual subjects. Table 1 suggests that the progressions were from stage I, II, or III at baseline. However, it is unknown whether any or many of the recipients who were in WHO stage I or II at baseline progressed to WHO stage IV or died of AIDS-related causes.

Table 2 shows the numbers of subjects whose conditions at the end of follow-up belonged to five categories. The numbers of subjects in the vitamin A alone–group at baseline and at end of follow-up are displayed in Table 7.2 for the purpose of this example.

Of the numbers shown in Table 7.2, only the number of subjects whose WHO stages increased ≥ stage II is a description of the progressions of individual subjects. The others are descriptions of the conditions of the subjects at the end of follow-up. They are not descriptions of progressions. It is unknown, for instance, how many of the subjects whose WHO stages at baseline were I, or II died.

Example 7.1.5 Olschewski (347, 5)

A study randomly assigned 203 subjects with severe pulmonary arterial hypertension and chronic thromboembolic pulmonary hypertension (New York Heart Association functional class III or IV) to receive repeated daily inhalation of iloprost (101 subjects) or placebo (102 subjects) for 12 weeks. One outcome was an improvement in the NYHA (New York Heart Association) functional class in the

Table 7.3 Descriptions of changes in severity of heart failure presented in Table 2 of Olschewski and Others (2002)

	Change in NYHA class							
	Improved By two classes	Improved By one class	Unchanged	Worsened	Died	Data missing	Other[a]	SUM
Iloprost	1.0% (1)	23.8% (24)	64.4% (65)	5.9% (6)	1.0% (1)	1.0% (1)	3.0% (3)	100.1% (101)
Placebo	0.0% (0)	12.7% (13)	65.7% (67)	7.8% (8)	3.9% (4)	0.0% (0)	9.8% (10)	99.9% (102)

[a]Treatment discontinued or withdrawn

absence of a deterioration in the clinical condition or death during 12 weeks of follow-up. Revelation of this outcome was depicted in Olschewski and Others (2002) as follows on one occasion:

> More patients in the iloprost group than in the placebo group had an improvement in the severity of heart failure, as assessed by the NYHA class ($P = 0.03$) (Table 2).

Table 2 shows the percentages of subjects whose NYHA classifications changed in four ways (improved by two classes, improved by one class, unchanged, and worsened) and the percentages of subjects who died. The percentages are displayed in Table 7.3 for the purpose of this example. They reveal that, compared with the placebo group, the iloprost group had a higher percentage of subjects whose NYHA classifications improved by one class (23.8% vs. 12.7%) and a lower mortality rate (1.0% vs. 3.9%). The percentages of subjects whose NYHA classifications remained unchanged were similar (64.7% and 65.7%). These percentages are valuable but partial descriptions of changes in the severity of heart failure. It is unknown, for instance, how many of the improvements were from IV to III or from III to II. The baseline NYHA classes of the subjects who died are also unknown.

Example 7.1.6

Shamim and Others (2002) presented the results of a study investigating the long-term effect of nonsurgical reduction of the septum on functional capacity and echocardiographic characteristics in patients with hypertrophic cardiomyopathy. Sixty-four consecutively qualified patients were studied. Assessments were performed before the procedure, at six weeks, and two years after the procedure. Some of the results were related as follows:

> There were significant improvements in NYHA class from before the procedure to six weeks after the procedure and during long-term follow-up ($P < 0.001$). Before the ablative procedure, 2 patients were in NYHA class I, 16 were in class II, 39 were in class III, and 7 were in class IV. Six weeks after the procedure, 50 patients were in NYHA class I, 9 were in class II, 3 were in class III, none were in class IV, 2 had no follow-up data. Four patients were lost to follow-up before the long-term follow-up visit. Of the remaining 60 patients, 57 were in NYHA class I, 3 were in class II, none were in class III or IV. Whereas 46 patients (72 percent) were classified in NYHA class III or IV before the procedure, none were in these categories two years after the procedure.

Table 7.4 Reported numbers (percentages) of subjects whose NYHA classes belonged to four NYHA classes

	I	II	III	IV	SUM
Before procedure	2 (3.1%)	16 (25.0%)	39 (60.9%)	7 (10.9%)	64 (99.0%)
6 weeks after	50 (80.6%)	9 (14.5%)	3 (4.8%)	0 (0.0%)	62 (99.0%)
2 years after	57(95.0%)	3 (5.0%)	0 (0.0%)	0 (0.0%)	60 (100.0%)

The numbers of subjects whose NYHA classes belonged to four classes at the three time points are shown in Table 7.4. They suggested that the NYHA classifications of many subjects improved. Six weeks after the procedure, the number of subjects with class I increased markedly from 2 to 50, and the numbers of subjects with class II, III, and IV declined substantially (16 to 9, 39 to 3, and 7 to 0, respectively). Two years after the procedure, the number of subjects in class I further increased to 57, the number of subjects in class II further declined to 3, and there were no subjects in class III or IV.

This is a special case. The number of subjects with NYHA class I increased markedly after the procedure; it seems that the conditions of many subjects improved. However, the numbers are descriptions of the conditions of the subjects at the three time points; they do not unveil how many of the subjects whose NYHA classes improved from IV to I, III to I, or from IV to II. It is unknown whether there was some worsening.

7.2 Distribution of Observation-Pairs

When paired data sets are qualitative, the categories of the observations specify a limited number of distinct types of observation-pairs. The percentages of observation-pairs belonging to the distinct types constitute the distribution of the observation-pairs and unveil the revelation of the data completely.

Definition: Distribution of Observation-Pairs of Paired Qualitative Data Sets

The distribution of the observation-pairs of paired qualitative data sets comprises the percentages of observation-pairs of the data sets belonging to the types of pairs specified by the categories among the observations.

One important property of paired qualitative data sets is that percentages of observation-pairs that comprise the distribution of the observation-pairs are exclusive to the given data sets and yield precise percentages of observations in the data sets that comprise the distributions of the data sets. The percentages of observations in the data sets belonging to categories, on the other hand, do not yield precise percentages of observation-pairs. There are several scenarios of the percentages of observation-pairs that yield the same percentages of observations in the data sets. In other words, the distribution of observation-pairs of paired qualitative data sets is exclusive to the data sets and yields precise delineations of the respective distributions of the data sets. The respective distributions of two paired qualitative data sets, on the other hand, are not exclusive to the data sets; they may be the results of several scenarios of the distribution of the observation-pairs.

- *Distribution of Observation-Pairs of Paired Dichotomous Data Sets*

Paired dichotomous data sets are a particularly important types of paired qualitative data sets. It is used in the following to exemplify properties of paired qualitative data sets.

Observations of paired dichotomous data sets belong to two categories and form four types of observation-pairs. The percentages of observations in the data sets belonging to the two categories comprise the distributions of the data sets. The percentages of the four types of observation-pairs comprise the distribution of observation-pairs.

For convenience, paired data sets are designated data set 1 and data set 2, and the two categories are designated YES and NO. The four types of observation-pairs are written as [YES, YES], [YES, NO], [NO, YES], and [NO, NO], where the first element of a doublet denotes the categories of observations of data set 1, and the second denotes categories of observations of data set 2. The percentages of the four types of observation-pairs are written as %[YES, YES], %[YES, NO], %[NO, YES], and %[NO, NO]. Percentages of YES and NO observations in data set 1 are denoted by %[YES|1] and %[NO|1], and percentages of YES and NO observations in data set 2 are denoted by %[YES|2] and %[NO|2.]. The numbers of the four types of observation-pairs are written as #[YES, YES], #[YES, NO], #[NO, YES], and #[NO, NO]. The numbers of YES and NO observations in data set 1 are denoted by #[YES|1] and #[NO|1], and the numbers of YES and NO observations in data set 2 are denoted by #[YES|2] and #[NO|2.]. The percentages and numbers are exhibited methodically in a table such as Table 7.5.

Table 7.5 is a contingency table for paired dichotomous data sets. The percentages %[YES, YES], %[YES, NO], %[NO, YES], and %[NO, NO] exhibited in the cells of its first two rows and first two columns are the percentages of the four types of observation-pairs that constitute the distribution of the observation-pairs. The percentages displayed in the cells of the last column, %[YES|1] and %[NO|1], are the percentages of YES and NO observations of data set 1 that constitute the distribution

Table 7.5 Percentages (numbers) of four types of observation-pairs of paired dichotomous data sets

		Data set 2		
		YES	NO	SUM
Data set 1	YES	%[YES, YES] (#[YES, YES])	%[YES, NO] (#[YES, NO])	%[YES|1] (#[YES|1])
	NO	%[NO, YES] (#[NO, YES])	%[NO, NO] (#[NO, NO])	%[NO |1] (#[NO |1])
	SUM	%[YES	2] (#(YES|2])	%[NO |2] (#(NO |2])	100% (# of Pairs)

of data set 1. The percentages displayed in the cells of the bottom row %[YES|2] and %[NO|2] are the percentages of YES and NO observations of data set 2 that constitute the distribution of data set 2. Numbers of observation-pairs and observations belonging to categories are exhibited in parentheses.

One feature of the table is that it shows how the percentages and numbers of YES and NO observations in the data sets are related to percentages and numbers of observation-pairs. It shows that:

- %[YES|1] = %[YES, YES] + %[YES, NO] and %[NO |1] = %[NO, YES] + %[NO, NO]
- %[YES|2] = %[YES, YES] + %[NO, YES] and %[NO |2] = %[YES, NO] + %[NO, NO]

Similarly,

- #[YES|1] = #[YES, YES] + #[YES, NO] and #[NO |1] = #[NO, YES] + #[NO, NO]
- #[YES|2] = #[YES, YES] + #[NO, YES] and #[NO |2] = #[YES, NO] + #[NO, NO]

Example 7.2.1

The set of tonsillectomy histories of the 85 cases of Hodgkin's disease of Johnson and Johnson (1972) and the set of tonsillectomy histories of their sibling controls are paired dichotomous data sets. There are four types of observation-pairs characterizing four types of case–control pairs. Table 7.6 is a two-way table for paired data sets that presents a methodical description of the paired dichotomous data sets. It shows percentages and numbers of the four types of case–control pairs as well as percentages and numbers of cases and controls who did and did not have a history of tonsillectomy.

The percentages (numbers) displayed in the main body of Table 7.6, the cells of the first two rows and first two columns, are percentages (numbers) of the four types of case–control pairs.

- 30.6% (26) is the percentage (number) of case–control pairs of which the cases and control both underwent tonsillectomy.
- 17.6% (15) is the percentage (number) of case–control pairs of which the cases underwent tonsillectomy and the control did not.
- 8.2% (7) is the percentage (number) of case–control pairs of which the cases did not undergo tonsillectomy and the control did.

Table 7.6 Tonsillectomy histories of 85 cases of Hodgkin's disease and their matched controls

		Matched control		
		YES	NO	SUM
Case	YES	30.6% (26)	17.6% (15)	48.2% (41)
	NO	8.2% (7)	43.6% (37)	51.8% (44)
	SUM	38.8% (33)	61.2% (52)	100.0% (85)

- 43.6% (35) is the percentage (number) of case–control pairs of which the cases and controls did not undergo tonsillectomy.

These percentages comprise the distribution of the 85 observation-pairs and fully manifest the revelations of the tonsillectomy data of the 85 cases and their sibling controls.

The percentages exhibited in the rightmost column (48.2% and 51.8%) are percentages of cases who did and did not have a history of tonsillectomy. They comprise the distribution of the observations of the cases. The percentages exhibited in the bottom row (38.8% and 61.2%) are percentages of controls who did and did not have a history of tonsillectomy. They comprise the distribution of the observations of the controls.

The table shows that the percentages and numbers of cases and controls who did and did not have a history of tonsillectomy are summations of percentages and numbers of appropriate types of observation-pairs. Indeed:

- The percentage (number) of cases with a history of tonsillectomy 48.2% (41) equals the summation of the percentage (number) of case–control pairs of which both cases and controls had a history of tonsillectomy and the percentage (number) of case–control pairs of which the cases had a history of tonsillectomy but the control did not (48.2% = 30.6% + 17.6% and 41 = 26 + 16).
- The percentage and number of cases without a history of tonsillectomy 51.8% and 44 equal the summation of the percentage and number of case–control pairs of which the cases did not have a history of tonsillectomy but the controls did and the percentage and number of case–control pairs of which the cases and control both did not have a history of tonsillectomy (51.8% = 8.2% + 43.6% and 44 = 7 + 37).
- The percentage and number of controls with a history of tonsillectomy 38.8% and 33 equal the summation of the percentage and number of case–control pairs of which both had a history of tonsillectomy and the percentage and number of case–control pairs of which the cases did not have a history of tonsillectomy but the controls did (38.8% = 30.6% + 8.2% and 33 = 26 + 7).
- The percentage and number of controls without a history of tonsillectomy 61.2% and 52 equal the percentage and number of case–control pairs of which the cases did not have a history of tonsillectomy but the controls did and the percentage and number of case–control pairs of which both cases and controls did not have a history of tonsillectomy (61.2% = 17.6% + 43.6% and 52 = 15 + 37).

The distribution of the 85 observation-pairs is exclusive to the 85 case–control pairs of Johnson and Johnson (1972), but the distributions of the observations of the cases and controls are not. There are several scenarios of the distribution of the observation-pairs that yield the distributions of the observations of the cases and the controls. One is shown in Table 7.7, which shows the same percentages and numbers of cases and controls with and without a history of tonsillectomy as the case and controls of Johnson and Johnson (1972) but a decidedly different percentage and number of case–control pairs. It yields the same odds ratio for unpaired dichotomous

Table 7.7 A scenario of the percentages of four types of case–control pairs that yield percentages of cases and controls of the 85 cases and 85 controls of Johnson and Johnson (1972)

		Matched control		
	Tonsillectomy	YES	NO	SUM
Case	YES	37.6% (32)	10.6% (9)	48.2% (41)
	NO	1.2% (1)	50.6% (43)	51.8% (44)
	SUM	38.8% (33)	61.2% (52)	100.0% (85)

data sets (41/44)/(33/52) = 1.47 but a decidedly larger odds ratio for paired dichotomous data sets (9/1 = 9 vs. 15/7 = 2.14). This would suggest that the risk of Hodgkin's disease in the 33 subjects who had a history of tonsillectomy is as much as 9 times, instead of 2.14 times, of the risk in the 52 subjects who did not have a history of tonsillectomy.

Example 7.2.2 Madhi (371, 10)

Madhi and Others (2014) (Example 7.1.2) used percentages of recipients who had seroprotective HAI titers (≥1:40) before and after vaccination to assess the effects of the IIV3 vaccine and placebo. The percentages are descriptions of the commonness of seroprotective HAI titers before and after vaccination. They unveiled how the commonness of seroprotective titers in the two groups changed but not how the titers of the recipients changed individually. The percentage of recipients whose HAI titers improved from <1:40 to ≥1:40 and the percentage of recipients whose HAI titers worsened from ≥1:40 to <1:40 are unknown.

The HAI titers of a recipient before and after vaccination constitute an observation-pair. How the titers of a group of recipients changed after vaccination is indicated by their observation-pairs. Whether the titer of a recipient is seroprotective is a dichotomous observation; there are four types of observation-pairs characterizing four types of changes. How the titers of a group of recipients changed is indicated by the percentages of the four types of observation-pairs, not by the percentages of recipients whose titers were seroprotective before and after vaccination.

Using change in the percentages of seroprotective titers before and after vaccination to assess the effect of the vaccine has two inherent flaws. One is that the percentages are assessments of the prevalence of seroprotective titers before and after vaccination; they do not unveil how the titers of the recipients changed individually. The other is that the percentages and their differences are not exclusive to the given data; there are several scenarios of the percentages of the four types of observation-pairs that yield the same percentages of seroprotective titers before and after vaccination. This is demonstrated by the two scenarios of the titers of the 142 recipients of the A/H3N5 strain of the IIV3 vaccine displayed in Table 7.8 as examples.

The two scenarios show the same percentages and numbers of seroprotective titers before and after vaccination as those shown in Table 3 of Madhi and Others (2014) but distinct percentages and numbers of observation-pairs. Scenario

Table 7.8 Two scenarios of percentages of A/H3N2 recipients whose HAI titers changed in four ways

Scenario 1				Scenario 2			
After				After			
Titer ≥ 1:40	YES	NO	SUM	Titer ≥ 1:40	YES	NO	SUM
YES	2.8% (4)	20.4% (29)	23.2% (33)	YES	22.5% (32)	0.7% (1)	23.2% (33)
Before				Before			
NO	76.1% (108)	0.7% (1)	76.8% (109)	NO	56.3% (80)	20.4% (29)	76.8% (109)
SUM	78.9% (112)	21.1% (30)	100.0% (142)	SUM	78.8% (112)	21.1% (30)	99.9% (142)

1 suggests that the effect of the IIV3 vaccine is relatively capricious. Titers of as many as 76.10% of recipients improved from <1:40 to ≥1:40, but those of 20.4% worsened from ≥1:40 to <1:40. Scenario 2 suggests that the effect of vaccine is rather unfailing. Titers of 56.3% of the recipients improved to seroprotective after vaccination, and those of only 0.7% worsened.

Example 7.2.3 Bullen and Others (1985)

Example 7.1.3 noted that the percentages of the 16 subjects in the weight loss group whose hormonal conditions belonged to three types are descriptions of the group of subjects during two consecutive menstrual cycles. They are not descriptions of the evolutions of hormonal conditions of individual subjects during two menstrual cycles.

The hormonal conditions of a subject during two menstrual cycles constitute an observation-pair. The observations of the two menstrual cycles are paired. How the conditions of a subject evolved is indicated by their observation-pairs. The observations belong to three categories: normal luteal function, abnormal luteal function, and loss of luteinizing hormone surge. There are nine types of observation-pairs characterizing nine change patterns. How the conditions of the 16 subjects evolved is indicated by the percentages of the nine change patterns and not by the percentages of subjects whose conditions belonged to the three categories during the two cycles.

Using the percentages of subjects in the three conditions during two consecutive menstrual cycles to assess the effect of the strenuous training had two flaws. One is that the percentages are appraisals of changes in the commonness of the conditions between the menstrual cycles; they are not appraisals of changes in conditions of the subjects between two menstrual cycles individually. The other is that there are several scenarios of the nine types of change patterns that yield the same percentages during the two cycles.

To determine how the conditions of the subjects evolved, the article was reviewed to look for percentages or numbers of the nine change patterns. The following narrative was found:

Table 7.9 A likely scenario of percentages of subjects in the weight loss group whose hormonal phenomena changed in nine ways

		Cycle II			
		Normal luteal function	Abnormal luteal function	Loss of LH surge	SUM
Cycle I	Normal luteal function	6% (1)	0% (0)	0% (0)	6% (1)
	Abnormal luteal function	6% (1)	13% (2)	44% (7)	63% (10)
	Loss of LH surge	0% (0)	0% (0)	31% (5)	31% (5)
	SUM	12% (2)	13% (2)	75% (12)	100% (16)

> The mutually exclusive nature of the hormonal phenomena (loss of the midcycle surge in luteinizing hormone and formation of a normally functioning corpus luteum) permitted a direct comparison of the distribution of cycle classes in members of each weight group over time (exercise cycles I and II). The participants in the weight-maintenance group did not have a uniform trend of changes in hormonal dysfunction over the course of the study. However, seven participants in the weight-loss group (44 per cent) were found to proceed from abnormal luteal function in exercise cycle I to loss of the surge in luteinizing hormone in cycle II. This progression in the severity of the hormonal abnormality was significant by McNemar's test ($P < 0.01$).

This suggests that the percentage and number of one type of change pattern—worsening from abnormal luteal function to loss of the surge in luteinizing hormone—are 44% and 7%, respectively.

There are several scenarios of the percentages of the nine change patterns that yield the reported percentages of subjects in the three conditions during the two cycles. One scenario that is consistent with the results reported by Bullen and Others (1985) is shown in Table 7.9. It shows 44% and 7 the percentage and number of one type of change pattern—worsening from abnormal luteal function to loss of the surge in luteinizing hormone—and the same percentages and numbers of subjects whose hormonal disturbance belonged to the three types during cycle I and cycle II as those displayed in Table 4 of the article.

If Table 7.9 were factual, it would be an enlightening description of the evolutions of hormonal conditions of the 16 women. Indeed, it would reveal the following:

- The strenuous training induced abnormal luteal function in 63% (10) and loss of the luteinizing hormone surge in 31% (5) of the subjects during cycle I.
- As training continued from cycle I to cycle II, the hormonal conditions of 44% (7) of the subjects worsened from abnormal luteal function to loss of the luteinizing hormone surge. The conditions of 50% (8) did not change: 6% (1) stayed as normal luteal function, 2 (13%) stayed as abnormal luteal function, and 5 (31%) stayed as loss of luteinizing hormone surge.
- The condition of only 6% (1) improved from abnormal during cycle I to normal luteal function during cycle II.

Table 7.9 also provides a plausible explanation for the perplexing result: "*In the weight-loss group, abnormal luteal function occurred significantly more often* *during exercise cycle I than exercise II (P<0.01).*" The reason that the percentage of women with abnormal luteal function was lower during cycle II than during cycle I (12% vs. 63%) is that the conditions of seven of the ten women with abnormal luteal function in cycle I worsened to the more severe disturbance: loss of the luteinizing hormone surge in cycle II.

Table 7.10 One scenario of percentages (numbers) of the 15 change patterns in the vitamin A group

		End of follow-up					
	WHO stage	1	2	3	4	Death	SUM
Baseline	1	2.6% (7)	36.4% (99)	19.5% (53)	3.7% (10)	15.8% (43)	77.8%[a] (212)
	2	0.0% (0)	0.4% (1)	8.8% (24)	4.8% (13)	5.5% (15)	9.6%[a] (53)
	3	0.0% (0)	0.0% (0)	0.0% (0)	0.0% (0)	2.6% (7)	2.6% (7)
	SUM	2.6% (7)	36.8% (100)	28.3% (77)	8.5% (23)	23.9% (65)	100.0%[a] (272)

[a]Differs from sum due to rounding off

Example 7.2.4 Fawzi (351, 1)

Example 7.1.4 noted that the numbers presented in Table 2 of Fawzi and Others (2004) yield limited useful information regarding progressions in the conditions of the subjects from baseline to end of follow-up. Only the numbers of subjects whose WHO stages increased ≥ stage II at the end of follow-up are descriptions of the progressions of individual subjects.

Observations of a subject at baseline and at the end of follow-up constitute a before–after observation-pair. The observations at baseline belonged to three categories: WHO stages I, II, and III; those at the end of follow-up belonged to five categories: WHO stages I, II, III, IV, and died from AIDS-related causes. There are 15 types of observation-pairs characterizing 15 change patterns. How the conditions of a subject progressed is indicated by the observation-pair of the subject; how the conditions of a group of subjects progressed is portrayed by percentages of the 15 change patterns. As percentages and numbers of the 15 change patterns were not reported, it is unknown how the conditions of a group of subjects evolved.

There are several scenarios of the numbers of the 15 change patterns that yield the percentage shown in Tables 1 and 2 of the article. One likely scenario of the vitamin A group is shown in Table 7.10.

Table 7.10 shows the following:

1. The same percentages of subjects whose WHO stages were I, II, and III at baseline as those shown in Table 1

2. The same number of subjects belonging to the category death from AIDS-related causes as the one shown in Table 2 (65 = 43 [I to death] + 15 [II to death] + 7 [III to death])
3. The same number of subjects belonging to the category progression to stage IV as the one shown in Table 2 (23 = 10 [I to IV] + 13 [II to IV] + 0 [III to IV])
4. The same number of subjects belonged to the category progression to ≥stage III as shown in Table 2 (165= 53[I to III] + 24[II to III] + 10[I to IV] + 13[II to IV] + 43[I to death] + 15[II to death] + 7[III to death]
5. A slightly larger number of subjects belonged to the ≥stage II increase category (141) than the reported number (134). (53 [I to III] + 10 [I to IV] + 43 [I to Death] +13[II to IV] + 15[II to Death] +7[III to Death] = 141)
6. A slightly larger number of subjects belonged to the category progression to stage IV or death from AIDS-related causes (88) than the reported number (79) (23 [Progression to stage IV] + 65 [Death from AIDS-related causes] = 88)

If the scenario depicted in Table 7.10 were factual, it would reveal valuable additional information regarding disease progression in the vitamin A–alone group including the following:

1. The disease stages of 97% (264) of the subjects worsened, and those of only 3% (8) remained unchanged (7 remained stage I, and 1 remained stage II).
2. All seven subjects who were in WHO stage III at baseline died from AIDS-related causes.
3. Among the 53 subjects who were in WHO stage II at baseline, 15 (5.5% of 272) died from AIDS-related causes, 13 (4.8% of 272) progressed to stage IV, and 24 (8.8% of 272) progressed to stage III. Only 1 (0.4% of 272) remained at stage II.
4. Among the 212 subjects whose WHO stages were I at baseline, 43 (15.8% of 212) died from AIDS-related causes, 10 (3.7% of 212) progressed to stage IV, 53 (19.5% of 212) progressed to stage III, and 99 (36.4% of 212) progressed to stage II. The disease stages of 7 (2.6%) remained at stage I.

The following would also be clear:

1. The number of subjects belonging to the category progression to stage IV (23) included 10 who progressed from I and 13 who progressed from II.
2. The number of subjects belonging to the category progression to ≥stage III (165) included 53 who progressed from I to III, 10 from I to IV, 43 from I to death, 24 from II to III, 13 from II to IV, 15 from III to IV, 15 from II to death, and 7 from III to death.

Example 7.2.5 Olschewski (347, 5)

The percentages of subjects whose NYHA classification changed in four ways (improved by two classes, improved by one class, unchanged, and worsened) and the percentages of subjects who died shown in Table 2 of Olschewski and Others (2002) are valuable descriptions of the changes in the subjects of the two treatment groups. However, some important details were left out.

Table 7.11 A scenario of percentages (numbers) of 14 types of observation-pairs of the iloprost group

		12 weeks after treatment							
		NYHA class				Death	Data missing	Other[a]	SUM
		I	II	III	IV				
Baseline	III	0.0% (0)	0.0% (0)	52.5% (53)	5.9% (6)	0.0% (0)	1.0% (1)	0.0% (0)	59.4% (60)
	IV	0.0% (0)	1.0% (1)	23.8% (24)	11.9% (12)	1.0% (1)	0.0% (0)	3.0% (3)	40.6% (41)
	SUM	0.0% (0)	1.0% (1)	76.2% (77)	17.8% (18)	1.0% (1)	1.0% (1)	3.0% (3)	100.0% (101)

[a]Treatment discontinued or withdrawn

The observations of a subject at baseline and 12 weeks after treatment form an observation-pair. How the condition of the subject changed is indicated by the observation-pair of the subject. The baseline observations belonged to either of two categories (NYHA class III or IV), and the after-treatment observations belonged to one of seven categories (NYHA classes I, II, II, IV, death, missing data, and others). There are 14 types of observation-pairs. The percentages of observation-pairs belonging to the 14 types constitute the distribution of the observation-pairs and unveil how the conditions of a group of subjects changed in detail. The percentages shown in Table 2 of Olschewski and Others (2002) are valuable synopses of the percentages of the 14 types of observation-pairs. If percentages of the 14 types of observation-pairs were available, it would unveil some valuable additional details.

A likely scenario of the percentage of 14 types of observation-pairs that comprise the distribution of the observation-pairs of the iloprost group is shown in Table 7.11. The scenario yields the percentages of subjects whose NYHA classification changed in four ways and the percentages of subjects who died shown in Table 2 of Olschewski and Others (2002) and suggests additional information including the following:

1. The NYHA classes of 23.8% (24) of the subjects improved from IV to III.
2. The NYHA classes of 52.5% (53) of the subjects stayed at III, and 11.9% (12) stayed at IV.
3. Only one subject died; the NYHA class of the subject was IV.

Example 7.2.6 Shamim (347, 17)

Shamim and Others (2002) (Example 7.1.6) reported that the number of subjects whose NYHA classes were I increased radically from II before nonsurgical reduction of the septum to 50 six weeks after treatment and to 57 two years after treatment. The number of subjects whose NYHA classifications were II decreased from 16 before nonsurgical reduction of the septum to 9 six weeks after the procedure and to 3 two years after the procedure. These numbers are descriptions of the conditions of subjects at three time points: before procedure, six weeks after procedure, and two

Table 7.12 Assumed numbers (percentages) of subjects in NYHA classes at three time points

NYHA class	I	II	III	IV	SUM
Before procedure	2 (3.3%)	16 (26.7%)	36 (60.0%)	6 (10.0%)	60 (100.0%)
6 weeks after	48 (80.0%)	9 (15.0%)	3 (5.0%)	0 (0.0%)	60 (100.0%)
2 years after	57 (95.0%)	3 (5.0%)	0 (0.0%)	0 (0.0%)	60 (100.0%)

Table 7.13 One scenario of the progressions of NYHA classes in 60 subjects

[IV, III, II]	[IV, III, I]	[IV, II, I]	[III, II, I]	[III, I, I]	[II, I, I]	[I, I, I]	Others	SUM
5% (3)	0% (0)	5% (3)	10% (6)	50% (30)	27% (16)	3% (2)	0%(0)	100% (60)

years after procedure. They are not descriptions of progressions of the conditions of individual subjects. They submit that the NYHA classifications of many subjects improved but do not unveil how the NYHS classes of the subjects improved individually.

The NYHA classes of a subject at the three time points form an observation-series. How the NYHA classes of a subject progressed is indicated by the observation-series of the subject. There are 64 types of observation-series characterizing 64 change patterns. The NYHA classes of 60 subjects were known at all time points. There are 60 observation-series. How the conditions of the 60 subjects progressed is indicated by the percentages of observation-series belonging to the 64 types.

Numbers of subjects in NYHA class I, II, III, and IV among the 60 subjects whose classes were known at all three time points were not reported. They are assumed to be the ones displayed in Table 7.12 for the purpose of this example.

When the observation-series are written as triplets in order of time, Table 7.13 presents a curtailed description of one likely scenario of the percentages of the 64 types of observation-series that yields the assumed percentages shown in Table 7.12.

Table 7.13 yields the same numbers of subjects whose NYHA classes were I, II, III, and IV as the ones shown in Table 7.12. It, if factual, would be an informative description of the progressions of the 60 subjects. It unveils the following:

1. The NYHA classes of the two subjects whose baseline classes were I did not change.
2. The NYHA classes of the six subjects whose baseline classes were IV all improved, three from IV to III then to II ([IV, III, II]), and three from IV to II then to I ([IV, II, I]).
3. The NYHA classes of the 36 subjects whose baseline classes were III all improved, 6 improved to II six weeks after treatment and then to I two years after treatment ([III, II, I]); 30 improved to I and then stayed at I ([III, I, I]).

4. The NYHA classes of the 16 subjects whose baseline classes were II improved to I six weeks after treatment and stayed at I two years after treatment ([II, I, I]).

Note Table, Row, and Column Percentages

The percentages exhibited in the cells of a paired data two-way table are computed by using the total number of observation-pairs exhibited in the rightmost bottom cell of the table as their denominators. They are table percentages. The percentages displayed in the cells of an unpaired data two-way table, on the other hand, may be row percentages or column percentages. They are row percentages if the percentages displayed in the cells of a row are calculated by using the total number of observations in the data set displayed in the rightmost cell of the row as their denominators. They are column percentages when the percentages displayed in the cells of a column are calculated by using the total number of observations in the data set displayed in the bottom cell of the column as their denominators.

Note In this book, paired data two-way tables display percentages of YES first and percentages of NO second. Tables printed by computers generally display percentages of NO first and percentages of YES second. When paired data two-way tables are reviewed, it is important to keep track of the order of the YES and NO categories.

7.3 Synoptic Descriptions of Paired Qualitative Data Sets

Revelations of two paired qualitative data sets are manifested by distributions of observation-pairs. They are proficiently highlighted by percentages of pertinent types of observation-pairs. Percentages of observations yield limited useful information. They are not exclusive to the given data sets. There are scenarios for the percentages of observation-pairs that yield the same percentages of observations.

7.3.1 Paired Dichotomous Data Sets

When paired data sets are dichotomous, there are four types of observation-pairs. Two are discordant, [YES, NO] and [NO, YES] pairs. Revelations of paired dichotomous data sets are highlighted by percentages of discordant pairs. The ratio of the percentages of discordant pairs is a useful single synoptic measure. It is exclusive to the given data. There are other synoptic measures. They are not exclusive to the given data.

When the percentages and numbers of observation-pairs and the percentages and numbers of YES and NO observations in paired dichotomous data sets are denoted by those exhibited in Table 7.2. Synoptic measures are computed as follows:

$$\text{Ratio of percentages of discordant observation-pairs} = \frac{\%[\text{YES, NO}]}{\%[\text{NO, YES}]} = \frac{\#[\text{YES, NO}]}{\#[\text{NO, YES}]} \tag{7.3.1}$$

$$\text{Difference of percentages of discordant observation-pairs} = \%[\text{YES, NO}] - \%[\text{NO, YES}] \tag{7.3.2}$$

$$\text{Ratio of percentages of YES} = \frac{\%[\text{YES}|1]}{\%[\text{YES}|2]} = \frac{\#[\text{YES}|1]}{\#[\text{YES}|2]} \tag{7.3.3}$$

$$\text{Difference of percentages of YES} = \%[\text{YES} \mid 1] - \%[\text{YES} \mid 2] \tag{7.3.4}$$

$$\text{Odds ratio for unpaired data sets} = \frac{\%[\text{YES}|1]/\%[\text{NO}|1]}{\%[\text{YES}|2]/\%[\text{NO}|2]} \tag{7.3.5}$$

The ratio of percentages of discordant observation-pairs (Eq. 7.3.1) is dubbed the odds ratio for paired dichotomous data sets. The percentages of YES and NO observations in paired dichotomous data sets are not exclusive to the given data. There are scenarios of the percentages of observation-pairs that yield the same percentages of YES and NO observations. The ratio of percentages of YES, difference of percentages of YES, and odds ratio for unpaired data sets (Eqs. 7.3.3, 7.3.4, and 7.3.5) have the flaw that they are not exclusive to the given data. Their values are identical among the scenarios of the percentages of observation-pairs that yield the same percentages of YES and NO observations in the given data.

Example 7.3.1.1

The estimated relative risk suggested by Pike and Smith (1973) 15/7 = 2.14 is an odds ratio for paired dichotomous data sets (Eq. 7.3.1). The numbers 15 and 7 are numbers of discordant observation-pairs. 15 is the number of case–control pairs of which the cases underwent tonsillectomy but the controls did not; 7 is the number of case–control pairs of which the cases did not undergo tonsillectomy but the controls did. Pike and Smith (1973) suggested that it is the correct estimate of the relative risk of interest, the ratio of the risk of Hodgkin's disease among the subjects with a history of tonsillectomy relative to the risk among the subjects without. It insinuates that the risk of Hodgkin's disease among the subjects who underwent tonsillectomy is approximately 2.14 times that among the subjects who did not.

Table 7.14 Values of synoptic measures computed from Tables 7.6 and 7.7

	Table 7.6	Table 7.7
Odds ratio for paired dichotomous data sets	17.6%/8.2% = 2.14	0.6%/1.2% = 8.83
Difference of percentages of discordant case–control pairs	17.6% − 8.2% = 9.4%	10.6% − 8.2% = 9.4%
Difference of percentages of cases and controls with a history of tonsillectomy	48.2% − 38.8% = 9.4%	48.2% − 38.8% = 9.4%
Ratio of the percentages of cases and controls with a history of tonsillectomy	48.2%/38.8% = 1.24	48.2%/38.8% = 1.24
Odds ratio for unpaired dichotomous	$\left(\frac{48.2\%}{51.8\%}\right)/\left(\frac{38.8\%}{61.2\%}\right) = 1.45$	$\left(\frac{48.2\%}{51.8\%}\right)/\left(\frac{38.8\%}{61.2\%}\right) = 1.45$

Table 7.15 Values of synoptic measures computed from two scenarios of percentage of four change patterns among 148 A/H3N2 recipients of Madhi and Others (2014)

	Scenario 1	Scenario 2
Ratio of percentages of discordant observation-pairs	76.1%/20.4% = 3.7	56.3%/0.7% = 80.4
Difference in the percentages of discordant observation-pairs	76.1% − 20.4% = 55.7%	56.3% − 0.7% = 55.6%
Ratio of before and after vaccination percentages of seroprotective titer	78.9%/23.2% = 3.4	78.9% = 3.4
Difference of before and after vaccination percentages of seroprotective titer	78.9% − 23.2% = 55.7%	78.9% − 23.2% = 55.7%
Odds ratio for unpaired dichotomous	$\left(\frac{78.9\%}{21.1\%}\right)/\left(\frac{23.2\%}{76.8\%}\right) = 12.3$	$\left(\frac{78.9\%}{21.1\%}\right)/\left(\frac{23.2\%}{76.8\%}\right) = 12.3$

The odds ratio for paired data sets: 15/7 = 2.14 is exclusive to the data of the 85 case–control pairs of Johnson and Johnson (1972). The other synoptic measures are not. There are several scenarios of the percentages and numbers of the four types of case–control pairs that yield the same percentages of cases and controls with and without a history of tonsillectomy as those of the data of Johnson and Johnson (1972). This is exemplified by Table 7.14, which shows values of synoptic measures computed from the data of the 85 case–control pairs of Johnson and Johnson (1972) and those computed from the conjectural scenario of the percentages of the four types of case–control pairs shown in Table 5.3.

Example 7.3.1.2 Madhi (371, 10)

Table 7.8 presents two scenarios of the percentages of four change patterns among 142 recipients of the A/H3N2 variant of the IIV3 vaccine reported by Madhi and Others (2014). The suggestions of the two scenarios differed distinctly.

Values of synoptic measures of the two scenarios are shown in Table 7.15. The two scenarios yield drastically distinct values of the odds ratio for paired data sets (3.7 vs. 80.4) but identical values for the other synoptic measures.

The odds ratio for paired dichotomous data sets of scenario 1: 76.1%/20.4% = 3.7 suggests that the likelihood of being seropositive after vaccination was 3.7 times that before. This seems to suggest that the vaccine was effective. However, it is important to note that although the titers of 76.1% of recipients improved, those of 20.4% worsened.

The odds ratio for paired dichotomous data sets of scenario 2: 56.3%/0.7% = 80.4 suggests that the likelihood of being seropositive after vaccination was 80.4 times that before vaccination. However, it is important to note that the conditions of as many as 42.9% of the recipients remained the same after vaccination.

7.3.2 Paired Polytomous Data Sets

When paired qualitative data sets are polytomous, there are more than two types of discordant pairs. Revelations of paired polytomous data sets are highlighted by percentages of selected types of observation-pairs.

Example 7.3.2.1 Bullen (312, 21)

The hormonal disturbance data of the 16 subjects in the weight loss group of Bullen and Others (1985) (Example 7.1.3) during two menstrual cycles are paired polytomous data sets. There are nine types of observation-pairs. One way to highlight the revelation of the paired polytomous data sets is to cite percentages of selected types of observation-pairs.

Table 7.9 shows a likely scenario for the percentages of the nine types of observation-pairs. The indications of the scenario may be highlighted by noting that the conditions of seven (44%) subjects worsened from abnormal luteal function during cycle I to loss of LH surge during cycle II, and that the condition of 6% (1) of the subjects improved from abnormal luteal function to normal luteal function.

Example 7.3.2.2 Fawzi (351, 1)

Table 7.10 shows one scenario of the percentage and numbers of the change patterns of the 272 subjects in the vitamin A group of Fawzi and Others (2004). One way to highlight the indication of the scenario is to stress the following:

1. Among the 212 subjects who were in WHO stage I at baseline, 10 progressed to stage IV and 43 died.
2. Among the 53 subjects who were in WHO stage II at baseline, 13 progressed to stage IV and 15 died.
3. All 7 subjects who were in WHO stage III at baseline died.

7.4 Intelligent Reading and Informative Reporting

Revelations of paired qualitative data sets are often depicted by percentages or numbers of observations in the data sets belonging to categories. These percentages yield limited information. Revelations of paired qualitative data sets are manifested by percentages of observation-pairs and not by percentages of observations. The percentages of observation-pairs constitute the distribution of the observation-pairs and are exclusive to the given data. The percentages of observations are not exclusive to the given data. There are several scenarios of the percentages of observation-pairs that yield the same percentages of observations.

To read intelligently descriptions of paired qualitative data sets, it is critical to look for percentages or numbers of observation-pairs and examine their suggestions. If percentages or numbers of observation-pairs were not found, likely scenarios or conflict scenarios are valuable references. To report informatively, it is productive to articulate suggestions of percentages of observation-pairs.

Example 7.4.1 Speich (370, 7)

The study reported by Speich and Others (2014) (Example 3.5.2.3) assessed the risks of adverse events and related symptoms. Table 3 shows the numbers and percentages of children who had adverse events before treatment, 3 and 24 hours after the first treatment, and 3 and 24 hours after the second treatment. The numbers and percentages are integrated descriptions of the conditions of the children at the five time points. They unveiled how the commonness of adverse events in groups of subjects progressed after treatment; they did not unveil how the conditions of the children progressed over the five time points individually. The table shows that, for instance, among the 119 children in the oxantel pamoate–albendazole group, adverse symptoms were observed in 10.1% (12) at baseline, 7.6% (9) and, 15.1% (18) at 3 hours and 24 hours after the first treatment, and 12.6% (15) and 12.8% (15) 3 hours and 24 hours after the second treatment. These percentages and numbers are descriptions of the commonness of the conditions in the group of 119 children at the five time points. They do not unveil how the conditions of 119 children progressed individually.

There are several scenarios of the numbers and percentages of the 32 types of progressions that yield the reported numbers and percentages presented in Table 3. To read intelligently, it is productive to review some likely scenarios. One is shown in Table 7.16, which uses N and Y to denote having and not having adverse events or related symptoms and lists them in order of time.

The observations of a child regarding occurrence of adverse events at the five time pints form an observation-series. How the condition of a child progressed is indicated by the observation-series of the child. Whether adverse events occurred is a dichotomous observation. There are 2×2×2×2×2 = 32 types of observation-series specifying 32 progression patterns. How the conditions of the 119 children progressed is indicated by the percentages of the 32 progression patterns. Several

Table 7.16 A Scenario of percentages of progression patterns in the oxantel pamoate–albendazole group

Type of progression	[N,N,N,N, N]	[N,N,Y,Y, Y]	[Y,N,Y,N, N]	[Y,Y,Y,Y, Y]	Others	SUM
Percentage (number)	84.9% (101)	5.0% (6)	2.5% (3)	7.6% (9)	0.0% (0)	100.0% (119)

scenarios of the percentages of the 32 types of observation series yield the reported percentages of adverse events or related symptoms at the 5 points in time. To read intelligently, it is productive to use some as reference. One is shown in Table 7.16, which uses Y and N to denote having or not having adverse events or relates symptoms and list them in order of time. If it is factual, it would suggest the following:

1. Adverse events or related symptoms were not noted at all time points in 84.9% (101) and noted at all five time points in 7.6% (9) of the 119 children.
2. Adverse events or related symptoms were noted in 5.0% (6) of the 119 children until 3 months after the first treatment and 3 months and 24 months after the second treatment.
3. One child who had adverse events or related symptoms at baseline were free of adverse events or related symptoms after treatments.

To report informatively, it is enlightening to use percentages of these types of progressions to articulate progressions of the children.

Example 7.4.2 Thakar (347. 17)

Thakar and Others (2002) presented the results of a study that compared the effects of subtotal abdominal hysterectomy and total abdominal hysterectomy in women with respect to bladder, bowel, and sexual functions. Women referred for hysterectomy because of benign disease were randomly assigned to receive subtotal or total hysterectomy. The abstract of the article stated:

> The rates of urination frequency (urination more than seven times during the day) were 33 percent in the subtotal hysterectomy group and 31 percent in the total hysterectomy group before surgery, and they fell to 24 percent and 20 percent, respectively, at 12 months ($P = 0.03$ for the change over time within each group; $P = 0.84$ for the interaction between the treatment assignment and time.

To read intelligently, it is critical to note that the rates of frequent urination (urination more than seven times during the day) are descriptions of the commonness of the condition in the two groups of subjects before and 12 months after surgery. The declines in the rates are not descriptions of changes in the conditions of individual subjects. Indeed, the differences $33\% - 24\% = 9\%$ and $31\% - 21\% = 11\%$ revealed only that the percentage of subjects with frequent urination declined 9 and 11 percentage points after the procedures. The percentages of subjects whose conditions improved and the percentage of subjects whose conditions worsened are unknown.

Whether a subject had frequent urination is a dichotomous observation. The observations of a subject before and after surgery form an observation-pair. There are four types of observation-pairs characterizing four change patterns. The effect of being in a treatment group is fully unveiled by the percentages of the four types of observation-pairs in the group; the before and after procedure percentages of frequent urination yield limited information. To read intelligently, it is important to note that there are several scenarios of the percentages of the four types of observation-pairs that yield the reported before and after procedure percentages. It is productive

Table 7.17 Scenario A for changes in frequent urination that yields the before and after rates reported by Thaker and others (2002)

Subtotal hysterectomy				Total hysterectomy			
After surgery				After surgery			
Frequent urination	YES	NO	SUM	Frequent urination	YES	NO	SUM
YES	23% (27)	10% (12)	33% (39)	YES	1% (1)	30% (37)	31% (38)
Before surgery				Before surgery			
NO	1% (1)	66% (79)	67% (80)	NO	19% (23)	50% (60)	69% (83)
SUM	24% (28)	76% (91)	100% (119)	SUM	20% (24)	80% (97)	100% (121)

Table 7.18 Scenario B for changes in frequent urination that yields the before and after rates reported by Thaker and Others (2002)

Subtotal hysterectomy				Total hysterectomy			
After surgery				After surgery			
Frequent urination	YES	NO	SUM	Frequent urination	YES	NO	SUM
YES	1% (1)	32% (38)	33% (39)	YES	19% (23)	12% (15)	31% (38)
Before surgery				Before surgery			
NO	23% (27)	45% (53)	67% (80)	NO	1% (1)	68% (82)	69% (83)
SUM	24% (28)	77%[a] (91)	100% (119)	SUM	20% (24)	80% (97)	100% (121)

[a]Differs from reported rates slightly (77% vs. 76%)

to consider markedly different scenarios. Two scenarios with contrasting suggestions are shown in Tables 7.17 and 7.18.

If the scenario shown by Table 7.17 were factual, it would suggest the following:

- The effect of being in subtotal hysterectomy was rather weak. The conditions of only 10% (12) of the subjects improved from frequent urination to not frequent urination after the procedure. The conditions of as many as 23% (27) remained frequent urination, and 1% (1) worsened from not frequent urination to frequent urination after the procedure.
- The effect of being in the total hysterectomy group was equivocal. The conditions of 30% (37) improved from frequent urination to not frequent urination after the procedure. However, the conditions of 19% (23) worsened from not frequent urination to frequent urination after the procedure.

If the scenario shown by Table 7.18 were factual, it would suggest the following:

- The effect of being in the subtotal hysterectomy group was equivocal. The conditions of 32% (38) of the subjects improved from frequent urination to not frequent urination after the procedure. However, the conditions of as much as 23% (27) worsened from not frequent urination to frequent urination.
- The effect of being in the total hysterectomy group is rather weak. The conditions of only 12%(13) improved from frequent urination to not frequent urination after the procedure. The condition of 1 (1%) subject worsened.

To report informatively, it is more constructive to use percentages of the four change patterns to depict the effects of being assigned to the two treatment groups and the distinction in the effects.

Example 7.4.3 Schiffman (317, 19)

The results of a study assessing the effect of aspartame on the incidence of headache and related neurologic symptoms are presented by Schiffman and Others (1987). The study enrolled 40 individuals who had a history of headache and related neurologic symptoms within 24 hours after consuming products containing aspartame. Subjects were identified by their prior complaints of products containing aspartame to the FDA or manufacturers. Each subject was challenged for two days. On the first day, a subject was given either aspartame or placebo. The other substance was given after a one-day wash-out period. The order of receiving aspartame and placebo was determined randomly.

The incidence of headache while receiving aspartame and while receiving placebo are recounted in Schiffman and Others (1987) as follows on one occasion:

> Eight participants had headaches while receiving aspartame but not placebo. Twelve participants had headache while receiving placebo but not aspartame. Six participants had headaches during both treatments. When these participants were included, the incidence of headache was 35 percent with aspartame and 45 percent with placebo. The incidence of adverse symptoms with placebo was equivalent to that with aspartame (Table 3).

This is an informative description of two paired dichotomous data sets. The observations of a subject while receiving aspartame and while receiving placebo constitute an observation-pair. The set of observations of the subjects while receiving aspartame and the set of observations of the participants while receiving placebo are paired. There are 40 observation-pairs. Whether a subject reported headache is a dichotomous observation; there are four types of observation-pairs. The numbers 8, 12, and 6 are the numbers of three types of observation-pairs; they yield that the number of the fourth type is 14. The numbers unveil the following:

1. 20% (8) of participants reported headaches while receiving aspartame but did not while receiving placebo.
2. 30% (12) of participants did not report headaches while receiving aspartame but did while receiving placebo.
3. 15% (6) of participants reported headaches while receiving aspartame and while receiving placebo.
4. 35% (14) of participants did not report headaches while receiving aspartame and while receiving placebo.

The four percentages comprise the distribution of the observation-pairs. They present a comprehensive account of the distinction between the effects of aspartame and placebo on the 40 subjects with respect to headache.

The percentage of subjects who reported headaches while receiving aspartame but did not while receiving placebo (20%) was lower than the percentage of subjects who did not report headaches while receiving aspartame but did while receiving placebo (30%). They suggest that as far as the 40 subjects of the study are concerned, the odds of having headache are lower while receiving aspartame than the odds while receiving placebo.

The percentage of the four types of participants yield that the percentages of subjects who reported headaches while receiving aspartame and while receiving placebo are 35% and 45%, respectively. They are descriptions of the responses of the individual participants to aspartame and placebo and are not exclusive to the data of the 40 subjects. There are other scenarios for the percentages of the four types of participants that yield 35% and 45% as the percentages of participants who reported headache while receiving aspartame and while receiving placebo.

One feature of Schiffman and Others (1987) is that it uses one single table, Table 4 (Table 7.19), to present comprehensive descriptions of the effects of aspartame and placebo on as many as 11 adverse symptoms. Each row of the table displays the numbers of the four types of observation-pairs with respect to one symptom. The numbers may be used to compute the percentages of four types of observation-pairs that constitute the distribution of the observation-pairs of two paired dichotomous data sets.

Table 7.19 Table 3 of Schiffman and Others (1987)

Table 3 Numbers of subjects with adverse symptoms according to treatment[a]

Symptom	Aspartame	Placebo	Both	Neitku
Headache	8	12	6	14
Dizziness	3	3	1	33
Fatigue	3	3	0	34
Nausea	4	5	0	31
Numbness	0	1	0	39
Tinnitus	I	1	0	38
Visual impairment	2	1	2	35
Anxiety	3	2	0	35
Disorientation	1	1	0	38
Other symptoms	8	12	6	14
Any symptom except headache	11	13	8	8

[a]Headache occurred with both treatments, neither treatment, aspartame and not placebo, and placebo and not aspartame. P-values for McNemar's test in the exact form ranged from 0.50 for headache to 1.00 for the symptoms that occurred less frequently. The 95% confidence interval for the difference in incidence rates between aspartame and placebo was −35 to +12%.

Example 7.4.4 Janerich (323, 10)

Janerich and Others (1990) presented the results of a case–control study that studies 191 nonsmoking lung cancer cases and 191 lung cancer-free controls. Each control was identified by matching with a specific case in terms of age (within five years), sex and county of residence. Household exposure to tobacco smoke of a subject was measured by smoker-years, the product of the number of years the subject lived in the household and the number of smokers in the household. The association between the risk of lung cancer and exposure to tobacco smoke during three periods of life was evaluated. One description of the revelations of the smoker-years is presented in the article as follows:

> Table 2 shows the odds ratios for developing lung cancer in relation to the degree of exposure to tobacco smoke in the household for the 191 nonsmoking case–control pairs. The data are stratified by levels of exposure (measured in smoker-years) and by the period of life when the exposure occurred. Exposure during childhood and adolescence was defined as exposures that occurred when the participants were less than 21 years of age. Exposure during adulthood includes all household exposures from 21 years of age to the time of diagnosis. Although the odds ratios for the higher exposure categories are somewhat higher than those for the lower categories, no clear dose–response relation is evident, and most of the 95 percent confidence intervals include 1.0. For exposure in childhood and adolescence, the highest level of exposure is associated with the greatest elevation in risk, and the 95 percent confidence interval excludes the null value (odds ratio, 2.07; 95 percent confidence interval, 1.16 to 3.68).

To read intelligently, it is useful to review Table 2 (Table 7.20), which shows the numbers and percentages of cases and controls whose smoker-years belonged to categories, odds ratios, and 95% confidence intervals. A footnote of Table 2 indicates: *Odds ratios are shown for a person with the exposure specified as compared with a person with no exposure (0 smoker-years).* This suggests that the odds ratios are assessments of distinctions in risks of lung cancer in subjects whose smoker-years belonged to a level relative to the risk of the subjects whose smoker-years were zero. The odds ratio 2.07 is displayed in the row showing the numbers and percentages of cases and controls whose exposures during childhood and adolescence were $\geq$25 smoker-years. It is the ratio of the odds of being a lung cancer case among the subjects whose childhood and adolescence exposures were $\geq$ 25 smoker-years relative to the subjects who were not exposed to household tobacco smoke during childhood and adolescence and suggests that the risk of lung cancer of the subjects whose childhood and adolescence exposure were $\geq$ 25 smoker-years is 2.07 times the risk of the subjects who were not exposed to household tobacco smoke during childhood and adolescence. The 95% confidence interval of the odds ratio 1.16 to 3.68 excludes the null value of odds ratio 1.0 and suggests that the odds ratio 2.07 may be declared statistically significant. However, the interval is wide. Its boundaries are 56% and 178% of the odds ratio 2.07 and suggest that if the study were replicated a score of times, the odds ratios of some replicated studies might be as little as 56% or as much as 178% of the reported odds ratio. The reproducibility of the odds ratio 2.07 is inadequate. Although the odds ratio 2.07 may be declared statistically significant, it is astute to limit it to the 191 cases and 191 controls of the study.

Table 7.20 Table 2 of Janerich and Others (1990)

Table 2 Relation of smoker-years of exposure to environmental tobacco smoke to the risk of lung cancer among persons who never smoked more than 100 cigarettes[a]

No of smoker-years	Case patients	Controls	Odds ratio (95% CI)
	no. (%)		
Childhood and adolescence[b]			
0	57 (29.8)	68 (35.6)	–
1–24	82 (42.9)	94 (49.2)	1 09 (0.68-1.73)
≥25	52 (27.2)	29(15.2)	2.07 (1.16-3.68)
Adulthood			
0	44 (23.0)	39 (20.4)	–
1–24	37 (19.4)	48 (25.1)	0.64(0.34-1.21)
25–49	46 (24.1)	50 (26.2)	0.81 (0.45-1.45)
50–74	36 (18.9)	32 (16.8)	1.00 (0.52-1.93)
≥75	28 (14.7)	22(11.5)	1.11 (0.56-2.20)
Lifetime			
0	32 (16.8)	33 (17.3)	–
1–24	20 (10.5)	27 (14.1)	0.78 (0.36-1.67)
25–49	35 (18.3)	46(24.1)	0.80 (0.43-1.50)
50–74	44 (23.0)	40 (20.9)	1.19 (0.63-2.27)
75–99	33 (17.3)	21 (11.0)	1.80 (0.83-3.90)
≥100	27 (14.1)	24 (12.6)	1.13 (0.56-2.28)

[a]Based on 191 matched case–control pairs. CI denotes confidence interval. Odds ratios arc shown for a person with the exposure specified as compared with a person with no exposure (0 smoker-years). Because of rounding, percentages do not always total 100
[b]Less than 21 years of age

The Methods section states:

> Statistical techniques appropriate for the analysis of individually matched case–control studies were used. For clarity of presentation, percentages were tabulated for case patients and control participants separately, rather than for matched pairs. However, odds ratios were computed on the basis of the matched pairs.

The controls were identified by matching with specific cases individually. Each case and its matched control constitute a case–control pair. The childhood and adolescence smoker-years were stratified into three categories; they specify nine types of case–control pairs. The odds ratio 2.07 was determined from percentages of case–control pairs and not percentages of cases and controls whose childhood and adolescence smoker-years belonged to the three categories that are shown in Table 2. The presentation of the numbers and percentages of cases and controls whose childhood and adolescence smoker-years were 0, 1–24, and ≥ 25 smoker-years is clear. However, they are not directly related to the odds ratios. It is more informative to present the percentages or numbers of the 9 types of case–control pairs.

Review Questions

1. Do percentages of YES among before and among after treatment observations unveil informatively how the conditions of a group of subjects changed individually?
2. Do percentages of before–after observation-pairs unveil informatively how the conditions of a group of subjects changed individually?
3. Do percentages of YES and NO observations among before and among after treatment observations yield precise values of percentages of before–after observation-pairs?
4. Do percentages of before–after observation-pairs yield precise values of the percentages of YES and NO observations among the before and among the after observations?
5. To depict revelations of paired dichotomous data sets synoptically, what is the merit of the ratio of percentages of discordant pairs?
6. Why are revelations of paired dichotomous data sets depicted by percentages of YES and NO observations, but statistical significance is tested by procedures for paired dichotomous data sets?

Exercise

7.E.1 Suppose that the tonsillectomy rates of 100 Hodgkin's disease cases of Vianna and Others (1971) and their matched controls are 67% and 43%, respectively.

(a) Compute the ratio and difference of the two tonsillectomy rates and elaborate their suggestions.

(b) Make up two scenarios for the percentages of four types of case–control pairs that yield 67% and 43% as the tonsillectomy rates of the cases and the controls. One scenario shows that the percentage of case–control pairs in which the case did not undergo tonsillectomy but the control did is 1%, and the other shows that the percentage is 32%.

(c) Elaborate the relative advantages of using odds ratios for paired dichotomous data sets (Eq. 7.3.1) to underscore the revelations of the tonsillectomy data of the cases and their matched controls.

7.E.2 Table 3 of Madhi and Others (2014) shows that the numbers (percentages) of 142 IIV3 recipients who had seroprotective HAI titers before and after receiving the A(H1N1)pdmb09 strain were 73 (51.4%) and 133 (93.7%), respectively.

(a) Discuss whether the numbers and percentage unveil how the HAI titers of the recipients changed after vaccination individually.

(b) Make up two disagreeing scenarios of the percentages of observation-pairs that yield the reported percentages. Elaborate the insinuations of the two scenarios.

(c) Compute the five synoptic measures defined by Eqs. 7.3.1 to 7.3.5 and discuss their usefulness.

7.E.3 Review Table 4 of Bullen and Others (1985) (Table 7.1).
  (a) Elaborate the suggestions of the numbers and percentages of subjects who had clinical disorders during the two menstrual cycles.
  (b) Discuss whether the numbers and percentages unveil how the conditions of the subjects changed between the two cycles. Why?
  (c) Make up one scenario of the percentages of change patterns that yield the reported percentages during two menstrual cycles.
  (d) Elaborate the suggestion of the scenario.

7.E.4 Table 1 of Fawzi and Others (2004) (Example 7.1.4) shows that among the 268 women in the multivitamins + vitamin A group, the percentages of subjects whose WHO disease stages were I, II, and III at baseline were 80.4%, 18.1%, and 1.5%, respectively. Table 2 shows that at the end of follow-up, 70 progressed to stage IV or death from AIDS-related causes, 60 to death from AIDS-related causes, 22 to stage IV, 163 to ≥stage III, and 133 to ≥stage II increase.
  (a) Discuss suggestions of the numbers of subjects displayed in the two tables.
  (b) Use a paired data two-way table to present a likely scenario or the percentages and numbers of progression patterns of the 268 women that would yield the percentages and numbers shown in Table 1 and Table 2.
  (c) Articulate the suggestions of the scenario.

7.E.5 Table 1 of Olschewski and Others (2002) (Example 7.1.5) shows that in the placebo group, the NYHA classes of 59 (57.8%) of the subjects were III and those of 43 (42.2%) were IV. Table 7.3 shows percentages and numbers of subjects of the placebo group whose conditions changed in five ways that were displayed in Table 2 of Olschewski and Others (2002). Suggest a scenario for the percentages of change patterns of the 102 subjects that yield the percentages of subjects whose NYHA classes improved by one class, by two classes, worsened, and unchanged. Elaborate the suggestions of the scenario.

7.E.6 Table 3 of Schiffman and Others (1987) (Table 7.16) shows number of subjects who reported fatigue. Use a paired data two-way table to present a comprehensive description of the data pertaining to reporting fatigue and elaborate the suggestions of the data.

7.E.7 Table 3 of Speich and Others (2014) (Example 7.4.1) shows that among the 120 children in the oxantel pamoate group, adverse events were observed in 17.5% (21) at baseline, 13.2% (16) at 3 hours, and 16.5% (20) at 24 hours after the first treatment.
  (a) Elaborate what the percentages suggest.
  (b) Suggest a scenario for the percentages of progression patterns that yield the reported percentages.
  (c) Elaborate the suggestions of the scenario.

References

Bullen, B. A., et al. (1985). Induction of menstrual disorders by strenuous exercise in untrained women. *The New England Journal of Medicine, 312*(21), 1349–1353.

Fawzi, W. W., et al. (2004). A randomized trial of multivitamin supplements and HIV disease progression and mortality. *The New England Journal of Medicine, 351*(1), 23–32.

Janerich, D. T., et al. (1990). Lung cancer and exposure to tobacco smoke in the household. *The New England Journal of Medicine, 323*(10), 632–636.

Johnson, S. K., & Johnson, R. E. (1972). Tonsillectomy history in Hodgkin's disease. *The New England Journal of Medicine, 315*(17), 1122–1125.

Madhi, S. A., et al. (2014). Influenza vaccination of pregnant women and protection of their infants. *The New England Journal of Medicine, 371*(10), 918–931.

Olschewski, H., et al. (2002). Inhaled Iloprost for severe pulmonary hypertension. *The New England Journal of Medicine, 347*(5), 322–329.

Pike, M. C., & Smith, P. G. (1972). Lancet.

Pike, M. C., & Smith P. G. (1973). Tonsillectomy and Hodgkin's disease. *The Lancet, 301*(7800), 434.

Schiffman, S. S., et al. (1987). Aspartame and susceptibility to headache. *The New England Journal of Medicine, 317*(19), 1181–1185.

Shamim, W., et al. (2002). Nonsurgical reductions of the interventricular septum in patients with hypertrophic cardiomyopathy. *The New England Journal of Medicine, 347*(17), 1326–1333.

Speich, B., et al. (2014). Oxantel pamoate-albendazole for *Trichuris trichiura*. *The New England Journal of Medicine, 370*(7), 610–620.

Thakar, R., et al. (2002). Outcomes after total versus subtotal abdominal hysterectomy. *The New England Journal of Medicine, 347*(17), 1318–1325.

Vianna, N. J., & Davies, J. N. (1971). Tonsillectomy and Hodgkin's disease: The lymphoid tissue barrier. *Lancet, 1*(7696), 431–432.

Chapter 8
Relationship Between Two Quantitative Variables

Evaluating how observations on two quantitative variables relate is an important task in medical research.

This chapter demonstrates that observations on two quantitative variables may relate in various ways, and how observations on two quantitative variables relate is eloquently manifested by scatterplots that depict observations graphically. Least-squares equations of regression analyses are often presented to supplement manifestations of scatterplots. Values of correlation coefficients are cited. Statistical significance is declared when *P*-values of statistical significance tests are small. Statistically significant relationships are frequently oversimplifications or distractions. The suggestions of correlation coefficients are technical and sketchy.

Section 8.1 uses examples to demonstrate that observations on two quantitative variables may relate in many ways. Use of least-squares equations of regression analyses and correlation coefficients to supplement manifestations of scatterplots is examined in Sect. 8.2. Section 8.3 illustrates that "significant relationships" are often oversimplifications, distractions, or both. Intelligent reading and informative reporting are illustrated by examples in Sect. 8.4.

8.1 Examples

This section reviews examples of descriptions of relationships between observations on two quantitative variables.

Example 8.1.1
Leonard and Others (2004) present the results of a study that evaluated the effect of glucocorticoids on growth and nutritional status. The study performed dual energy ray absorptiometry of the whole body and spine in 60 children and adolescents with glucocorticoid-sensitive nephrotic syndrome and 195 without it.

P. C. Chang, *Data Analysis of Medical Studies*,
https://doi.org/10.1007/978-3-031-49984-5_8

Fig. 8.1 Figure 1 of Leonard and Others (2004)

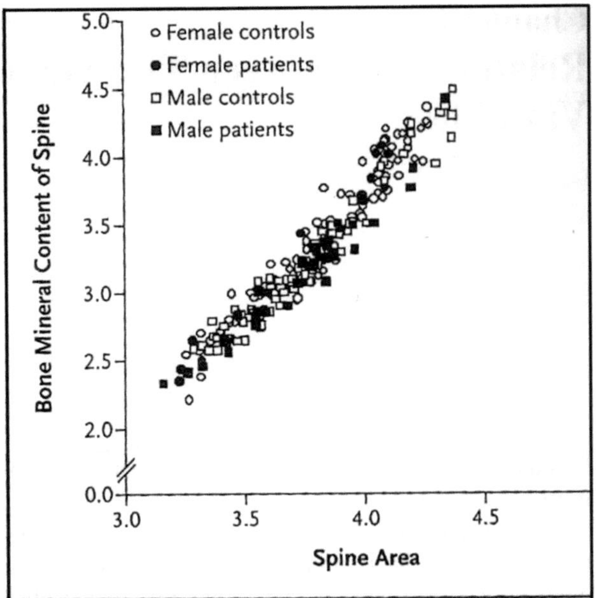

Figure 1. Bone Mineral Content of the Lumbar Spine Relative to Bone Area in Patients with Glucocorticoid-Sensitive Nephrotic Syndrome and Control Subjects. Values have been log-transformed.

The bone mineral content of the spine and the spine area of a subject form an observation-pair. Figure 1 of the article (Fig. 8.1) uses dots to denote pairs of logarithms of the bone mineral contents of the spine and logarithms of the spine areas of the 255 subjects. The height of a dot signifies the logarithm of bone mineral content in accordance with labels marked along a vertical line, and the distance of a dot from the vertical line signifies the logarithm of spine area in accordance with labels marked along a horizontal line.

Pairs of logarithms of bone mineral contents of spine and logarithms of areas of spine of female and male patients and controls are denoted by dots of different symbols. The four types of dots are well mixed. The logarithms of the bone mineral contents of the spines vary in narrow ranges, and the ranges are higher when logarithms of spine areas are larger. They impart the image of a narrow strip and suggest a relatively close relationship. The bone mineral contents of the spine of the subjects tend to be larger when their areas of spine are larger.

Example 8.1.2

Boyd and Others (2002) present the results of a study that collected mammogram data from 353 pairs of monozygotic twins and 246 pairs of dizygotic twins from Australia and 218 pairs of monozygotic twins and 134 pairs of dizygotic twins from Canada and the United States. The total area of the breast and the area of dense tissue

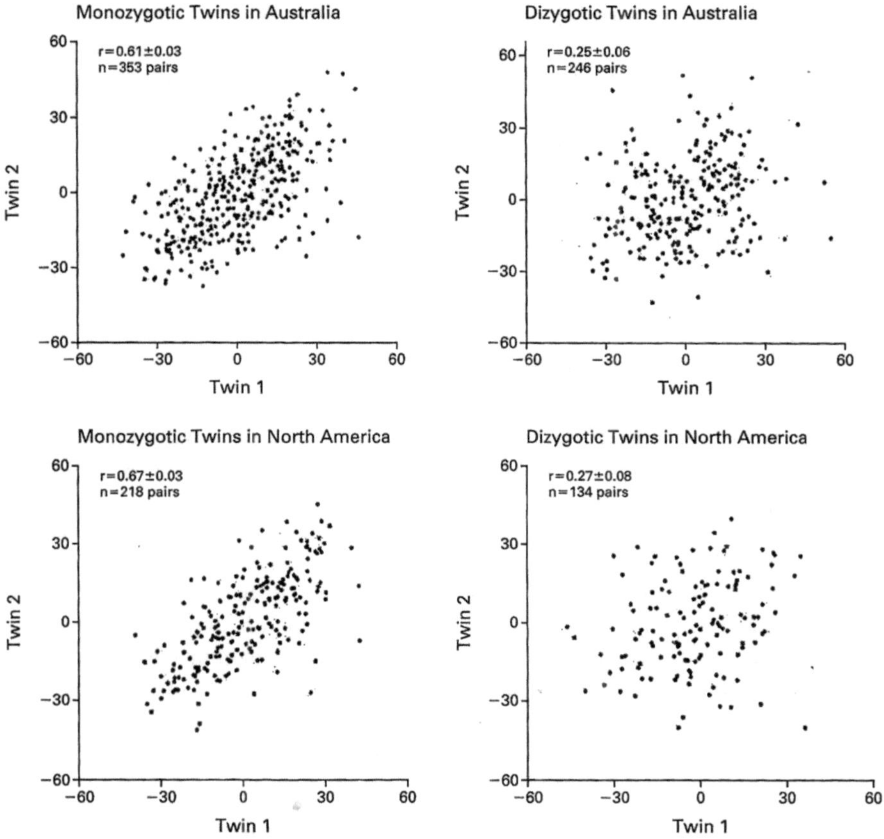

Figure 3. Correlations in the Percentage of Dense Tissue for Paris of Twins in Australia and North America. Plus-minus values are estimates ±SE.

Fig. 8.2 Figure 3 of Boyd and Others (2002)

that appeared on the mammogram were measured to calculate the percentage of dense tissue.

Figure 3 of the article (Fig. 8.2) uses dots to denote percentages of tense tissues of pairs of twins. The two twins of a pair are designated twin 1 and twin 2. Percentages of dense tissues of twin 2s are signified by heights of dots in accordance with labels marked along a vertical line, and percentages of dense tissues of twin 1s are signified by distances of dots from the vertical axis in accordance with labels marked along a horizontal line, the horizontal axis. There are four assortments of dots; they show how the percentages of tense tissues in each of the four groups of twins relate.

For instance, the top left panel suggests that the percentages of dense tissues of the twin 2s of the 353 homozygotic twins from Australia vary in moderately wide ranges of increasing heights when the percentages of twin 1s are larger. The assortment of dots imparts an image of American football and suggests that the percentages of dense tissues of the 353 homozygotic twins are moderately related.

The panel shows $r = 0.61 \pm 0.03$ and $n = 353$ pairs. The symbol r denotes the correlation coefficient. Its value of 0.61 is moderately close to 1.0 and confirms the indication of the assortment of dots that the percentages of dense tissues of the 353 pairs of homozygotic twins from Australia are moderately related. The value following the ± sign is the standard error of the correlation coefficient; it is an improvised estimate of the standard deviation of the correlation coefficients of replicates of the study if the study replicated a score of times, and suggests that the correlation coefficients of most replicates of the study might vary between 0.52 and 0.67 approximately.

The top right panel suggests that the percentages of dense tissues of the twin 2s of the 246 dizygotic twins from Australia vary in wide ranges of similar heights whether the percentages of twin 1s are smaller or larger. The assortment of dots imparts the image of a ragged basketball and suggests that the percentages of dense tissues of the 246 dizygotic twins are not related.

The panel shows $r = 0.25 \pm 0.06$ and $n = 246$ pairs. The symbol r denotes the correlation coefficient. Its value of 0.25 is relatively close to 0 and confirms the indication of the assortment of dots that the relationship of the percentages of dense tissues of the 246 pairs of dizygotic twins from Australia is negligible. The value 0.06 is the standard error of the correlation coefficient; it is an improvised estimate of the standard deviation of the correlation coefficients of replicates of the study if the study were replicated a score of times, and suggests that the correlation coefficients of most replicates of the study might vary between 0.13 and 0.37 approximately.

Example 8.1.3

A study investigated the use of urinary anion gap (sodium plus potassium minus chloride) in the evaluation of hyperchloremic metabolic acidosis in 38 patients with altered distal urinary acidification, 8 patients with diarrhea, and 7 normal subjects receiving ammonium chloride. Results of the study are reported by Battle and Others (1988). One result is described as follows:

> When normal subjects receiving ammonium chloride and all patients were considered together, there was a significant inverse correlation between urinary ammonium (y) and the urinary anion gap (x): y = -0.42x + 23.6 (r = 0.72, P<0.001). Thus, the higher the anion gap, the lower the urinary ammonium concentration (Fig. 3)

The assertion of a significant inverse correlation is corroborated by $y = -0.42x + 23.6$ ($r = 0.72$, $P < 0.001$) and Fig. 3 (Fig. 8.3). The equation $y = -0.42x + 23.6$ is a description of the relationship between the mean of the urinary ammonium concentrations and the urinary anion gaps of 53 subjects. The notation $r = 0.72$ suggests that the correlation coefficient equals −0.72. It is not close to −1.0 and does not suggest that the equation $y = -0.42x + 23.6$ and the urinary anion gaps of the 53 subjects yield accurate appraisals of the urinary ammonium concentrations of the subjects.

Figure 3 uses positions of dots to denote the 53 pairs of urinary ammonium concentration and urinary anion gap. Values of urinary ammonium concentrations

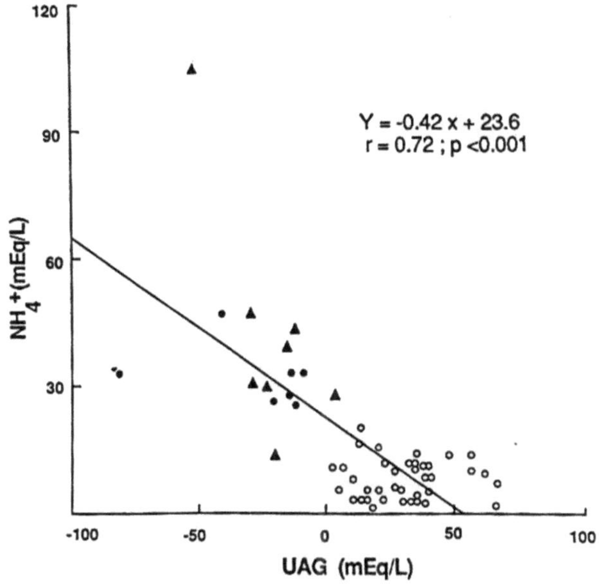

Fig. 8.3 Figure 3 of Battle and Others (1988)

Figure 3. Urinary Ammonium (NH_4^+) in Relation to the Urinary Anion Gap (UAG).

The 38 patients with altered distal urinary acidification are represented by open circles; the 7 normal subjects receiving ammonium chloride, by closed circles; and the 8 patients with hyperchloremic metabolic acidosis associated with diarrhea, by triangles.

are signified by heights of dots in accordance with labels marked along a vertical line; values of urinary anion gaps are signified by distances of dots from the vertical line in accordance with labels marked along a horizontal line. A graphical display of the equation $y = -0.42x + 23.6$ is depicted.

$P < 0.001$ is an improvised estimate of the probability that the correlation coefficient deviates from 0 as much as -0.72 or more if chance was the explanation. It is smaller than 0.05 and suggests that the correlation coefficient (-0.72) could be declared statistically significant.

Example 8.1.4

Rivkees and Others (1988) present the results of a study that treated 18 girls and 6 boys with severe primary hypothyroidism with levothyroxine to maintain normal thyroid function. One outcome of the study is was related as follows:

> The loss in adult height (the difference between the height predicted at diagnosis, based on bone age, and the actual adult height) correlated significantly with the duration of untreated hypothyroidism and with the height standard deviation score at diagnosis (Fig. 3).

Figure 3 (Fig. 8.4) uses the positions of dots to denote the 16 pairs of loss of predicted mature height and duration of hypothyroidism. The heights of dots signify magnitudes of loss of predicted mature height in accordance with labels marked

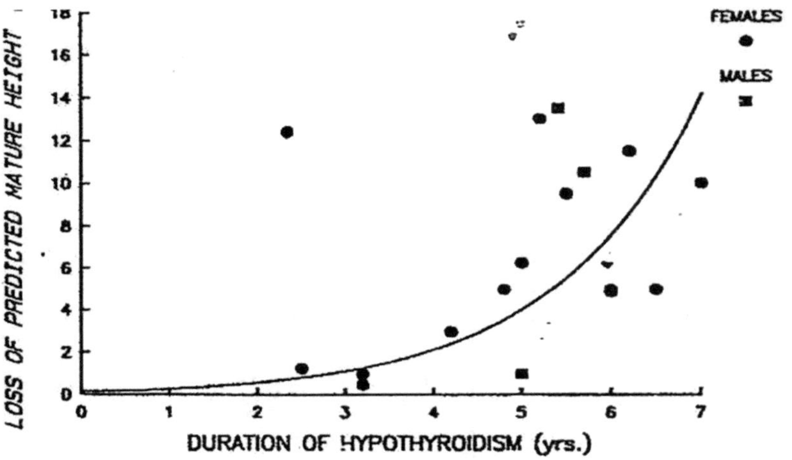

Figure 3. Relation between Loss in Adult Height of Treated Children with Hypothyroidism (Predicted Adult Height at Diagnosis Minus Actual Mature Height) and Duration of Hypothyroidism at Diagnosis (Chronologic Age Minus Bone Age). ($y = 0.18e^{0.06x}$; $r = 0.76$; $P<0.01$).

Fig. 8.4 Figure 3 of Rivkees and Others (1988)

along a vertical line; distances of dots from the vertical line signify lengths of duration of hypothyroidism in accordance with labels marked along a horizontal line. The dots show that the losses of predicted mature height of subjects whose durations of hypothyroidism are longer vary in higher ranges.

A curve is displayed to underscore the manifestation of the dots. The caption of the figure suggests that it is a graphical display of the exponential curve $y = 0.18e^{0.6x}$, which is a description of the relationship between the mean of loss of predicted mature height and duration of hypothyroidism. The caption of the figure also shows $r = 0.76$ and $P < 0.01$. The value 0.76 is probably the coefficient of determination of the exponential equation $y = 0.18e^{0.6x}$. It is not far below 1.0 and suggests that the exponential equation is a relatively useful characterization of the relationship demonstrated by the 16 pairs of loss of predicted adult height and duration of hypothyroidism.

$P < 0.01$ suggests that 0.76 may be declared statistically significant.

Example 8.1.5

Battle and Others (1988) (Example 8.1.3) used its Figure 2 (Fig. 8.5) to depict how 20 pairs of urinary pH level and urinary sodium concentrations of subjects with diarrhea relate. The height of a dot represents the value of urinary pH in accordance with the labels marked along a vertical line, and the distance of a dot from the vertical line represents the value of urinary sodium concentration in accordance with the labels marked along a horizontal line. A curve is exhibited to underscore the

Fig. 8.5 Figure 2 of Battle and Others (1988)

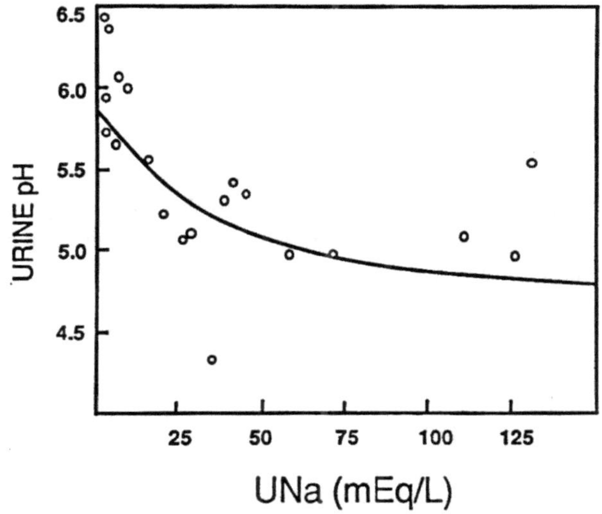

Figure 2. Urinary pH in Relation to Urinary Sodium Concentration in Eight Patients with Diarrhea.

Urinary sodium was increased by administration of either furosemide or sodium chloride in only three patients. The relation between urinary pH (y) and urinary sodium (x) could be expressed as a curvilinear line, according to the following equation: y = −0.16 ln(x) + 5.8 (r = 0.75, P<0.001).

manifestation of the dots. The footnote of the figure suggests that the curve is a graphical display of the equation $y = -0.16\ \ln(x) + 5.6$. The footnote also shows $r = 0.75$ and $P < 0.001$. The value 0.75 is probably the coefficient of determination of the equation $y = -0.16\ \ln(x) + 5.6$. It is relatively close to 1.0 and confirms the indication of the figure that most dots are not far from the curve. $P < 0.001$ suggests that the coefficient of determination may be declared statistically significant.

Manifestation of the scatterplot was articulated candidly by the following account:

> The urinary pH was related to the urinary sodium concentration, in that when urinary sodium was very low (less than 25 mm per liter approximately), urinary pH could not be reduced below 5.3, but when urinary sodium increased, urinary pH fell below 5.3 in all but one patient (Fig. 2).

This is a candid description of the relationship between urinary pH levels and urinary sodium concentrations in the 38 subjects.

8.2 Regression Analysis and Correlation Coefficient

The above examples demonstrate that observations on two quantitative variables may relate in various ways, and how they relate is informatively manifested by scatterplots that depict the observations graphically. Least-squares equations of regression analyses or values of correlation coefficients are often presented to supplement the manifestation of scatterplots. The least-squares equations may be oversimplifications or distractions.

- *Scatterplot*

The observations on two quantitative variables of the same observational unit form an observation-pair. A scatterplot uses the positions of symbols to signify observation-pairs. One variable is designated the outcome, response, or dependent variable, and the other is designated the explanatory, predictor, or independent variables. The heights of the symbols signify the values of the outcome variable in accordance with labels marked along a vertical line, and the distances of the symbols from the vertical line signify the values of the explanatory variables in accordance with labels marked along a horizontal line. The lines are the vertical and horizontal axes of the plot.

The dots demonstrate how the observation of the two variable relate informatively.

Figures 8.1 to 8.5 are examples of scatterplots. They demonstrate how observations on two quantitative variables relate candidly and show that observations on two quantitative variables may relate in various ways.

- *Least-Squares Equation*

Manifestations of scatterplots are often underlined by least-squares equations of regression analysis. The line shown in Fig. 8.3 and the curves shown in Figs. 8.4 and 8.5 are graphical displays of least-squares equations.

When observations on two quantitative variables are analyzed to assess how they relate, one variable is designated the outcome (response or *dependent*) variable, and the other the explanatory (predictor or *independent*) variable. A regression analysis determines from observations an expression of a mathematical function that presumes how the two variable relate. The function is the regression function of the analysis, and the resulting expression is a characterization of the relationship. Usually, the expression is determined by the method of least-squares or maximum likelihood. In this book, the expression is dubbed a least-squares equation for convenience.

Whether the least-squares equation of a regression analysis embodies a straight line or a curve is determined by the regression function of the analysis. When the regression function presumes that the relationship is characterized by a straight line, it is called a linear regression analysis. Its least-squares equation embodies a straight line and is dubbed a least-squares line. When the regression function of a regression analysis presumes that the relationship is characterized by a curve, it is called a curvilinear regression analysis. Its least-squares equation embodies a curve and is dubbed a least-squares curve. Least-square equations are descriptions of the relationships between the mean of observations on the outcome variables and values of the explanatory variable.

The usefulness of the least-squares equation of a regression analysis is determined by the following two indications of scatterplot:

- Whether the least-squares equation is a literal characterization of the relationship between the means of the observation of the outcome variable and values of the explanatory variable
- How close the observation-pairs are to the least-squares equation.

A least-squares equation is misleading if it is not a literal characterization of the relationship between the means of the observations on the outcome variable and values of the explanatory variable. It is an oversimplification if many observation-pairs are distant from it.

For instance, if the regression function of a regression analysis presumes that the relationship between loss of predicted adult height and duration of hypothyroidism is characterized by a straight line, the data of Rivkees and Others (1988) would yield a least-squares line.

- *Coefficient of Determination*

An important result of regression analysis is the coefficient of determination of its least-squares equation. If the least-squares equation of a regression analysis is used to appraise values of observations of the outcome variable from values of observations on the explanatory variable, the sum of the squares of the deviations between the appraisals by the least-squares equation and the observations on the outcome variable is a measure of the overall error of the appraisals. It is labeled an error sum of squares. The sum of the squares of the deviations between the observations on the outcome variable and their mean is a measure of the overall error of the rudimentary appraisal that all observations on the outcome variable are identical and equal their mean. It is labeled a total sum of squares. The error sum of squares is smaller than or equal to the total sum of squares. Their difference is labeled the regression sum of squares. When the total sum of squares, error sum of squares, and regression sum of squares of a least-squares equation are written as SST, SSE, and SSR, SST = SSR + SSE. The coefficient of determination of the equation, written as R^2, is:

$$R^2 = 1 - \frac{\text{SSE}}{\text{SST}} = \frac{\text{SSR}}{\text{SST}} \tag{8.2.1}$$

It relates to accuracy if the least-squares equation and observations on the explanatory variable are used to appraise the observations on the outcome variables. It ranges between 0 and 1.0. Close to 1.0 suggests that the least-squares equation yields relatively accurate appraisals, and close to 0 suggests that the equation yields appraisals that are nearly as erroneous as those of the rudimentary appraisal that all observations on the outcome variable are identical and equal their mean.

One way to assess the suggestion of the coefficient of determination of a least-squares equation more specifically is to note that its difference from 1.0 ($1.0 - R^2$) is a measure of the overall error of using the equation and observations on the explanatory variable to appraise observations on the outcome variable relative to the overall error of rudimentary appraisal that all observations on the outcome variable are identical and equal their mean.

The error sum of squares (SSE) is a measure of the overall error of the appraisals of the observations on the outcome variable by the least-squares equation and observations on the explanatory variable, and the total sum of squares (SST) is a measure of the overall error of the rudimentary appraisal that all observations on the outcome variable are identical and equal their mean. The fraction SSE/SST $= 1.0 - R^2$ is a measure of the overall error of the appraisals of the observations on the outcome variable by the least-squares equation and observations on the explanatory variable relative to the overall error of the rudimentary appraisal that all observations on the outcome variable are identical and equal their mean.

When the coefficient of determination of a least-squares equation is $R^2 = 0.40$, $1.0 - R^2 = 0.60$ suggests that the overall error of the appraisals of the observations on the outcome variable by the least-squares equation and observations on the explanatory variable is 60% of the overall error of the rudimentary appraisal that all observations on the outcome variable are identical and equal to their mean. When the coefficient of determination of a least-squares equation is $R^2 = 0.70$, $1.0 - R^2 = 0.30$ suggests that the overall error of the appraisals of the observations on the outcome variable by the least-squares equation and observations on the explanatory variable is 30% of the overall error of the rudimentary appraisal that all observations on the outcome variable are identical and equal to their mean.

- *Correlation Coefficient*

Correlation coefficients are often presented to corroborate narratives of relationships between observations on two quantitative variables. Its indication is technical and subtle. Its value relates to the closeness of observation-pairs to the least-square line of linear regression analysis and is useful only if the relationship between observations on two quantitative variables is characterized by a straight line. It also relates to the slope of the line.

The correlation coefficient is usually denoted by r. It is close to 1.0 or -1.0 if all observation-pairs are close to the least-squares line and are close to 0 if most observation-pairs are distant from the least-squares line and the line is nearly horizontal.

One way to gauge the suggestion of a correlation coefficient is to note that its square is the coefficient of determination of a least-squares line and that one minus the coefficient of determination is a measure of the overall error of using the least-squares line and observations on the explanatory variable to appraise the observations on the outcome variable relative to the overall error of the rudimentary appraisal that all observations on the outcome variables are identical and equal their mean.

For instance, a correlation coefficient of 0.40 or -0.40 suggests that the coefficient of determination of the least-squares line is $R^2 = 0.16$. $1 - R^2 = 0.84$ suggests that the overall error of the appraisals of observations on the outcome variable by the least-squares line and observations on the explanatory variable is as much as 84% of the overall error of the rudimentary appraisal that all observations on the outcome variable are identical and equal the mean of the observations. A correlation coefficient of 0.70 or -0.70 suggests that the coefficient of determination of the least-squares line is $R^2 = 0.49$. $1 - R^2 = 0.51$ suggests that the overall error of the appraisals of observations on the outcome variable by the least-squares line and observations on the explanatory variable is 51% of the overall error of the rudimentary appraisal that all observations on the outcome variable are identical and equal the mean of the observation.

- *P-Values of Statistical Significance Tests*

P-values of statistical significance tests are cited frequently. Relationships are declared statistically significant when *P*-values are smaller than 0.05. The small *P*-values suggest only that the deviations of coefficients of determination or correlation coefficients from 0 would be particularly unlikely if chance were the explanation. It is alright to dismiss the concern that the coefficients of determination or correlation coefficients are incidental. It is not an affirmation that the relationship is strong and clinically important. The relationship may be trivial. *P*-values larger than 0.05 suggest only that the deviations of coefficients of determination or correlation coefficients from 0 would not be particularly unlikely if chance were the explanation. It is not astute to dismiss the concern that the coefficients of determination or correlation coefficients are incidental.

Example 8.2.1
Figure 1 of Leonard and Others (2004) (Fig. 8.1) present a scatterplot. It shows clearly that the logarithms of bone mineral contents of spines and logarithms of spine areas of the 255 subjects are closely related.

Pairs of logarithms of the bone mineral contents of the spine and logarithms of the spine areas of 255 subjects are denoted by dots. The logarithm of the bone mineral content of the spine is the outcome variable, and the logarithm of the spine area is the explanatory variable. Labels are marked on a vertical line to specify values of logarithms of bone mineral content signified by heights of dots; labels are marked on a horizontal line to specify values of logarithm of spine areas by distances from the vertical line. The lines are the vertical and horizontal axes of the scatterplots.

The indication of the scatterplot is clear. Least-squares equation of regression analysis and correlation coefficient are not cited.

Example 8.2.2
The assortments of dots denoting percentages of dense tissues of twins displayed in Figure 3 of Boyd and Others (2002) (Fig. 8.2) are scatterplots. They unveil plainly how percentages of dense tissues of the twins relate. Correlation coefficients and their standard errors are exhibited to supplement the indications of the scatterplots.

The scatterplot of the top left panel shows that the percentages of dense tissues of the homozygotic twins from Australian are moderately related. The panel shows $r = 0.61 \pm 0.03$ and $n = 353$. The correlation coefficient 0.61 relates to the closeness of the 353 pairs of percentages of dense tissue to the least-squares line of linear regression analysis. Its square $0.61^2 = 0.37$ is the coefficient of determination of the least-square line of linear regression analysis. One minus the square of the correlation coefficient $1.0 - 0.61^2$ equals 0.63. It suggests that if the least-squares line and the percentages of dense tissue of twin 1s were used to appraise the percentages of dense tissue of twin 2s, the overall error of the appraisals would be as much as 63% of the overall error of the rudimental appraisal that the dense tissues of all twin 2s are identical and equal their mean.

The standard error: 0.03 is an improvised estimate of the standard deviation of the distribution of the correlation coefficients of replicates of the study if the study were replicated a score of times. It yields [0.55 to 0.67] an estimate of the region of the distribution of the correlation coefficients of replicates of the study that would include approximately 95% of the correlation coefficients. The boundaries of the region are within 10% of the correlation coefficient: 0.61. The standard error: 0.03 may be considered a suggestion that the correlation coefficient is adequately reproducible.

The scatterplot of the top right panel shows that the percentages of dense tissues of the 246 dizygotic twins from Australia scatter in similar wide spans of similar heights whether the dense tissues of twin 1 s are small or large. The percentages of dense tissues of the 246 dizygotic twins from Australia are not related. The panel shows $r = 0.25 \pm 0.06$ and $n = 246$. The correlation coefficient of 0.25 is relatively close to 0 and agrees with the indication of the scatterplot that the percentages of the dense tissues of the 246 pairs of dizygotic twins from Australia are not related. One minus the square of the correlation coefficient $1.0 - 0.25^2$ equals 0.94. This suggests that if the least-squares line of linear regression analysis and the percentages of dense tissue of twin 1 s were used to appraise the percentages of dense tissue of twin 2 s, the overall error of the appraisals would be as much as 94% of the overall error of the rudimental appraisal that the dense tissues of all twin 2 s are identical and equal their mean.

The standard error 0.06 is an improvised estimate of the standard deviation of distribution of the correlation coefficients of replicates of the study if the study were replicated a score of times. It yields [0.13 to 0.37] as an estimate of the region of the distribution of the correlation coefficients of replicates of the study that would include 95% of the correlation coefficients. The correlation coefficients of most replicates of the study would be small and agree with the correlation coefficient of the study that the percentages of dense tissue of the dizygotic twins from Australia are not related.

Example 8.2.3

Figure 3 of Battle and Others (1988) (Fig. 8.3) uses a scatterplot to show how urinary ammonium concentrations and urinary anion gaps of 53 subjects relate. It uses positions of dots to denote the 53 pairs of urinary ammonium concentration and urinary anion gap. The urinary ammonium concentration is the outcome variable, and the urinary anion gap is the explanatory variable. Labels are marked on a vertical line to specify values of urinary ammonium concentrations signified by heights of dots; labels are marked on a horizontal line to specify values of urinary anion gaps specified by distances of dots from the vertical line.

The figure shows: $Y = -0.42x + 23.6$, $r = 0.72$, and $p < 0.001$. These are the results of linear regression analysis. The regression function of the analysis presumes that the mean of urinary ammonium concentrations relates to values of urinary anion gap by a straight line. The equation: $Y = -0.42x + 23.6$ is the least-squares equation of the analysis. The symbol Y denotes mean of urinary ammonium concentration, and the symbol x denotes value of urinary anion gap. That the equation embodies a straight line is a result of the presumption that the mean of urinary ammonium concentrations relates to values of urinary anion gap by a straight line. The value -0.42 is the slope (rate of change) of the line, and 23.6 is the height of the line when the urinary anion gap is 0. They are results of the observations. A graphical display of the equation $Y = -0.42x + 23.6$ is shown.

The notation $r = 0.72$ suggests that the correlation coefficient of the least-square line is -0.72. It is not distant from -1.0 and suggests that, if the least-squares line and the urinary anion gaps were used to appraise the urinary ammonium concentrations of the 53 subjects, the overall error of the appraisals is 48% of the overall error of the rudimentary appraisal that the urinary ammonium concentrations of the 53 subjects are identified and equal to their mean.

$P < 0.001$ suggests that the correlation coefficient: -0.72, may be declared statistically significant, and the concern that it may be incidental may be dismissed.

Figure 3 of Battle and Others (1988) uses different symbols to denote subjects in the three groups. Open circles denote subjects with altered distal urinary acidification, and closed dots denote subjects without altered distal urinary acidification. The assortment of open circles is lower than and located to the right of the assortment of closed circles and close triangles. They unveiled that the urinary anion gaps of the subjects with altered distal urinary acidification are all positive and those of the subjects without altered distal urinary acidification are all negative, and that the urinary ammonium concentrations of the subjects with altered distal urinary acidification are lower than those of the subjects without altered distal urinary acidification.

The assortment of open circles disperses haphazardly in spans of similar heights when urinary anion gaps are small and large. It does not demonstrate a discernible relationship. The assortment of closed circles and closed triangles disperses haphazardly when urinary anion gaps are distant or only slightly below 0. It does not demonstrate a discernible relationship. The urinary ammonium concentrations and urinary anion gaps are not related if the subjects with and those without altered urinary acidification are evaluated separately.

The urinary anion gaps and urinary ammonium concentrations of the subjects with and without altered distal urinary acidification differ. The urinary anion gaps of the subjects with altered distal urinary acidification (open circles) are all positive, and their urinary ammonium concentrations are all below 20. The urinary anion gaps of the subjects without altered distal urinary acidification (closed circles and closed triangles) are all negative, and their urinary ammonium concentrations, with only one exception, are all above 20.

The regression analysis was performed by using data from 53 subjects. The least-squares line $Y = -0.42 + 23.6$, correlation coefficient $r = -0.72$, and $P < 0.001$, to a considerable extent, are the results of the distinction between the subjects with and without altered distal urinary acidification. It is more constructive to note that the urinary anion gaps and urinary ammonium concentrations are not related when the subjects with and without altered distal urinary acidification are evaluated separately.

Example 8.2.4
The scatter plot of Figure 3 of Rivkees and Others (1988) (Fig. 8.4) shows that losses of predicted mature height tend to be larger when durations of hypothyroidism are longer. The loss of predicted mature height is the outcome variable, and the duration of hypothyroidism is the explanatory variable. A vertical line marks values of loss of predicted adult height signified by heights of dots, and a horizontal line mark values of duration of hypothyroidism signified by distances from the vertical line. These are the vertical and horizontal axes of the scatterplot.

A curve is exhibited. The caption of the figure suggests that the curve is a graphical display of the exponential equation $y = 0.18e^{0.08x}$, which is the least-squares equation of a regression analysis. The regression function of the analysis presumes that the relationship between loss of predicted adult height and duration of hypothyroidism is characterized by an exponential curve of the form $y = \alpha\ e^{\beta x}$, where x denotes duration of hypothyroidism and Y mean of losses of mature height of subject whose duration of hypothyroidism is x. The values 0.18 and 0.08 are values of α and β determined from the 16 pairs of observations.

The caption of the figure also shows $r = 0.76$ and $P < 0.01$. The value 0.76 is probably the coefficient of determination of the least-squares equation $y = 0.18e^{0.08x}$. It submits that if the exponential equation was used to appraise the losses of mature height of the 16 subjects from their durations of hypothyroidism, the overall error of the appraisal is approximately 24% of the overall error of the rudimentary appraisal that the losses of all 16 subjects are identical and equal to their mean. This is consistent with the demonstration of Figure 3 that most pairs of loss of predicted mature height and duration of hypothyroidism are relatively close to the curve.

$P < 0.01$ suggests that $r = 0.76$ may be declared statistically significant. It is alright to dismiss the concern that the least-squares equation is incidental.

Example 8.2.5
The scatterplot of Figure 2 of Battle and Others (1988) (Fig. 8.5) shows clearly how urinary pH and urinary sodium concentration of eight subjects with diarrhea relate. Urinary pH levels are higher than 5.3 (5.3 to 6.5) when urinary sodium is below 25 mm per liter but lower than 5.3 (5.0 to 5.3) when urinary sodium concentrations are larger than 25 mm per liter. Urinary pH is the outcome variable, and urinary sodium concentration the explanatory variable. The vertical line that marks values of urinary pH signified by heights of dots is its vertical axis, and the horizontal line that marks values of urinary sodium concentration signified by distances from the vertical line is its horizontal axis.

A curve is exhibited to underscore the relationship demonstrated by the dots. The footnote of the figure suggests that the curve is a graphical display of the equation $y = -0.16\ \ln(x) + 0.56$. It also shows $r = 0.75$ and $P < 0.001$. The curve is a graphical display of the equation $y = -0.16\ \ln(x) + 0.56$, which is the least-squares equation of a regression analysis and a description of the relationship between the mean of urinary pH and urinary anion gap. The regression function of the analysis presumes that the relationship between the mean urinary pH and the urinary sodium concentration of subjects with diarrhea is characterized by a curve of the form *Mean of* $Y = \beta \ln(x) + \alpha$, where x denotes the urinary sodium concentration and Y urinary pH. The values −0.16 and 5.8 are the values of β and α determined from the 20 pairs of observations.

The value 0.75 is probably the coefficient of determination of the least-squares equation $y = -0.16 \ln(x) + 0.56$. If the equation $y = -0.16 \ln(x) + 0.56$ were used to appraise the urinary pH values of the 20 subjects from their urinary sodium concentrations, the overall error of the appraisals would be approximately 25% of the overall error of the rudimentary appraisal that the urinary pH values of all 20 subjects are identical and equal to their mean. This is consistent with the demonstration of Figure 2 that some pairs of loss of urinary pH and urinary sodium concentration are relatively distant from the curve.

$P < 0.001$ suggests that $r = 0.75$ may be declared statistically significant. It is alright to dismiss the concern that the least-squares equation is incidental.

8.3 Significant Relationships

Relationships between observations on two quantitative variables are often dubbed "significant." A relationship between observations on two quantitative variable is dubbed "significant" when its correlation coefficient or least-square equation characterizing the relationship between the mean of the response variable and values of the explanatory variable is declared statistically significant. The "significant" relationship may be trivial or misleading.

Correlation coefficients and least-squares equations are dubbed statistically significant when their *P*-values are smaller than 0.05. *P*-values of correlation coefficients and least-squares-equations relate to numbers of observation. The *P*-value of same correlation coefficient and least-squares equation is smaller if the correlation coefficient and least-squares equation are results of larger number of observations. Table 8.1 shows the numbers of observation-pairs that are sufficiently large so that *P*-values of correlation coefficients are below 0.05. The table shows, for instance, that the *P*-value of a correlation coefficient as small as 0.30 would be smaller than 0.05 if it were computed from 50 or more observation-pairs. The *P*-value of a

Table 8.1 Number of observation-pairs and statistical significance of correlation coefficient ($P \leq 0.05$)

Correlation coefficient	±0.1	±0.2	±0.3	±0.4	±0.5	±0.6	±0.7	±0.8	±0.9
Number of observation-pairs	400	100	50	25	20	12	8	6	5

correlation coefficient as close to 0 as −0.20 would be smaller than 0.05 if it were computed from 100 or more observation-pairs.

The statistical significance of the correlation coefficient and that of the slope of the least-squares line of linear regression analysis are closely related. When the *P*-value of a correlation coefficient is smaller than 0.05, the *P*-value of the slope of its corresponding least-squares line is also smaller than 0.05.

Example 8.3.1

Gross and Others (2002) (Example 1.1.2) uses the following account to relate the relationship between 1999 smoking rates and expenditures for tobacco control programs of the 50 US states:

> States with higher smoking rates had significantly lower expenditures for tobacco control programs (Spearman's rho = -0.38, P = 0.007) (Table 2 and Fig. 2).

Figure 2 (Fig. 8.6) uses a scatterplot to depict the 50 pairs of expenditures for tobacco control programs and smoking rates. The plot shows that the expenditures disperse haphazardly in wide ranges whether smoking rates are low or high. The expenditures and smoking rates do not demonstrate a discernible relationship. The assertion that states with higher smoking rates had significantly lower expenditures for tobacco control programs is supported by the scatterplot.

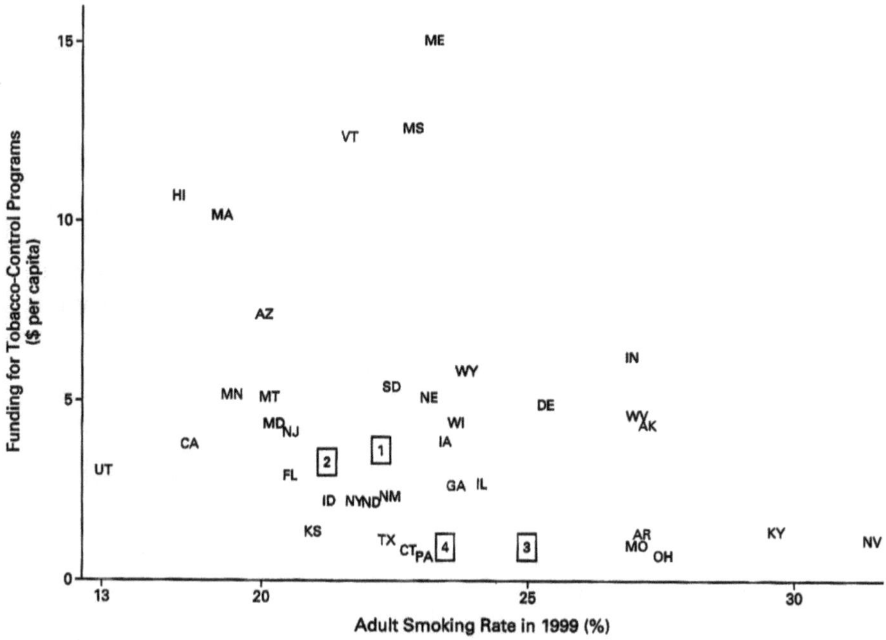

Figure 2. State Funding for Tobacco-Control Programs According to State Smoking Rates.
Several groups of states overlapped on the graph and are represented by the following boxed numbers: 1 — Colorado, Washington, Rhode Island, and New Hampshire; 2 — Oregon and Virginia; 3 — Tennessee, Michigan, North Carolina, and Oklahoma; and 4 — Louisiana, South Carolina, and Alabama.

Fig. 8.6 Figure 2 of Gross and Others (2002)

Spearman's rho is the correlation coefficient computed by using ranks of observations instead of values of observations. It (−0.38) is not distant from 0 and not a suggestion of a close relationship between the ranks of expenditures on tobacco control programs and smoking rates of the states. One minus its square equals 0.86. This suggests that if the least-squares line determined from the ranks of the expenditures and the ranks of smoking rates were used to appraise the ranks of expenditures, the overall error of the appraisals would be as much as 86% of the overall error of the rudimentary appraisal that the ranks of expenditures of all 50 states are identical and equal 25.

$P = 0.007$ suggests that if the 50 states were elements of a random sample, the probability that Spearman's rho deviates from 0 as much as −0.38 or more would be only 0.007 if chance were the explanation. It is smaller than 0.05 and suggests that Spearman's rho −0.38) may be declared statistically significant, and the concern that Spearman's rho (−0.38) is incidental may be dismissed. Although Spearman's rho −0.38 may be declared statistically significant, it is not a certification that states with higher smoking rates had significantly lower expenditures for tobacco control programs.

It is more constructive to articulate the indication of Figure 2 that the expenditures for tobacco control programs and smoking rates of the states do not demonstrate a discernible relationship.

The 50 states are not elements of a random sample. The smoking rates and expenditures of tobacco control programs are descriptions of the states. Whether the spearman's rho may be declared statistical significant is not an issue.

Example 8.3.2

Gustafson and Others (1987) present the results of a study that analyzed serum samples obtained from students at two secondary schools eight days after the onset of the first case of the outbreak of measles in Corpus Christi, Texas, in the spring of 1985. The relationship between the titer levels of ELISA for measles antibody and the interval since immunization of 580 students was evaluated. These students received one vaccination before they were two years old and were evaluated 11–17 years after their immunizations. The relationship between titer level and time since immunization between 11 and 17 years is articulated as follows:

> These 580 students were all immunized between 1968 and 1974, or 11 to 17 years before being tested. There was a weak (r = -0.09) but statistically significant (P = 0.03, t test for slope) decline in titer with time. The slope of the log-linear regression line was -0.022 ln (T + 0.914) per year (Fig. 3).

Figure 3 (Fig. 8.7) uses a scatterplot to depict the 580 pairs of normalized log-transformed titer levels (IgG titer [LN(ΔO.D.)]) and intervals since immunization. It suggests that the normalized log-transformed titer levels scatter haphazardly in comparably wide spans when the years since immunization are 11 years or shortly longer or close to 17 years. The 580 pairs of normalized log-transformed titer levels and years since immunization do not demonstrate a discernible relationship.

A descending line is exhibited. It is a graphical display of linear regression analysis and a description of the relationship between the means of normalized

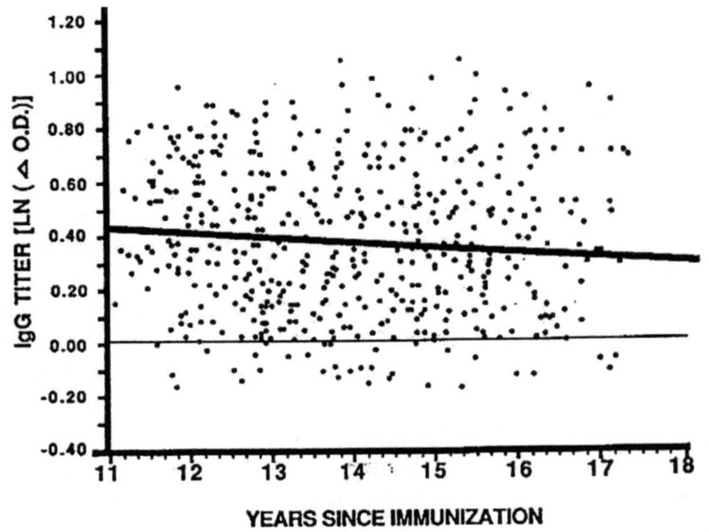

Figure 3. Results of ELISA for Measles Antibody According to the Interval since Immunization among 580 Students Immunized Once before the Age of Two Years.

Values indicating seronegativity appear below the thin line. The thick line represents the log-linear regression curve.

Fig. 8.7 Figure 3 of Gustafson and Others (1987)

log-transformed titer levels and the interval since immunization. The dots disperse haphazardly below and above the line between −0.10 and 1.10 whether intervals since immunization are close to 11 years or 17 years. The line is an oversimplification when it is used to depict the relationship between the normalized log-transformed titer levels and intervals since immunization of the 580 students. It is a distraction. It would be more obvious that the normalized log-transformed titer levels and intervals since immunization of the 580 students do not demonstrate a discernible relationship if the line were not exhibited.

The correlation coefficient −0.09 is close to 0 and suggests that the normalized log-transformed titer levels and intervals since immunization of the 580 students are not related. One minus the square of the correlation coefficient $1.0 - (-0.09)^2 = 0.9919$ suggests that if the displayed descending line were used to appraise the normalized log-transformed titer levels of the 580 students from their intervals since immunization, the overall error of the appraisals would be as much as the rudimentary appraisal that the normalized log-transformed titer levels of all students were identical and equal their mean.

$P = 0.03$ suggests that the slope of the least-squares line deviating from 0 as much as −0.022 would be particularly unlikely if chance were the explanation. The slope may be declared statistically significant. It also suggests that the correlation coefficient of −0.09 may be declared statistically significant.

Although the slope of the least-square line may be declared statistically significant, both the correlation coefficient of −0.09 and the scatterplot suggest that the normalized log-transformed titer levels and years since immunization of the 580 students are not related. It is astute to read with care the assertion that there was a weak but statistically significant decline in titer with time. It is more constructive to stress the indication of the scatterplot that the normalized log-transformed titer levels and years since immunization of the 580 students do not demonstrate a discernible relationship.

Example 8.3.3

Pierard and Lancellotti (2004) present the results of a study that administered quantitative Doppler echocardiography to 28 patients with acute pulmonary edema and left ventricular dysfunction and 46 patients without a history of acute pulmonary edema during exercise. Exercise-induced changes in the effective regurgitant orifice area and the transtricuspid pressure gradient were evaluated in subjects with and without acute pulmonary edema.

Figure 1 of the article (Fig. 8.8) uses positions of dots to depict the effective regurgitant orifice areas and transtricuspid pressure gradients of the 74 subjects. The

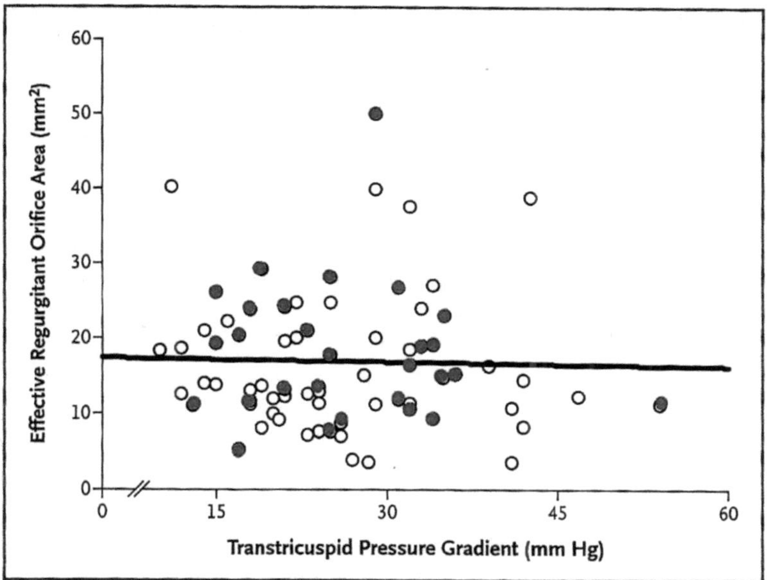

Figure 1. Correlation between the Effective Regurgitant Orifice Area and the Transtricuspid Pressure Gradient at Rest.
The correlation between the variables was not significant (r=−0.02). Red circles indicate patients who had pulmonary edema, and open circles patients in the comparison group, with no pulmonary edema. Some data points in the comparison group indicate values for more than one patient.

Fig. 8.8 Figure 1 of Pierard and Lancellotti (2004)

dots disperse haphazardly in wide ranges of comparable heights whether the transtricuspid pressure gradients of the subjects are small or large. They do not demonstrate a discernible relationship between the effective regurgitant orifice areas and transtricuspid pressure gradients of the 74 subjects.

A barely descending line is exhibited. It is a graphical display of the least-squares line determined from the 74 pairs of observations and a description of the relationship between means of effective regurgitant orifice areas and transtricuspid pressure gradient values. It is an oversimplification. For many pairs of the effective regurgitant orifice area and transtricuspid pressure gradient are distant from the line. It is also a distraction. That the effective regurgitant orifice areas and transtricuspid pressure gradients of the 74 subjects do not demonstrate a discernible relationship would be more evident if it were not exhibited.

Footnote of Figure 1 states: "*The correlation between the variables was not significant (r = −0.02).*" Although the correlation coefficient $r = -0.02$ was not declared statistically significant, it is useful. It is close to 0 and confirms the manifestation of the scatterplot that the effective regurgitant orifice areas and transtricuspid pressure gradients of the subjects do not demonstrate a discernible relationship.

Figure 3 of the article (Fig. 8.9) uses a scatterplot to depict the relationship between exercise-induced changes in effective regurgitant orifice area and

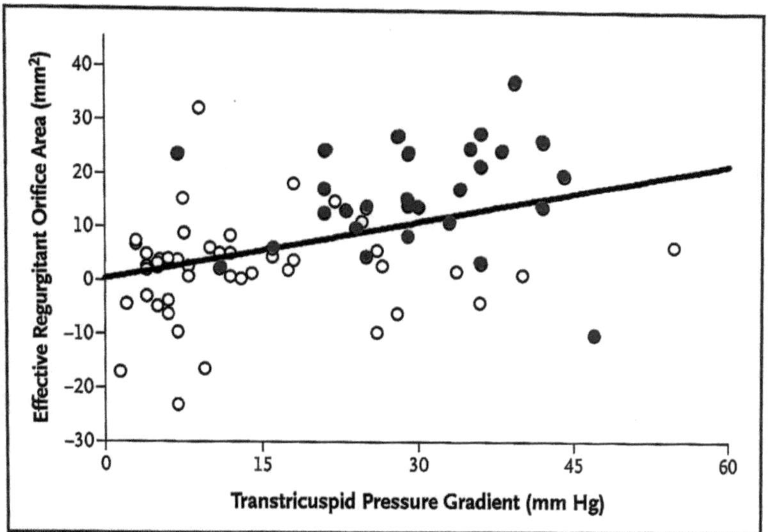

Figure 3. Correlation between Exercise-Induced Changes in the Effective Regurgitant Orifice Area and the Transtricuspid Pressure Gradient.
The correlation between the variables was significant (r=0.4, P<0.001). Red circles indicate patients who had pulmonary edema, and open circles patients in the comparison group, with no pulmonary edema. Some data points in the comparison group indicate values for more than one patient.

Fig. 8.9 Figure 3 of Pierard and Lancellotti (2004)

transtricuspid pressure gradients of the subjects. The dots disperse haphazardly in wide ranges of similar heights whether the transtricuspid pressure gradients of the subjects are small or large. They do not demonstrate a noteworthy relationship.

An ascending line is exhibited. It is a graphical display of the least-squares line determined from the 74 pairs of observations and a characterization of the relationship between means of exercise-induced changes in effective regurgitant orifice area and transtricuspid pressure gradient values. Many pairs of exercise-induced changes in effective regurgitant orifice area and transtricuspid pressure gradients are distant from the line. The line is an oversimplification. It is also a distraction. That the exercise-induced changes in effective regurgitant orifice area and transtricuspid pressure gradients of the 74 subjects do not demonstrate a noteworthy relationship would be more evident if it were not exhibited.

Footnote of Figure 3 states: "*The correlation between the variables was significant ($r = 0.4$, $P < 0.001$).*" $P < 0.001$ is below 0.05 and suggests that the correlation coefficient (0.4) may be declared statistically significant. However, the correlation coefficient (0.4) is relatively close to 0 and suggests that the least-squares line of linear regression analysis and the transtricuspid pressure gradients of the subjects do not yield accurate appraisals of the exercise-induced changes in effective regurgitant orifice areas of the subjects. One minus its square $1.0 - 0.4^2 = 0.84$ suggests that the overall error of using transtricuspid pressure gradients and the leas-squares line to appraise exercise-induced changes in the effective regurgitant orifice area is as much as 86% of the overall error of the rudimentary appraisal that all changes are identical and equal their mean.

The fault of using statistical significance as certification of importance is exemplified by Figure 1 and Figure 3. Both do not demonstrate noteworthy relationships, particularly if the graphical displays of least-squares lines are ignored. The manifestation of Figure 1 is deemed "not significant," but that of Figure 3 is deemed "significant." This is not a contradiction if statistical significance is interpreted correctly. Not declaring statistically significant only means that it is not astute to dismiss the concern that the correlation coefficient $r = -0.02$ is incidental, and declaring statistically significant only means that the concern that the correlation coefficient $r = 0.4$ is incidental may be dismissed. The correlation coefficients are close to 0; they suggest that the observations do not demonstrate noteworthy relationship. It is more productive to articulate indications of the scatterplots that the effective regurgitant orifice areas and exercise-induced changes in the effective regurgitant orifice area and the transtricuspid pressure gradients of the subjects do not demonstrate noteworthy relationships.

Example 8.3.4

Lockley and Others (2004) present the results of a study that assessed work hours, sleep hours, and attentional failures in intensive care units during a traditional schedule and an intervention schedule. The traditional schedule included extended work shifts; the intervention schedule included shifts of 16 or fewer consecutive hours. The following is a narrative of the relationship between weekly duration of sleep and weekly duration of work:

Fig. 8.10 Figure 3C of Lockley and Others (2004)

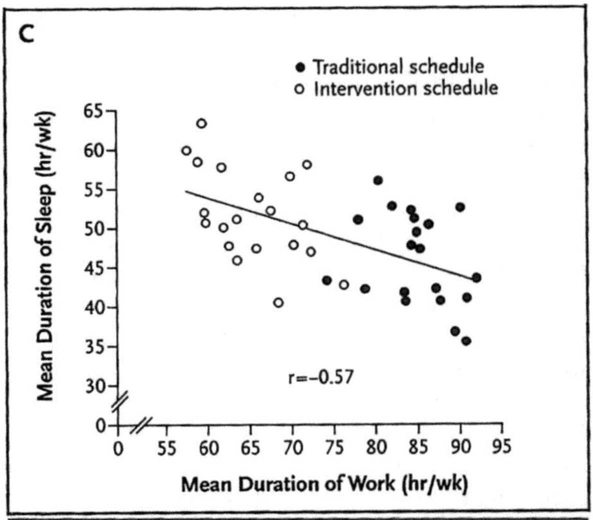

Figure 3. Subjective Mean Hours of Work per Week (Panel A), Duration of Sleep (Panel B), and the Relationship between the Duration of Work and the Duration of Sleep (Panel C) for 20 Interns during the Traditional Schedule and the Intervention Schedule.

All subjects worked less during the intervention schedule than during the traditional schedule (mean decrease, 19.5 hours per week) (Panel A). All but three subjects worked more than 80 hours per week during the traditional schedule, whereas the maximal number of hours worked during the intervention schedule was 76.3 hours. All but three subjects slept more during the intervention schedule, with the group averaging 5.8 hours more sleep per week (Panel B). The duration of work and the duration of sleep were inversely correlated (r=−0.57, P<0.001) (Panel C) during the traditional and intervention schedules, with the best-fit regression predicting a 19.2-minute loss of sleep per week for every additional hour of work per week.

> The weekly durations of sleep and work were significantly inversely correlated (r = -0.57, P<0.001), with a predicted loss of 19.2 minutes of work per week (Fig. 3).

The assertion that the weekly durations of sleep and work were significantly inversely correlated is corroborated by $r = -0.57$, $P < 0.001$, and Fig. 3.

Figure 3 (Fig. 8.10) uses dots to depict pairs of mean duration of sleep and the mean duration of work of the 20 interns during the two schedules. A descending line is displayed. The line coins the notion that the weekly durations of sleep and work are inversely correlated. It is the least-squares line determined from the mean durations of sleep and mean durations of work of the 20 interns during the two procedures.

One feature of Fig. 3C is that it uses open circles to denote the 20 pairs of mean duration of sleep and mean duration of work during the intervention schedule and close circles to denote the 20 pairs during the traditional schedule. The open circles scatter haphazardly and do not suggest a discernible relationship; the closed circles also scatter haphazardly and do not suggest a discernible relationship. The descending line is a distraction. That the mean durations of sleep and mean durations of work of the interns during each schedule are not related would be more apparent if the line were not displayed.

The assortment of open circles and the assortment of closed circles are separated and unveil that, with only one exception, the mean durations of work of the 20 interns during the intervention schedule are shorter than their mean durations of work during the traditional schedule, and that the mean durations of sleep of some interns during the intervention schedule are larger than their mean durations of sleep during the traditional schedule. The correlation coefficient $r = -0.57$, $P < 0.001$, and the descending line were determined from the 40 pairs of mean durations. They are misleading when they are used to describe the relationship between mean durations of sleep and mean durations of work of the 20 interns during either schedule. It is more judicious to articulate the indications of the two assortments of dots that the mean durations of sleep and work of the 20 interns are not related during each schedule.

Example 8.3.5

Leonard and Others (2004) (Example 8.1.1) use the following elegant statement to depict the relationship between the lifetime cumulative dose of glucocorticoids and height:

> The z score for height was significantly and inversely correlated with the lifetime cumulative dose of glucocorticoids in milligrams (r = -0.28, P=0.03) and milligrams per kilogram (r = -0.38, P=0.003).

The assertion that the z score for height was significantly and inversely correlated with the lifetime cumulative dose of glucocorticoids is substantiated by $r = -0.28$, $P = 0.03$ and $r = -0.38$, $P = 0.003$. The P-values suggest that the correlation coefficients could be declared statistically significant. However, the correlation coefficients $r = -0.28$ and $r = -0.38$ are relatively close to 0 and suggest questionable relationships. Their squares are 0.08 and 0.14. If least-squares lines were determined and used to appraise the z score for height from the lifetime cumulative dose of glucocorticoids, the overall error of the appraisals would be as much as 92% and 86% of the rudimentary appraisal that the z scores of all subjects were identical and equal their mean.

$P = 0.03$ and $P = 0.003$ are smaller than 0.05; the correlation coefficients may be declared statistically significant, and the concern that they are incidental may be dismissed. They are not the certification of close relationships.

It is more informative to use a scatterplot to depict the pairs of z scores for height and lifetime cumulative dose of glucocorticoids graphically. It then would be clear how useful or how feeble the relationship is.

8.4 Intelligent Reading and Informative Reporting

Narratives of relationships between observations on two quantitative variables are often stylish but indistinct or misleading. To read intelligently, it is prolific to consider the following remarks.

- *Intelligent Reading*

  1. How observations on two quantitative variables relate is informatively manifested by properly drawn scatterplots.
  2. Correlation coefficients are useful measures of closeness of relationships only when the relationships are literally characterized by straight lines.
  3. Least-squares equations of regression analysis may be oversimplifications or distractions. It is essential to scrutinize whether they are valid supplements of demonstrations of scatterplots.
  4. Small *P*-values and statistical significance are not certification of clinical importance. They suggest only that it is alright to dismiss the concern that relationships demonstrated by data are incidental.
  5. Statistically significant relationships may be trivial or misleading.
  6. If correlation coefficients, *P*-values, or both are the only descriptions of relationships, probe the suggestions of scatterplots and the correlation coefficients. Note that correlation coefficients do not suggest close relationships unless they are relatively close to 1.0 or −1.0.
  7. Petty relationships may be statistically significant when the numbers of observations are large.
  8. If observations are obtained from groups of subjects in different conditions or at different points in time, it is essential to examine how the groups of subjects differ. Relationships demonstrated by the combined data may be reflections of the distinctions among the different groups.

- *Informative Reporting*

  1. Use scatterplots to depict how observations on two quantitative variables relate. If data were obtained from subjects in different conditions, with different traits, or at different time points, use different symbols to denote observation-pairs in different sets. Articulate indications of scatterplots plainly.
  2. Use least-squares equations to highlight relationships only if they are literal descriptions of the relationship demonstrated by scatterplots.
  3. Exhibit graphical displays of least-squares equations only if they are candid characterizations of manifestations of scatterplots.

4. Do not simply state relationships are "significant" or "not significant." Describe the relationships plainly by articulating manifestations of scatterplots.
5. 95% confidence intervals of correlation coefficients may be used to assess the reproducibility of correlation coefficients.

Example 8.4.1

Adams and Others (2018) present the results of a study that randomly assigned patients with hereditary transthyretin amyloidosis with polyneuropathy to receive intravenous patisiran or placebo. The primary end point is the change at 18 months from baseline in the modified neuropathy impairment score+7 (mNIS+7), which ranges from 0 to 304 with higher scores indicating more impairment. It states:

> A correlation was observed between the degree of reduction in transthyretin levels from baseline and the change in the mNIS+7 at 18 months (Fig. 3).

Figure 3 (Fig. 8.11) uses circles and triangles to denote pairs of degrees of reduction in transthyretin levels from baseline and changes in mNIS+7 levels.

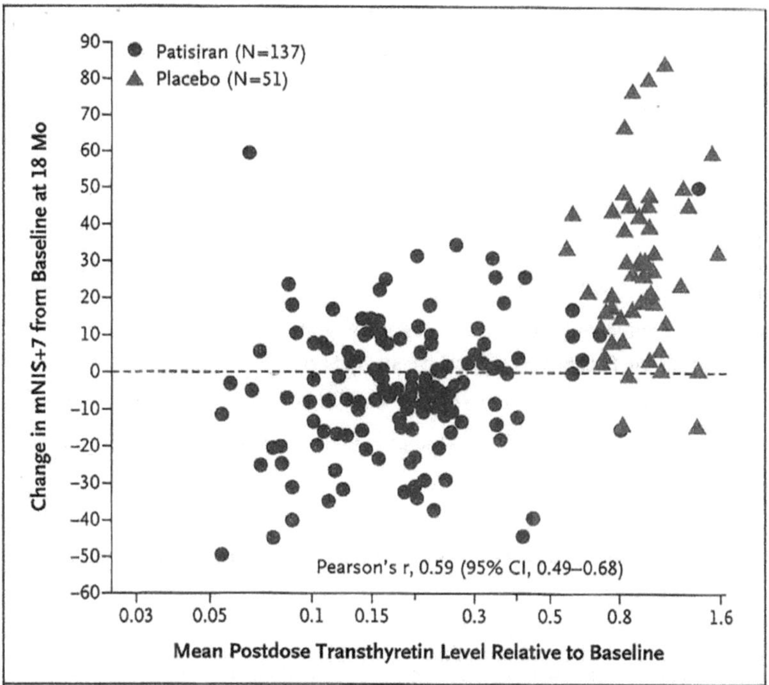

Figure 3. Correlation of Reduction in Transthyretin Levels with Change in mNIS+7 from Baseline at 18 Months.

The analysis included 188 patients with nonmissing mNIS+7 assessments at month 18.

Fig. 8.11 Figure 3 of Adams and Others (2018)

Pearson's *r*, 0.59 and 95% CI, 0.49 to 0.68) are shown. Pearson's r is the correlation coefficient, and 95% CI stands for the 95% confidence interval.

The correlation coefficient, 0.59, is not close to 1.0. This suggests that if the least-squares line is determined from the 188 pairs of changes in mNIS+7 and the degree of reduction in transthyretin level, the line would not yield accurate appraisals of the changes in mNS+7. One minus the square of 0.59 equals 0.65. The overall error of using the least-squares line and reductions in transthyretin level to appraise changes in mNIS+7 would be as much as 65% of the overall error of the rudimentary appraisal that the changes of all 188 subjects were identical and equal their mean. The relationship between the 188 pairs of change in mNIS+7 and reduction in transthyretin level is dubious.

The 95% confidence interval [0.49 to 0.68] is not wide and suggests that the correlation coefficient of 0.59 may be moderately reproducible. The boundaries of the interval are 83% and 115% of the correlation coefficient 0.59. They suggest that if the study were replicated a score of times, the correlation coefficients of most replicates would vary between 83% and 115% of the reported correlation coefficient 0.59.

One feature of Figure 3 is that it uses circles and triangles to denote observation-pairs of subjects in the two treatment groups. The assortment of circles suggests that the changes in mNIS+7 of the 137 subjects of the patisiran group disperse in wide spans of comparable heights whether reductions in transthyretin levels are smaller or larger. The assortment of triangles suggests that the changes in mNIS+7 of the 51 subjects of the placebo group also disperse in wide spans of comparable heights whether reductions in transthyretin levels are smaller or larger. The two assortments of dots do not demonstrate discernible relationships.

The circles are located to the left and are lower than many triangles. The reductions in transthyretin levels of the subjects in the patisiran group are smaller than those of the subjects in the placebo group. The changes in mNIS+7 of many subjects in the patisiran group are negative and smaller than those of nearly all subjects in the placebo group which mostly are positive. The correlation coefficient of 0.59 was computed from the data of 188 subjects in the two treatment groups. Its value of 0.59, to a considerable extent, is a result of the distinction between the two treatment groups. The reported correlation between the degree of reduction in transthyretin dose and the change in mNIS+7 is not validated by the data of the subjects in the patisiran group or the placebo group.

To read intelligently, it is critical to note that the asserted correlation is a result of the distinction between the two treatment groups. The changes in the mNIS+7 from baseline at 18 months and the reductions in transthyretin level from baseline do not demonstrate a discernable relationship when the two groups of subjects are evaluated separately. To report informatively, it is productive to stress the indication of Figure 3. Articulate how the two treatment groups of subjects differ and underscore that the data of the two groups of subjects do not demonstrate a discernable relationship when they are evaluated separately.

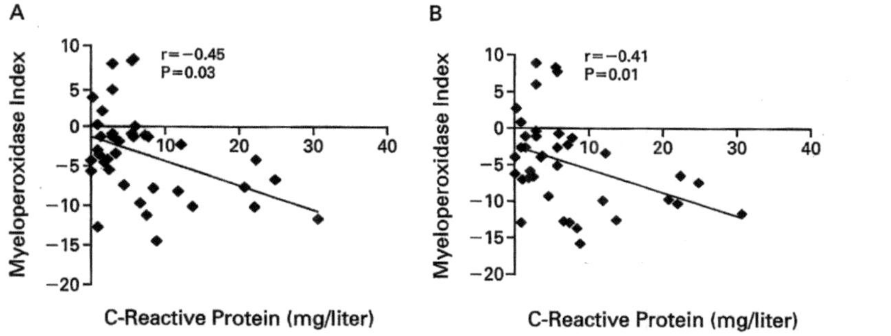

Figure 3. Correlation between Systemic Values for C-Reactive Protein and the Change in the Myeloperoxidase Content in Blood from the Aorta and the Great Cardiac Vein.

C-reactive protein values were significantly and inversely correlated with the myeloperoxidase content of blood from the aorta (Panel A) and the great cardiac vein (Panel B). The diagonal lines are the regression lines.

Fig. 8.12 Figure 3 of Buffon and Others (2002)

Example 8.4.2

Buffon and Others (2002) present the results of a study that measured the neutrophil myeloperoxidase content in the cardiac and femoral circulation in 65 patients (24 with unstable angina and a left coronary lesion, 9 with unstable angina and a right coronary lesion, 13 with chronic stable angina, 13 with variant angina and recurrent ischemia, and 6 controls). One result is related as follows:

> Overall, in the five groups, a significant correlation was found between systemic levels of C-creative protein and the aortic neutrophil myeloperoxidase content (r = -0.45, P = 0.03), as well as between systemic levels of C-creative protein and the neutrophil myeloperoxidase content in blood from the great cardiac vein (r = -0.41, P = 0.01) (Fig. 3).

The ground of the assertion that significant correlations were found is the values of correlation coefficients and their *P*-values. The correlation coefficients are not close to −1.0 and do not suggest close relationships. The scatterplots of Fig. 3 (Fig. 8.12) do not suggest discernable relationships. Least-squares lines are displayed. The lines are not literal characterizations of the manifestation of the scatterplots.

To read intelligently, it is critical to note that although the correlation coefficients were declared statistically significant, they are not close to 1.0 and do not suggest close relationships. More importantly, Fig. 3 (Fig. 8.13) shows that the least-squares lines are not literal characterizations of manifestations of scatterplots. Many dots scatter widely and are distant from the lines.

A close examination of panel A of Fig. 3 revealed that there are basically two assortments of dots. The assortment of dots denoting subjects whose changes in C-reactive protein are less than 10 mg/liter vary widely from approximately −15 to +8. They suggest that the aortic myeloperoxidase indices of these subjects are not related to their changes in C-reactive protein. The assortment of dots denoting subjects whose C-reactive protein levels are larger than 10 mg/liter are all negative and vary between −15 and 0. They suggest that the aortic myeloperoxidase indices

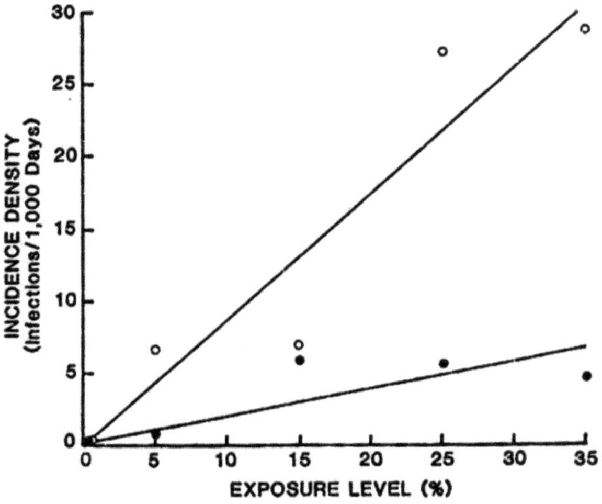

Figure 1. Rise in Incidence Density of New Nosocomial RSV Infections with Increasing Levels of Exposure to Hospitalized Patients Shedding Virus, per 1000 Patient-Days.

Open circles denote the incidence densities of nosocomial infections during the period before the intervention. The equation for the regression line for this group is $y = 0.86x + 0.39$, with $r^2 = 0.86$. H_0; slope = 0, rejected ($P<10^{-9}$).

Closed circles denote the incidence densities of nosocomial infections during the period after the intervention. The equation for the regression line for this group is $y = 0.19x + 0.10$, with $r^2 = 0.68$. H_0; slope = 0, rejected ($P<0.05$).

The ratio of the slopes of the incidence densities of the two groups was 4.5 ($P<0.001$). The equation for the regression line for both patient groups combined is $y = 0.44x + 0.95$, with $r^2 = 0.88$. H_0; slope = 0, rejected ($P<10^{-5}$).

Fig. 8.13 Figure 1 of Leclair and Others (1987)

of these subjects are not related to their changes in C-reactive protein. Panel B also shows that there are two assortments of dots. The assortment of dots denoting subjects whose changes in C-reactive protein are less than 10 mg/liter suggest that the femoral myeloperoxidase indices and changes in C-reactive protein of these subjects are not related. The assortment of dots denoting subjects whose changes in C-reactive protein are greater than 10 mg/liter suggest that the femoral myeloperoxidase indices and changes in C-reactive protein of these subjects are not related.

The descending lines and the correlation coefficients −0.45 and −0.41 are distractions. They are results of linear regression analyses that presume straight line relationships. If they are not presented, it would be more evident that the myeloperoxidase index and C-reactive protein are not related if subjects whose C-reactive protein are below and above 10 mg/liter are evaluated separately.

To report informatively, it is constructive to stress the distinction between the subjects whose C-reactive protein was below and above 10 mg/liter. Use different symbols to depict the subjects in the five groups without the descending line and stress the distinction between the subjects whose C-reactive protein are below and above 10 mg/liter. The different symbols would unveil valuable information, particularly if subjects whose C-reactive protein are below and above 10 mg/liter belonged to different groups.

Example 8.4.3

A longitudinal intervention trial was conducted during three nosocomial respiratory syncytial virus (RSV) seasons to assess whether increased compliance with a policy of glove and gown isolation precautions could reduce the high RSV infection rate in infants and toddler wards. A description of the relationship between the incidence rate of RSV infection and levels of exposure is presented in Leclair and Others (1987) as follows:

> Linear-trend analysis of the incidence density of all cases of nosocomial RSY infection over the five levels of exposure showed a strong overall association of increasing infection rate with increasing level of exposure ($P<10^{-5}$). When the data from before and after the intervention were analyzed separately, a stronger trend was found for the low compliance group ($P<10^{-9}$), and a weaker association was found for the high-compliance group ($P<0.05$).

To read intelligently, it is critical to note that $P < 10^{-9}$ and $P < 0.05$ are the results of linear regression analyses and suggest only that statistically significant may be declared. They are not certifications that the incidence rates and exposure levels are closely related.

How incidence rates and exposure levels relate are depicted in Figure 1 (Fig. 8.13). Incidence rates at five exposure levels during the period before intervention are denoted by open circles, and those during the period after intervention are denoted by closed circles. Manifestation of the open circles is underscored by a fast-rising line; manifestation of the closed circles is underscored by a slower rising line. The lines coin the notion that incidence density increased steadily as exposure level increased. The faster rising line suggests that the rate of increase is faster during the period before intervention than during the period after intervention.

The caption of the figure suggests that the faster rising line is a graphical display of $y = 0.86x + 0.39$, the coefficient of determination of the equation equals 0.86, and the P-value of the slope of the line is $<10^{-9}$. The slower rising line is a graphical display of $y = 0.19x + 0.10$, the coefficient of determination of the equation equals 0.68, and the P-value of the slope of the line is <0.05.

A close examination of the figure revealed that the infection rate did not increase steadily along a straight line but hopped in phases. During the period before intervention, infection rates hopped and showed three phases. The rate was 0 when the exposure level was 0, jumped to approximately 6 infections per 1000 days when the exposure levels were 5% and 15%, and jumped to approximately 25 or 26 infections per 1000 days when the exposure levels were 25% and 35%. During the period after intervention, there were basically two phases. The incidence rate was 0 or only 1 infection per 1000 days when exposure levels were 0% and 5% and was approximately 5 infections per 1000 days when exposure levels were 15%, 25%, and 35%. The lines are oversimplifications and distractions.

To read intelligently, it is astute to ignore the ascending lines, the correlation coefficient (−0.45), and *P*-values and note the hopping of the infection rates. To report informatively, it is productive to depict the pairs of infection rate and exposure rate without the least-squares line and stress the hopping of the infection rates.

Remark $P < 10^{-5}$ and $P < 10^{-9}$ are extraordinarily small considering that there are only ten and five pairs of observations, respectively.

Example 8.4.4

Giulian and Others (1987) present the results of a study that used an isoelectric-focusing procedure for measuring stable hemoglobin subunits to quantitate levels of hemoglobin F in blood samples of 59 patients with sudden infant death syndrome (SIDS) and 40 controls. The following is a narrative of a result:

> Figure 1 demonstrates the accuracy of the hemoglobin F determinations by means of hemoglobin-subunit analysis. Known relative amounts of hemoglobin F and hemoglobin A were compared from their relative proportions of γ- and β-globin chains as measured with the isoelectric-focusing protocol. Each of the points in Figure 1 represents the mean value from analyses of three separate gels, and the data showed good linearity (r = 0.9917) between the proportion of γ-globin chain and the total hemoglobin F between 0 and 97.5%.

Figure 1 (Fig. 8.14) uses dots to denote pairs of mean % HbF and mean %γ/(γ + β) values from analyses of three separate gels. It shows that all pairs are close to an

Fig. 8.14 Figure 1 of Giulian and Others (1987)

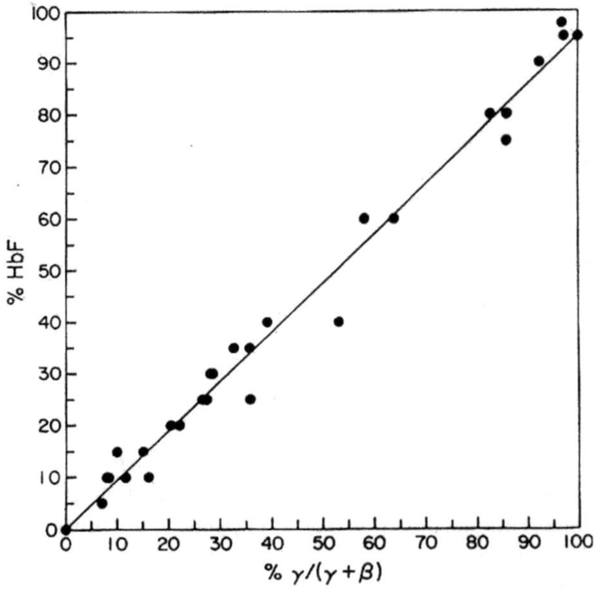

Figure 1. Determination of Levels of Hemoglobin F (HbF) with Hemoglobin-Subunit Analysis.

ascending line and suggests that the relationship between means of % HbF values and means of %γ/(γ + β) values is effectually portrayed by the least-squares line of a linear regression analysis. The correlation coefficient $r = 0.9917$ is close to 1.0 and confirms the indication of the figure that the means of %γ/(γ + β) values of three gels would yield accurate appraisals of means of % HbF values of three gels.

To read intelligently, it is important to note that each dot of the figure represents a pair of means of analyses of three separate gels. Figure 1 and the correlation coefficient are descriptions of the relationship between the means of %γ/(γ + β) values and means of % HbF values of three gels. They are not descriptions of the relationship between the %γ/(γ + β) values and % HbF values of analysis of individual gels. They are oversimplifications if the values of analyses of three gels varied widely.

An alternative is to use a scatterplot to depict the relationship between the values of % HbF and %γ/(γ + β) of single gels, and the correlation coefficient computed from the pairs of values of single gels was used to supplement the scatterplot.

Review Questions

1. What is the best way to show how observations on two quantitative relate?
2. Why are least-squares equations of regression analysis often oversimplifications or misleading?
3. Why are "significant" relationships often oversimplifications or misleading?
4. Is the correlation coefficient useful if a relationship is not literally characterized by a straight line?
5. Is 0.5 or −0.5 a suggestion of close relationship?
6. Are "significant" correlation coefficients certifications of close relationship?
7. Can a correlation coefficient as small as −0.1 be "significant?"
8. Why is it important to use dots of different symbols to denote observations on two variables obtained from subjects in different conditions?
9. Under what conditions are results of regression analyses valuable supplements to manifestations of scatterplots?

Exercise

8.E.1. Review Figure 2 of Leonard and Others (2004) (Fig. 8.15) and elaborate what it suggests. Suggest a likely value of the correlation coefficient.

8.E.2. Review the two lower panels of Figure 3 of Boyd and Others (2002) (Fig. 8.2) and elaborate their suggestions.

8.E.3. Review Figure 3B of Buffon and Others (2002) (Fig. 8.12).

(a) Elaborate the suggestions of $r = -0.41$ and $P = 0.01$.
(b) Discuss whether the descending line is a candid characterization of the indication of the scatterplot.
(c) Suggest a more candid narrative of the manifestation of the scatterplot.

Fig. 8.15 Figure 2 of Leonard and Others (2004)

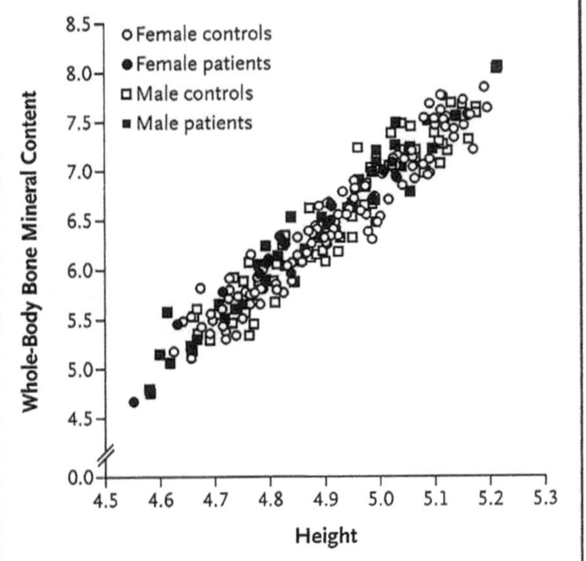

Figure 2. Whole-Body Bone Mineral Content Relative to Height in Patients with Glucocorticoid-Sensitive Nephrotic Syndrome and Control Subjects.
Values have been log-transformed.

8.E.4. Lal and Others (2011) present the results of a study that analyzed longitudinal clinical data of 86 patients with hemoglobin H disease; 60 had deletion of three or four α-globin genes (HbH), 23 had hemoglobin H constant spring (HCS) and 3 had other nonrelational forms of hemoglobin. The article stated: "*There was a significant correlation between the liver iron concentration and the serum ferritin level ($r = 0.54$, $P = 0.002$) ....*" Figure 4C (Fig. 8.16) presents a graphical display of the significant correlation.

(a) Elaborate the suggestion of $r = 0.54$ and $P = 0.002$.
(b) Elaborate the suggestion of Figure 4C if the descending line were not shown.
(c) Suggest a candid narrative of the relationship between liver iron concentration and serum ferritin level.

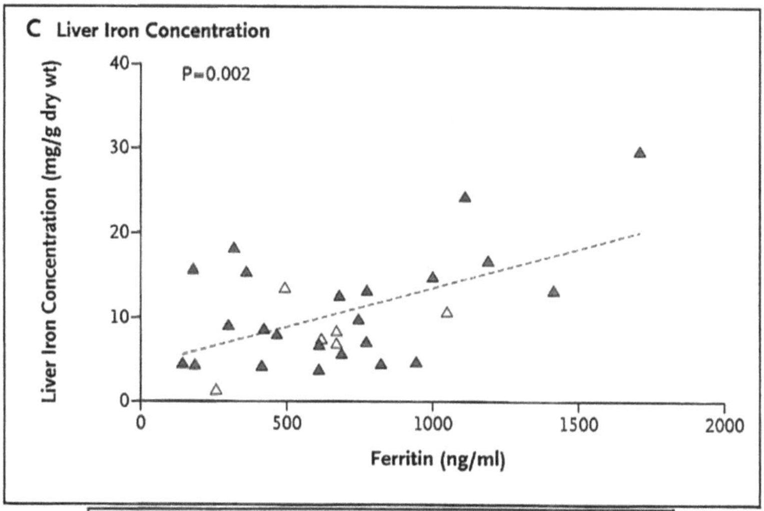

Figure 4. Serum Ferritin Levels in Patients with Deletional Hemoglobin H Disease (HbH) and Hemoglobin H Constant Spring Disease (HCS) and Correlation with Liver Iron Concentration.

The trend for ferritin levels according to age on the basis of linear regression (dashed line) increases after the age of 18 years in patients with HbH (Panel A) and increases from birth to the age of 30 years in those with HCS (Panel B). A significant correlation between the serum ferritin level and liver iron concentration is shown in patients with HbH and HCS, with the dashed line indicating the linear regression of liver iron concentration as compared with ferritin (Panel C).

Fig. 8.16 Figure 4C of Lal and Others (2011)

References

Adams, D., et al. (2018). Patisiran, an RNAi therapeutic, for hereditary transthyretin amyloidosis. *The New England Journal of Medicine, 379*(1), 11–21.

Battle, D. C., et al. (1988). The use of the urinary anion cap in the diagnosis of hyperchloremic metabolic acidosis. *The New England Journal of Medicine, 318*(10), 594–599.

Boyd, N. F., et al. (2002). Heritability of mammographic density, a risk factor for breast cancer. *The New England Journal of Medicine, 347*(12), 886–894.

Buffon, A., et al. (2002). Widespread coronary inflammation in unstable angina. *The New England Journal of Medicine, 347*(1), 5–12.

Giulian, G. G., et al. (1987). Elevated fetal hemoglobin levels in sudden infant death syndrome. *The New England Journal of Medicine, 316*(18), 1122–1126.

Gross, C. P., et al. (2002). State expenditure for tobacco-control programs and the tobacco settlement. *The New England Journal of Medicine, 347*(14), 1080–1086.

Gustafson, T. L., et al. (1987). Measles outbreak in a fully immunized secondary-school population. *The New England Journal of Medicine, 316*(13), 771–774.

Lal, A., et al. (2011). Heterogeneity of hemoglobin H disease in childhood. *The New England Journal of Medicine, 364*(8), 710–718.

Leclair, J. M., et al. (1987). Prevention of nosocomial respiratory syncytial virus infections through compliance with glove and gown isolation precautions. *The New England Journal of Medicine, 317*(6), 329–334.

Leonard, M. B., et al. (2004). Long-term, high-dose glucocorticoid and bone mineral content in childhood glucocorticoid-sensitive nephrotic syndrome. *The New England Journal of Medicine, 351*(9), 868–875.

Lockley, S. W., et al. (2004). Effect of reducing interns' weekly work hours on sleep and attentional failure. *The New England Journal of Medicine, 351*(18), 1829–1837.

Pierard, L. A., & Lancellotti, P. (2004). Ischemic mitral regurgitation and acute pulmonary edema. *The New England Journal of Medicine, 351*(16), 1627–1634.

Rivkees, S. A., et al. (1988). Long-term growth in juvenile acquired hypothyroidism: The failure to achieve normal adult stature. *The New England Journal of Medicine, 318*(10), 599–602.

Chapter 9
Association Between Two Qualitative Variables

The relationship between observations on two qualitative variables is often referred to as associations between the variables. Observations on two variables obtained from a cohort of subjects are analyzed. Like the evaluation of relationship between observations on two quantitative variables, one variable is designated the outcome, response, or dependent variable, and the other the explanatory, predictor, or independent variable. The cohort of subjects are divided into sub-cohorts by attributes of the explanatory variable. Association between the two variables is assessed by comparing the distributions of the observations on the outcome variable among sub-cohorts of subjects specified by attributes of the explanatory variable.

The task of evaluating the association of one qualitative outcome variable with a qualitative explanatory variable and the task of evaluating the distinction among groups of subjects with respect to observations on a qualitative outcome variable differ subtly. Both compare distributions of observations on among groups of subjects. They differ in how the groups are formed. When the association between two qualitative variables is evaluated, the groups compared are the results of using the explanatory variable to divide subjects into sub-cohorts. When distinction among groups of subjects with respect to observations on a quantitative variable is evaluated, the groups compared are the results of the assignment of subjects to treatment groups or enrollment of subjects according to the study protocol.

This chapter begins with a review of examples in Sect. 9.1. The use of measures of strength of association is demonstrated by examples in Sect. 9.2. Evaluating the reliability of diagnostic or prognostic procedures is a special case of association between two qualitative variables. Section 9.3 reviews the suggestions of measures of reliability. Examples of intelligent reading and informative reporting are presented in Sect. 9.4.

P. C. Chang, *Data Analysis of Medical Studies*,
https://doi.org/10.1007/978-3-031-49984-5_9

9.1 Examples

This section reviews the examples of association between two qualitative variables.

Example 9.1.1
Duncavage and Others (2018) presented the results of a study that sequenced bone marrow and skin samples of 90 adults with myelodysplastic syndrome (MDS) and underwent allogeneic transplantation. The article stated:

> With a cutoff point of at least 0.5% for the maximum variant allele frequency of mutation 30 days after allogeneic hematopoietic stem-cell transplantation (equivalent to heterozygous mutation cell in 100 cells) 21 of 32 mutation-positive patients (66%) and 14 of 54 mutation-negative patients (26%) had disease progression after transplantation.

This is a description of the association between two dichotomous variables demonstrated by the data of a cohort of 86 subjects. MDS progression is the outcome variable and mutation positivity the explanatory variable. Positive mutation is defined as at least 0.5% for the maximum variant allele frequency of mutation 30 days after allogeneic hematopoietic stem cell transplantation.

The cohort of 86 subjects were divided into a sub-cohort of 32 mutation-positive subjects and a sub-cohort of 54 mutation-negative subjects. The association of MDS progression with mutation positivity is described by the percentages of subjects whose MDS progressed in the sub-cohort of mutation-positive subjects and the sub-cohort of mutation-negative subjects (66% and 26%).

Example 9.1.2
Callaghan and Others (2004) presented the results of a study that discontinued anticonvulsant drugs in patients who had been free of seizures during two years of treatment with a single drug. An electroencephalogram was obtained in 89 patients before the start of treatment and then repeated before the withdrawal of treatment. The article stated:

> The relapse rates related to electroencephalographic classifications are summarized in Table 1. The highest relapse rates occurred in classes 3 and 4.

This is a description of the association between seizure relapse and electroencephalographic (EEG) classification demonstrated by the data of a cohort of 89 subjects. Seizure relapse is the outcome variable and EEG classification the explanatory variable. The cohort of 89 subjects were divided into four sub-cohorts by EEG classes. The association of seizure relapse with electroencephalographic (EEG) classification is depicted by seizure relapse rates of the four sub-cohorts of subjects specified by EEG class. Table 1 (Table 9.1) shows that the seizure relapse rate of the 35 subjects whose EEG classes belonged to class 2 (abnormal before treatment, normal before withdrawal) is the lowest (11.4%), and that he rate of 19 subjects whose EEG classes belonged to class 4 (abnormal before treatment, unchanged before withdrawal) is the highest (73.7%).

Table 9.1 Table 1 of Callaghan and Others (2004)

Table 1 Electroencephalographic (EEG) class and relapse rates

EEG class	Description	Relapse rate (%)	No. of patients relapsing/total
1	Normal before treatment and before withdrawal	35.5	11/31
2	Abnormal before treatment, normal before withdrawal	11.4	4/35
3	Abnormal before treatment, abnormal but improved before withdrawal	50.0	2/4
4	Abnormal before treatment, unchanged before withdrawal	73.7	14/19

Example 9.1.3 Quinn (318, 4)

Quinn and Others (1988) presented the results of a study that assessed the association of prevalence of human immunodeficiency virus (HIV) infection with risk factors; 2715 male and 1301 female patients attending inner-city clinics for sexually transmitted diseases in Baltimore were screened. The association of human immunodeficiency virus (HIV) infection with homosexual or bisexual activity was depicted as follows on one occasion:

> HIV seropositivity was significantly increased among men who reported participating in homosexual or bisexual activity since 1978, as compared with men who did not (Table 2).

This is a stylish description of the association between two dichotomous variables. HIV seropositivity is the outcome variable and participation in homosexual or bisexual activity the explanatory variable. Table 2 shows that the percentages of seropositivity were 34.7% of 193 in the sub-cohort of subjects who participated in homosexual or bisexual activity and 4.2% of 2031 subjects in the sub-cohort of subjects who did not participate in homosexual or bisexual activity. The odds ratio is 12.2 and *P*-value is <0.001.

The percentages suggest that the prevalence of HIV seropositivity among the 193 men who acknowledged homosexual or bisexual activity is higher than and 8.3 times of that among the 2031 men who did not. The odds ratio unveils that the odds of seropositivity for HIV among the 193 men who acknowledged homosexual or bisexual activity is 12.2 times the odds among the 2013 men who did not. *P* <0.001 suggests that the odds ratio may be declared statistically significant.

Example 9.1.4 (two explanatory variables)

Young and Others (1993) presented the results of a study that used the data of a random sample of 602 employed men and women 30–60 years old to evaluate the association of sleep-disordered breathing with sex and habitual snoring. The article stated:

> Table 3 shows the proportions of the habitual snorers and subjects who were not habitual snorers, according to the apnea-hypopnea score. Habitual snorers, both men and women, were more likely to have apnea-hypopnea scores of 15 or higher. The prevalence of mild sleep-disordered breathing (an apnea-hypopnea score of at least 5 but less than 15), however, was higher among habitual snorers for women only.

Table 9.2 Table 3 of Young and Others (1993)

Table 3. Sex-Specific Prevalence of Sleep-Disordered Breathing, According to Apnea–Hypopnea Score and Sampling Stratum.*

Group	Apnea–Hypopnea Score			Total
	<5	5–14	≥15	
	number of subjects (percent)			
Women (n = 250)				
Habitual snorers	105 (81)	16 (12)	9 (6.9)	130
Not habitual snorers	114 (95)	3 (2.5)	3 (2.5)	120
Men (n = 352)				
Habitual snorers	149 (66)	38 (17)	38 (17)	225
Not habitual snorers	106 (83)	17 (13)	4 (3.1)	127

*The habitual snorers reported snoring, snorting, or breathing pauses every night or almost every night, or extremely loud snoring. The rest of the survey subjects were considered not to be habitual snorers. Because of rounding, not all percentages total 100.

This is a description of the association of sleep-disordered breathing with sex and habitual snoring demonstrated by the data of 602 subjects. Sleep-disordered breathing is the outcome variable measured in three levels of apnea–hypopnea score (number of episodes of apnea and hypopnea per hour of sleep), and sex and habitual snoring are explanatory variables. The cohort of 602 subjects were divided into four sub-cohorts by sex (female or male) and habitual snoring (yes or no). The association of sleep-disordered breathing with the two explanatory variables is assessed by percentages of subjects whose apnea–hypopnea scores were mild, medium, and high in the four sub-cohorts.

Table 3 (Table 9.2) shows how the sleep-disordered breathing of the 602 subjects associated with habitual smoking and sex. The association with habitual smoking is manifested by the result that that the percentage of severe sleep-disordered breathing (apnea–hypopnea scores ≥15) is consistently higher among habitual snorers than among nonhabitual snorers whether the subjects are female (6.9% vs. 2.5%) or male (17% vs. 3.1%). The percentage of mild sleep-disordered breathing (apnea–hypopnea score 4 to 14 is also consistently higher among habitual snorers than that among nonhabitual snorers whether the subjects are female (12% vs. 2.5%) or male (17% vs. 13%). The association with sex is manifested by the result that the percentage of severe sleep-disordered breaching is consistently higher among the male subjects than the female subjects whether the subjects are habitual snorers (17% vs. 6.9%) or not (3.1% vs. 2.5%). The percentage of mild sleep-disordered breathing is consistently higher among the male subjects than among the female subjects whether the subjects habitual snorers (17% vs. 12%) or not (13% vs. 2.5%).

Example 9.1.5
A study examined 89 randomly selected children and adolescents with insulin-dependent diabetes to investigate the association of diabetic nephropathy with markers of risk for hypertension. One result of the study is presented in Krolewski and Others (1988) as follows:

> Having a parent with hypertension increased the risk of diabetic nephropathy almost four times above that in patients without hypertensive parents (odds ratio, 3.7; 95 percent confidence interval, 1.4 to 10.1).

This is a description of the association of diabetic nephropathy with parental hypertension demonstrated by the data of a cohort of 83 children. Diabetic nephropathy is the outcome variable and parental hypertension the explanatory variable. The strength of the association is measured by the odds ratio 3.7, ratio of odds of nephropathy in children having a parent with hypertension relative to those without.

Table 1 suggests that diabetic nephropathy was documented in 24 of the sub-cohort of 49 subjects with hypertensive parents and 7 of 34 subjects of the sub-cohort of subjects without. The numbers yield that the odds of having diabetic nephropathy are 24/25 among the 49 subjects with hypertensive parents and 7/27 among the 34 subjects without. Their ratio (24/25)/(7/27) = 3.7. It is a measure of the association of risk of nephropathy with hypertensive parents if risk is measured by odds. It suggests that the odds of nephropathy in subjects with hypertensive parents is 3.7 times of that in parents without.

The boundaries of the 95% confidence interval of the odds ratio: [1.4 to 10.1] are wide. Its boundaries are 38% and 270% of the odds ratio. They suggest that if the study replicated a score of times, there might be odds ratios as small as 38% and as larger as 270% of the odds ratio of the study. The reproducibility of the odds ratio 3.7 is inadequate. It is astute to limit the odds ratio 3.7 to the subjects of the study and consider it a preliminary indication only.

Example 9.1.6
Bjerregaard and Others (2018) presented the results of a study that analyzed the data of 62,565 Danish men whose weights and heights were measured at 7 and 13 years of age and in early adulthood (17–26 years of age). The weight status of these three periods were used to determine eight overweight patterns. The cohort of the 62,565 men were divided into sub-cohorts by the eight overweight patterns. Whether subjects received a diagnosis of type 2 diabetes at 30–60 years of age was ascertained. The article stated:

> Men who had been overweight at 7 years of age but had had remission of overweight by 13 years of age and had remained at a normal weight as young men had a risk of having type 2 diabetes diagnosed at 30 to 60 years of age that was similar to that among men who had

never been overweight (hazard ratio, 0.96; 95% confidence interval [CI], 0.75 to 1.21) (Fig. 1, and Table S2 in the Supplementary Appendix). Men who had been overweight only at 13 years of age or only at 7 and 13 years of age had a risk of having type 2 diabetes diagnosed at 30 to 60 years of age that was lower than that among men who had been persistently overweight but higher than that among men who had never been overweight (overweight only at 7 and 13 years of age vs. never overweight: hazard ratio, 1.47 [95% CI, 1.10 to 1.98]; persistently overweight vs. never overweight: hazard ratio, 4.14 [95% CI 3.57 to 4.79]).

This is a partial description of the association of having type 2 diabetes diagnosed at 30–60 years of age with a pattern of overweight. Having type 2 diabetes diagnosed at 30–60 years of age is the outcome variable and the pattern of overweight the explanatory variable. The outcome variable is dichotomous and the explanatory variable is polytomous with eight categories. Hazard ratios are cited to assess distinctions in risks of having type 2 diabetes diagnosed at 30–60 years of age between the sub-cohort of subjects with an overweight pattern and the sub-cohort of subjects who had never been overweight.

The hazard ratio 0.96 suggests that the risk of having type 2 diabetes diagnosed at 30–60 years of age among men who had been overweight only at 7 years of age is about the same as the risk among men who had never been overweight. The boundaries of its 95% confidence interval [0.75 to 1.21] are 78% and 126% of the odds ratio 0.96. The odds ratio is moderately reproducible; it is astute to be cautious if it were used to make inference.

The hazard ratio 1.47 suggests that the risk of having type 2 diabetes diagnosed at 30–60 years of age among men who had been overweight only at 7 and 13 years of age is about 1.47 times the risk among men who had never been overweight. The boundaries of its 95% confidence interval [1.10 to 1.98] are 68% and 136% of the odds ratio 1.47. The odds ratio is inadequately reproducible; it is astute to limit it to the subjects of the study.

The hazard ratio 4.14 suggests that the risk of having type 2 diabetes diagnosed at 30–60 years of age among men who had been persistently overweight at all ages is about 4.14 times the risk among men who had never been overweight. The boundaries of its 95% confidence interval [3.57 to 4.79] are 86% and 115% of the odds ratio 4.14. The odds ratio is moderately reproducible; it is astute to be cautious if it were used to make inference.

9.2 Contingency Table

Like the tasks of comparing unpaired and paired qualitative data sets, contingency table is a valuable tool when the association between qualitative variables is assessed. The tables present comprehensive delineations of associations among qualitative variables methodically.

The same format is used in this book to present contingency tables depicting associations between qualitative variables. Headings of columns indicate categories

Table 9.3 Association of MDS progression with mutation 30 days after stem cell transplantation

		MDS progression		
		YES	NO	SUM
Positive mutation	YES	66% (21)	34% (11)	100% (32)
	NO	26% (14)	74% (40)	100% (54)

of the outcome variable, and headings of rows indicate categories of explanatory variable. Percentages or other measures of prevalence or incidence in sub-cohorts specified by categories of the explanatory variable are displayed in rows. The percentages are row percentages; the sum of the percentages in the same row is 100% or within rounding error of 100%.

Example 9.2.1
Duncavage and Others (2018) (Example 9.1.1) used percentages and numbers of subjects whose MDS progressed to depict the association between MDS progression and positive mutation (maximum variant allele frequency of mutation 30 days after allogeneic hematopoietic stem cell transplantation). Table 9.3 presents a methodical display of the percentages and numbers. It is a two-way (2 by 2) contingency table and presents a comprehensive description of the association between MS progression and positive mutation. MDS progression is the outcome variable and positive mutation the explanatory variable. The percentages and numbers of subjects whose MDS did and did not progress in the mutation-positive and mutation-negative sub-cohorts are exhibited in rows. The percentages are row percentages determined by using the number exhibited in the rightmost cell of a row, number of subjects in a sub-cohort, to divide the numbers shown in the first two cells of the row. They comprise the distribution of the observations on the outcome variable of a sub-cohort of subjects specified by an attribute of the explanatory variable.

Example 9.2.2
Table 1 of Callaghan and Others (2004) (Table 9.1) is a two-way contingency table. It presents a comprehensive delineation of the association of seizure relapse with EEG classification. Numbers and percentages of subjects in each of four sub-cohorts specified by the EEG class are shown. The percentages depict cogently how seizure relapse is associated with EEG class.

Example 9.2.3 Quinn (318, 4)
Quinn and Others (1988) used 34.7% and 4.2% to depict the association of HIV seropositivity with participation in homosexual or bisexual activities demonstrated by data of a cohort of 2224 male subjects. Table 9.4, is a two-way contingency table that presents a comprehensive description of the association and shows how the percentages were computed.

Example 9.2.4
Table 3 of Young and Others (1993) (Table 9.2) is a three-way contingency table that presents a comprehensive delineation of the association of sleep-disordered breathing with habitual snoring and sex. It shows how percentages and numbers of

Table 9.4 Association of HIV seropositivity with participation in homosexual or bisexual activities

		HIV seropositivity		
		YES	NO	SUM
Homosexual or bisexual activity	YES	34.7% (67)	65.3% (126)	100% (193)
	NO	5.2% (105)	94.8% (1,926)	100% (2,031)

Table 9.5 Association of diabetic nephropathy with parental hypertension

		Diabetic nephropathy		
		YES	NO	SUM
Parental hypertension	YES	49% (24)	51% (25)	100% (49)
	NO	21% (7)	79% (27)	100% (34)

subjects whose apnea–hypopnea scores were high, medium, and low differed between subjects who were and were not habitual smokers among female and male subjects.

Example 9.2.5
Krolewski and Others (1988) used odds ratio (3.7) to measure the association of diabetic nephropathy with parental hypertension. The odds ratio suggests that the odds of diabetic nephropathy among 89 young subjects (children and adolescents) with insulin-dependent diabetes who have a parent with hypertension was 3.7 times the odds among those who did not.

The odds ratio is a result of dividing the cohort of 83 young subjects into two sub-cohorts of subjects with and without a hypertensive parent and determining the numbers and percentages of subjects with diabetic nephropathy in the sub-cohorts. Table 9.5 displays the numbers and percentage that were used to compute the odds ratio. The table is a two-way contingency table and presents a comprehensive delineation of the association. It shows that the prevalence of diabetic nephropathy in the sub-cohort of the 49 subjects having a hypertensive parent (49%) is higher and 2.3 times of that in the sub-cohort of 34 subjects not having a hypertensive parent (21%). It is important to note that the ratio of the prevalence rates is noticeably lower than the odds ratio.

Example 9.2.6
Bjerregaard and Others (2018) (Example 9.1.6) used hazard ratios to assess distinction in risks of having type 2 diabetes diagnosed at 30–60 years of age between the sub-cohorts of subjects with each of the eight overweight patterns and the sub-cohort of subjects who never had been overweight. Table 2 of the article (Table 9.6) shows number of subjects who had type 2 diabetes diagnosed at 30–60 years of age and hazard ratios assessing the risk of having type 2 diabetes diagnosed at 30–60 years of age in sub-cohorts of subjects specified by eight overweight patterns relative to the sub-cohort of subject who had never been overweight. The table constitutes a partial

Table 9.6 Table 2 of Bjerregaard and Others (378, 14)

Table 2. Adjusted Model of Patterns of Overweight from Childhood to Early Adulthood and the Risk of Type 2 Diabetes at 30 to 60 Years of Age.*

Variable	No. of Cases	Hazard Ratio for Type 2 Diabetes (95% CI)
Pattern of overweight†		
Never	2798	Reference
7 yr only	70	0.99 (0.78–1.25)
13 yr only	78	1.70 (1.35–2.12)
7 and 13 yr only	45	1.51 (1.13–2.03)
Early adulthood only	451	3.24 (2.93–3.58)
7 yr and early adulthood only	48	2.55 (1.92–3.39)
13 yr and early adulthood only	186	3.87 (3.33–4.49)
All ages	191	4.00 (3.45–4.63)
Intelligence-test score‡		
Low	1604	Reference
Medium	1319	0.86 (0.80–0.93)
High	944	0.70 (0.63–0.77)
Education§		
Short	1204	Reference
Medium	1508	0.84 (0.78–0.91)
Long	1155	0.75 (0.67–0.83)
Age at conscription	3867	0.93 (0.91–0.95)

* Data were stratified according to year of birth; in total, there were 62,565 observations and 3867 cases of type 2 diabetes diagnosed between 30 and 60 years of age. CI denotes confidence interval.

† Overweight was defined with the use of age-specific cutoff values for BMI proposed by the Centers for Disease Control and Prevention for boys (for age 7 years, ≥17.38; 13 years, ≥21.82; and early adulthood, ≥25).

‡ The intelligence-test scores were divided into three strata according to percentile.

§ Education was defined as short (7 to 10 years of primary school, with or without finals), medium (skilled training in industry, trade, or craft), or long (9 to 12 years of middle and secondary school or higher education).

Table 9.7 Prevalence of type 2 diabetes diagnosed at 30–60 years of age

	Type 2 diabetes at 30–60 years of age		
Pattern of overweight	YES	NO	Total
Never	5.1% (2798)	94.9% (51,731)	100% (54,529)
7 yr only	4.9% (70)	95.1% (1367)	100% (1437)
13 yr only	8.7% (78)	91.3% (822)	100% (900)
7 and 13 yr only	7.6% (45)	92.4% (546)	100% (591)
Early adulthood only	16.1% (451)	83.9% (2356)	100% (2807)
7 yr and early adulthood only	12.8% (48)	87.2% (326)	100% (374)
13 yr and early adulthood only	19.5% (186)	80.5% (770)	100% (956)
All age	19.7% (191)	80.3% (780)	100% (971)

description of the association of having type 2 diabetes diagnosed at 30–60 years of age with overweight pattern. Assessments of risks in sub-cohorts of subjects in the eight overweight patterns are not shown. It is unknown, for instance, how low the risk among the sub-cohort of subjects who had never been overweight and how high the risk among the sub-cohort of subjects who had been overweight at all ages are.

An alternative is to use a contingent table to present the percentages of subjects who had type 2 diabetes diagnosed at 30 to 60 years of age in the sub-cohort of subjects specified the eight overweight patterns. Table 1 of the article shows the numbers of subjects in sub-cohorts specified by the overweight patterns; Table 2 shows the number of subjects in each sub-cohort who had type 2 diabetes diagnosed at 30–60 years of age. These numbers were used to compute percentages of subjects who had type 2 diabetes diagnosed at 30–60 years of age in the eight sub-cohorts The percentages are shown in Table 9.7 which is a two-way contingency table. The percentages are prevalence rates and assessments of commonness of having type 2 diabetes diagnosed at 30 to 60 years of age and presents a comprehensive description of the association of having type 2 diabetes diagnosed at 30–60 years of age with overweight patterns. They unveil that, for instance, the percentage of subjects who had type 2 diabetes diagnosed at 30–60 years of age is 5.1% among the sub-cohort of subjects who had never been overweight and 19.7% among the sub-cohort of subjects who had been overweight at all ages.

The percentages shown in the table may be used to determine assessments of distinction in risks between any two sub-cohorts of subjects. For instance, the ratio of the percentage of the sub-cohort of subjects who had been overweight at all ages and that of the sub-cohort of subjects who had never been overweight is 19.7%/ 5.1% = 3.86 which is close to the hazard ratio shown in Table 2 and suggests that the prevalence of the subjects who had been overweight at all ages is about four times that of the subjects who had never been overweight.

One important indication of the table is that the percentages of subjects who had not been overweight in early adulthood (17–26 years of age) are below 10% (4.9%–8.7%), and those of subjects who had been overweight in early adulthood are above 12% (12.8%–19.7%).

The table yields that the total number of subjects who had not been overweight in early adulthood is 54,529 + 1737 +900 + 591 = 60,448. Of these, 2991 subjects (2,798 + 70 + 78 + 45) had type 2 diabetes diagnosed at 30–60 years of age. The total number of subjects who had been overweight in early adulthood is 2,087 + 374 +956 + 971 = 5,108. Of these, 876 subjects (451 + 48 + 186 + 191) had type 2 diabetes diagnosed at 30–60 years of age. These numbers yield that the percentage of subjects who had type 2 diabetes diagnosed at 30–60 years of age among those who had not been overweight in early adulthood is 2991/60,448 = 4.9%, the percentage of subjects who had type 2 diabetes diagnosed at 30–60 years of age among those who had been overweight in early adulthood is 876/5,108 = 17.1%. Their ratio 17.4%/4.9% = 3.6 suggests that the risk prevalence rate of having type 2 diabetes diagnosed at 30–60 years of age among those who had been overweight during early adulthood is about 3.6 times the prevalence rate among those who had not been overweight during early adulthood.

It is of interest to note that the prevalence rates displayed in Table 9.7 show that the hazard ratios shown in Table 2 of Bjerregaard and Others (2018) are close to their corresponding ratios of prevalence rates.

9.3 Measures of Strength of Association Between Two Qualitative Variables

The strength of association between qualitative variables is assessed by the same measures that are used to assess the degree of distinction between unpaired qualitative data sets. This section reviews some examples.

Example 9.3.1

Duncavage and Others (2018) (Example 9.1.1) used 66% and 26% to depict the association of MDS progression with positive variant allele frequency mutation after allogeneic hematopoietic stem cell transplantation. These are percentages of subjects whose MDS progressed during follow-up in mutation-positive and mutation-negative sub-cohorts. They are average incidence rates. The strength of the association may be measured by their difference or ratio.

The difference of the two average incidence rates RD = 66% − 26% = 40% unveils that the incidence rate of MDS progression among the 32 subjects of the mutation-positive sub-cohort is 40 percentage points higher than the incidence rate among the 54 subjects of the mutation-negative sub-cohort. The ratio of the incidence rates 66%/26% = 2.5 unveils that the incidence of MDS progression among the 32 subjects of the mutation-positive sub-cohort is 2.5 times the incidence among the 54 subjects of the mutation-negative sub-cohort.

Example 9.3.2 Callaghan (318, 15w)

Callaghan and Others (2004) (Example 9.1.2) used seizure relapse rates (percentages of subjects whose seizures relapsed) of sub-cohorts of subjects whose EEG classifications belonged to four classes to depict the association between seizure

Table 9.8 Rate differences and rate ratios comparing seizure rate of class 2 with other classes

	EEG class	Rate difference	Rate ratio
1	Normal before treatment and before withdrawal	35.5% − 35.5% = 0	35.5%/35.5% = 1
2	Abnormal before treatment, normal before withdrawal	11.4% − 35.5% = −24.1%	11.4%/35.5% = 0.3
3	Abnormal before treatment, abnormal, but improved before withdrawal	50.0% - 35.5% = 14.5%	50.0%/35.5% = 1.41
4	Abnormal before treatment, unchanged before withdrawal	73.7% − 35.5% = 38.2%	73.7%/35.5% = 2.08

relapse and EEG classification. One way to assess the strength of the association is to compare the incidence rates.

Table 9.8 shows rate differences and rate ratios when class 1 (normal before treatment and before withdrawal) is used as the reference class. The rate differences unveil that as compared with the subjects whose EEG classifications were normal before treatment and before withdrawal of treatment.

- The seizure relapse rate of the subjects whose EEG classifications improved from abnormal before treatment to normal before withdrawal is 24.1 percentage points lower.
- The seizure relapse rate of the subjects whose EEG classifications were abnormal before treatment and abnormal but improved before withdrawal is 14.5 percentage points higher.
- The seizure relapse rate of the subgroup of the subjects whose EEG classifications were abnormal before treatment and unchanged before withdrawal is 38.2 percentage points higher.

Rate ratios unveil that, as compared with subjects whose EEG classification were normal before treatment and before withdrawal of treatment,

- The seizure relapse rate of the subjects whose EEG classifications were abnormal before treatment but normal before withdrawal is lower than and 3-tenth of the rate of the subjects whose EEG classifications were normal before treatment and before withdrawal.
- The seizure relapse rate of the subjects whose EEG classification were abnormal before treatment and abnormal but improved before withdrawal is 1.41 times the rate of the subjects whose EEG classifications were normal before treatment and before withdrawal.
- The seizure relapse rate of the subjects whose EEG classification was abnormal before treatment and unchanged before withdrawal is 2.08 times the rate of the subjects whose EEG classifications were normal before treatment and before withdrawal.

Example 9.3.3

Quinn and Others (1988) (Example 9.1.3) used percentages of HIV seropositive subjects (34.7% vs. 4.2%) to depict the association of HIV seropositivity with homosexual or bisexual activity. The strength of the association was measured by odds ratio 12.2, which suggests that the odds of HIV seropositivity among the 191 subjects acknowledged participating in homosexual or bisexual activity are 12.2 times the odds among the 2031 subjects who did not.

The strength of the association may also be measured by the difference or ratio of the percentages. The percentages are measures of prevalence. Their difference $34.7\% - 4.2\% = 30.5\%$ suggests that the prevalence rate of HIV seropositivity among the 191 male subjects who acknowledged homosexual or bisexual activity is 30.5 percentage points higher than that among the 2031 who did not. Their ratio $34.7\%/4.2\% = 8.3$ suggests that the prevalence rate of HIV seropositivity among the 191 male subjects who acknowledged homosexual or bisexual activity was 8.3 times that among the 2031 who did not.

Example 9.3.4

Young and Others (1993) (Example 9.1.4) used percentages of subjects whose apnea–hypopnea scores belonged to three categories to depict the association of sleep-disordered breathing with habitual snoring and gender. The strength of the association may be measured by rate differences or rate ratios. Table 9.9 shows differences and ratios of the percentages by sex and habitual snoring. The differences and ratio unveil the following:

- Percentages of high apnea–hypopnea scores (≥15) of habitual snorers are 13.9 percentage points higher than and 5.48 times the percentage of nonhabitual snorers among the 352 male subjects and 4.4 percentage points higher than and 2.76 times the percentage of nonhabitual snorers among the 250 female subjects.

Table 9.9 Association of sleep-disordered breathing with habitual snoring and gender

	Apnea–hypopnea score			
	<5	5 – 14	≥15	Sum
	% (No.)	% (No.)	% (No.)	% (No.)
Women				
Habitual snorer	80.8% (105)	12.3% (16)	6.9% (9)	100.0% (130)
Nonhabitual snorer	95.0% (114)	2.5% (3)	2.5% (3)	100.0% (120)
Rate difference[a]	−14.2%	9.5%	4.4%	
Rate ratio[b]	0.85	4.80	2.76	
Men				
Habitual snorer	66.0% (149)	17.0% (38)	17.0% (38)	100.0% (225)
Nonhabitual snorer	83.5% (106)	13.4[c] (17)	3.1% (4)	100.0% (127)
Rate difference[a]	−17%	3.6%	13.9%	
Rate ratio[b]	0.80	1.25	5.48	

[a]Habitual snorers minus nonhabitual snorers
[b]Nonhabitual snorers divided by habitual snorer
[c]Differs from the one shown in Table 3 of Young and Others (1993) slightly

- Percentages of medium apnea–hypopnea scores of habitual snorers are 3.6 percentage points higher than and 1.25 times the percentage of nonhabitual snorers among the 352 male subjects and 9.5 percentage points higher than and 4.80 times the percentage of nonhabitual snorers among the 250 female subjects.

Example 9.3.5
Krolewski and Others (1988) (Example 9.1.5) reported that the odds of nephropathy among the 49 subjects with hypertensive parent were 3.7 times that among the 34 subjects without.

Table 1 suggests that diabetic nephropathy was documented in 24 of the sub-cohort of 49 subjects with hypertensive parents and 7 of 34 subjects of the sub-cohort of subjects without. The numbers yield that the percentages of subjects with diabetic nephropathy are 24/49 = 49% among the 49 subjects with hypertensive parents and 7/34 = 21% among the 34 subjects without. The percentages are assessments of the prevalence of diabetic nephropathy. Their difference: 49%–21% = 28% unveils that the prevalence rate of diabetic nephropathy of the 49 subjects with hypertensive parent is 28 percentage points higher than that of the 34 subjects without. Their ratio 3.7 suggests that the prevalence rate of diabetic nephropathy of the 49 subjects with hypertensive parents is 2.3 times that of the 34 subjects without.

9.4 Reliability of Diagnostic and Prognostic Procedures

Evaluating the reliability of diagnostic and prognostic procedures is a special case of appraising the association between two qualitative variables. It has its own nomenclature. Often-used terms are demonstrated in this section by examples.

When the reliability of a diagnosis or prognosis procedure is evaluated, known states or results of a well-established procedure are used as true states (diseased or disease-free). The numbers of appraisals of the procedure that do and do not agree with the true states are determined and used to compute measures of reliability. The numbers are displayed in Table 9.10.

Table 9.10 Numbers of test results by true states

		Diseased (true state)		
		YES	NO	SUM
Test results	Positive	# (Correct positive)	# (False positive)	# (Positive)
	Negative	# (False negative)	# (Correct negative)	# (Negative)
	SUM	# (Diseased)	# (Number disease-free)	# (TOTAL)

Measures of reliability are computed as follows:

$$\begin{aligned}&\text{Overall accuracy}\\&=\frac{\text{Number of correct tests}}{\text{Number of tests}}\times 100\%\\&=\frac{\text{Number of correct positive tests}+\text{Number of correct negative tests}}{\text{Number of tests}}\times 100\%\end{aligned}\quad(9.4.1)$$

$$\text{Sensitivity}=\text{Correct positive rate}=\frac{\text{Number of correct positive tests}}{\text{Number of diseased subjects}}\times 100\%\quad(9.4.2)$$

$$\text{Specificity}=\text{Correct negative rate}=\frac{\text{Number of correct negative tests}}{\text{Number of disease-free cases}}\times 100\%\quad(9.4.3)$$

$$\text{Positive predictive value}=\frac{\text{Number of correct positive tests}}{\text{Number of positive tests}}\times 100\%\quad(9.4.4)$$

$$\text{Negative predictive value}=\frac{\text{Number of negative positive tests}}{\text{Number of negative tests}}\times 100\%\quad(9.4.5)$$

Overall accuracy is the percentage of correct test results among all results; sensitivity and specificity are percentages of correct test results among diseased cases and among disease-free subjects, and predictive values are percentages of correct results among positive tests and among negative tests.

The reliability of a diagnostic or prognostic procedure may be evaluated by applying it to the set of data from which the procedure was constructed and applying it to data sets that were not involved in its construction. The former is dubbed a circular, internal, or retrospective evaluation and the latter an external, prospective evaluation, or validation. The data used to construct the procedures are dubbed training data; the data used to validate the procedure externally are dubbed validating data.

Example 9.4.1

Goldman and Others (1988) presented the results of a study that used the data of 1379 patients with chest pain to construct a computer protocol for the diagnosis of myocardial infarction (MI). The reliability of the protocol was evaluated circularly and externally. The circular evaluation was performed by applying the protocol to the 1379 subjects from whose data it was developed. The external validation was performed by applying the protocol to 4770 subjects whose data were not involved in its construction. Measures of reliability were determined by using ultimate diagnoses according to elaborate and strict clinical criteria as true states. For convenience, these subjects are dubbed MI cases and MI-free subjects.

Table 9.11 Numbers of classifications used to compute measure of reliability of circular evaluation

		Ultimate diagnoses (true state)		
		MI	MI-free	SUM
Protocol	MI present	253 (Correct positive)	378 (False positive)	631 (Positive)
	MI absent	6 (False negative)	742 (Correct positive)	748 (Negative)
	SUM	259 (MI present)	1120 (MI-free)	1379 (Total)

Circular Evaluation The results of the circular evaluation were related as follows:

> When applied retrospectively to the training sample from which it was derived, the protocol correctly classified 253 of 259 patients with infarction (98 percent) and 742 of 1120 patients without infarction (66 percent) (Table 1).

The percentages 98% and 66% are sensitivity and specificity. They unveil that the protocol correctly identified 98% (253) of the 259 MI cases and 66% (742) of the 1120 MI-free subjects.

Table 9.11 shows the data used in the circular evaluation. The reliability measures were determined as follows:

$$\text{Sensitivity} = \text{Correct positive rate} = \frac{\text{Number of correct positive tests}}{\text{Number of MI cases}} = \frac{253}{259} = 98\%$$

$$\text{Specificity} = \text{Correct negative rate} = \frac{\text{Number of correct negative tests}}{\text{Number of disease-free subjects}} = \frac{742}{1120} = 66\%$$

$$\text{Positive predictive value} = \frac{\text{Number of correct positive test}}{\text{Number of positive tests}} = \frac{253}{631} = 40\%$$

$$\text{Negative predictive value} = \frac{\text{Number of correct negative tests}}{\text{Number of negative tests}} = \frac{742}{748} = 99\%.$$

$$\begin{aligned}&\text{Overall accuracy}\\ &= \frac{\text{Number of correct positive tests} + \text{Number of correct negative tests}}{\text{Total number of tests}}\\ &= \frac{253 + 742}{1379} = 72\%\end{aligned}$$

The sensitivity suggests that 98% of the MI cases were correctly identified, and the sensitivity suggests that only 66% of the MI-free subjects were correctly identified. The positive predictive value suggests that only 40% of the positive results of

Table 9.12 Numbers of classifications used to compute measure of reliability of circular evaluation

		Ultimate diagnoses (true state)		
		MI	MI-free	SUM
Protocol	MI present	507 (Correct positive)	1083 (False positive)	1590 (Positive)
	MI absent	69 (False negative)	3111 (Correct negative)	3180 (Negative)
	SUM	576 (MI cases)	4194 (MI-free)	4770 (Total)

the protocol were correct; the negative predictive value suggests that as much as 99% of the negative results of the protocol were correct. The overall accuracy unveils that 72% of the results of the protocol were correct.

External Validation The computer protocol was validated externally by using data of 4770 patients who were not involved in the construction of the protocol. The numbers used in this external validation are displayed in Table 9.12. The reliability measures were computed from the numbers as follows:

$$\text{Sensitivity} = \text{Correct positive rate} = \frac{\text{Number of correct positive tests}}{\text{Number of MI cases}} = \frac{507}{576} = 88\%.$$

$$\text{Specificity} = \text{Correct negative rate} = \frac{\text{Number of correct negative tests}}{\text{Number of disease-free subjects}} = \frac{3111}{4194} = 74\%$$

$$\text{Positive predictive value} = \frac{\text{Number of correct positive test}}{\text{Number of positive tests}} = \frac{507}{1590} = 32\%$$

$$\text{Negative predictive value} = \frac{\text{Number of correct negative tests}}{\text{Number of negative tests}} = \frac{3111}{3180} = 98\%.$$

$$\begin{aligned}&\text{Overall accuracy}\\ &= \frac{\text{Number of correct positive tests} + \text{Number of correct negative tests}}{\text{Total number of tests}}\\ &= \frac{507 + 3111}{4770} = 76\%.\end{aligned}$$

Table 9.13 shows the reliability measures of the circular evaluation and the external validation. It shows that the overall accuracies and negative predictive value of the two evaluations are relatively close (76% vs. 72% and 98% vs. 99%). The external validation, compared with the circular evaluation, had lower sensitivity (88% vs. 98%) and positive predictive value (32% vs. 40%) but higher specificity (74% vs. 66%).

Table 9.13 Measures of reliability of computer protocol determined by circular and external evaluations

	Overall accuracy	Sensitivity	Specificity	Positive predictive	Negative predictive
Circular	72% (995/1379)	98% (253/259)	66% (472/1120)	40% (253/631)	99% (742/748)
External	76% (3618/4770)	88% (507/576)	74% (3111/4194)	32% (507/1590)	98% (3111/3180)

Table 9.14 Reliability measures of indirect water derivation test and hypertonic saline–stimulated copeptin with >4.9 pmol/liter cutoff

	Diagnostic accuracy	Sensitivity	Specificity	Predictive value positive	Predictive value negative
Indirect water deprivation	76.6% (108/141)	86.4% (51/59)	69.5% (57/82)	67.1% (57/76)	87.7% (253/631)
Hypertonic saline–stimulated copeptin with >4.9 pmol/liter	97.1% (136/140)[a]	93.2% (55/59)	100.0% (81/81)	100.0% (55/55)	95.3% (81/85)

[a]The sum of the total number of tests is 140. The diagnostic accuracy equals 136/140 = 97.1% not the one shown in Table 2 and cited in the narrative 96.5% (136/141)

Example 9.4.2

Fenske and Others (2018) presented the results of a study that compared water deprivation test with hypertonic saline infusion test for the diagnosis of diabetes insipidus. The results of 141 subjects with hypotonic polyuria were analyzed. The primary outcome was the overall diagnostic accuracy of each test when final diagnoses by independent board-certified experts in endocrinology were used as true states. The following is one description of the accuracies of the tests:

> The overall diagnostic accuracy of the hypertonic saline infusion test was significantly higher than that of the indirect water-deprivation test (96.5%. [95% confidence interval [CI], 92.1 to 98.6] vs. 76.6% [95% CI, 68.9 to 83.2]; P < 0.001) (Table 2).

Table 2 suggests that the diagnostic accuracies 96.5% and 76.6% are overall accuracies, percentages of test results confirmed by final reference diagnoses when the procedures were used to distinguish central diabetes insipidus from primary polydipsia. The reliability measures of the two tests are shown in Table 9.14, which shows clearly that the hypertonic saline–stimulated copeptin test with >4.9 pmol/liter cutoff, as compared with indirect water deprivation test, had not only substantially higher overall accuracy (97.1% vs. 76.6%) but also the other reliability measures. (The overall diagnostic accuracy of the hypertonic saline infusion test cited in the above narrative: 96.5% was computed by using 141 as the total number of tests. As shown in Table 9.15, it is 140 and the overall diagnostic accuracy is 136/140 = 97.1%.)

Table 9.15 Results of hypertonic saline–stimulated copeptin test with >4.9 pmol/liter cutoff in distinguishing central diabetes insipidus from primary polydipsia

		True state (final reference diagnosis)		
		Central diabetes insipidus	Primary polydipsia	SUM
Test result	Primary polydipsia	55 (Correct positive)	0 (False positive)	55 (Total positive)
	Central diabetes insipidus	4 (False negative)	81 (Correct negative)	85 (Total negative)
	SUM	59 (Central diabetes insipidus)	81 (Primary polydipsia)	140 (Total tests)

Table 9.15 presents the numbers of test results that were used to compute measure of reliability of the hypertonic saline infusion test with >4.9 pmol/liter cutoff. The reliability measures of the test were computed from these numbers as follows:

$$\text{Diagnostic accuracy} = \frac{\text{Number of correct positive tests} + \text{Number of correct negative tests}}{\text{Total number of tests}} = \frac{55 + 81}{140} = 97.1\%.$$

$$\text{Sensitivity} = \text{Correct positive rate} = \frac{\text{Number of correct positive tests}}{\text{Number of central diabetes insipidus}} = \frac{55}{59} = 93.2\%.$$

$$\text{Specificity} = \text{Correct negative rate} = \frac{\text{Number of correct negative tests}}{\text{Number of primary polydipsia}} = \frac{81}{81} = 100\%$$

$$\text{Positive predictive value} = \frac{\text{Number of correct positive test}}{\text{Number of positive tests}} = \frac{55}{55} = 100\%$$

$$\text{Negative predictive value} = \frac{\text{Number of correct negative tests}}{\text{Number of negative tests}} = \frac{81}{85} = 95.3\%$$

9.5 Intelligent Reading and Informative Reporting

To read intelligently descriptions of association between two qualitative variables, it is essential to identify the outcome and the explanatory variables and probe how measures of prevalence or incidence of attributes of the outcome variable differ among sub-cohorts of subjects specified by attributes of the explanatory variable. To report informatively, it is vital to depict distinctly how the prevalence or incidence of attributes of the outcome variable are measured and how they differ among sub-cohorts of subjects specified by attributes of the explanatory variable.

Example 9.5.1
Duncavage and Others (2018) (Example 9.1.1) used average incidence rates (66% and 26%) to depict the association of MDS progression during follow-up with maximum variant allele frequency of a mutation 30 days after allogeneic hematopoietic stem cell transportation. It also used adjusted cumulative incidence rates and hazard ratio to depict the association of MDS progression during 1 year of follow-up with maximum variant allele frequency of a mutation 30 days after allogeneic hematopoietic stem cell transportation. The article stated:

> The presence of at least one mutation with a variant allele frequency of at least 0.5% 30 days after allogeneic hematopoietic stem-cell transplantation was associated with a higher risk of disease progression at 1 year than the absence of such a mutation, even after adjustment for conditioning regimen (53.1% vs. 13.0%; hazard ratio, 3.86; 95% confidence interval [CI], 1.96 to 7.62; P<0.001) (Fig. S4A in the Supplementary Appendix).

The percentages 53.1% and 13.0% and hazard ratio 3.86 are the result of adjusting for the conditioning regimen. To read intelligently, it is critical to note that they would be oversimplifications and misleading if the cumulative incidence rates and hazard ratios of subgroups of subjects specified by the conditioning regiment (reduced-intensity conditions and myeloablative conditioning) differed substantially.

Figure 3A (Fig. 9.1) suggests that the adjusted cumulative incidence rates and hazard ratios are oversimplifications. It suggests that the one-year cumulative incidence rate of the mutation-positive subjects differed markedly (75% vs. 30% approximately) between the subjects who received the reduced-intensity conditioning regimen (red solid lines) and the subjects who received the myeloablative conditioning regimen (red dashed lines). The adjusted cumulative incidence rate of the mutation-positive subjects (53.1%) is in the middle and differs from the rates of the two subgroups of subjects (75% vs. 30%) substantially. It is an oversimplification and is misleading when it is applied to subjects who received either reduced-intensity or myeloablative conditioning regimen.

The one-year cumulative incidence rate of the mutation-negative subjects differed noticeably (15% vs. 10% approximately) between the subjects who received the reduced-intensity conditioning regimen (blue solid lines) and the subjects who received the myeloablative conditioning regimen (blue dashed lines). The adjusted cumulative incidence rate (13.0%) is in the middle of the incidence rates of the two

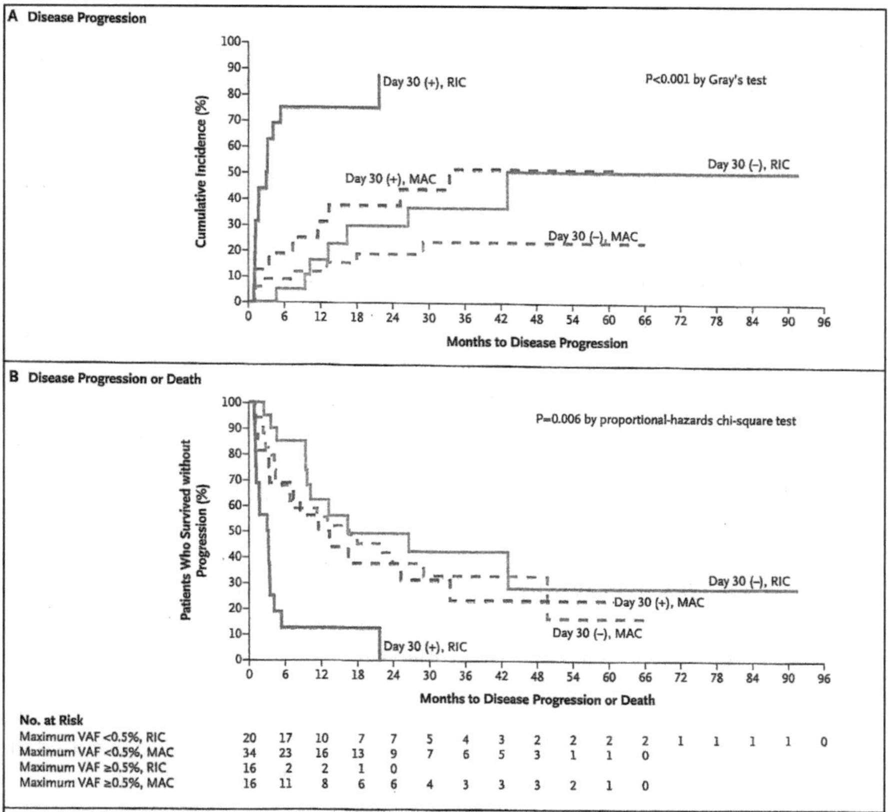

Figure 3. Association of Mutation Clearance with Outcomes.
The VAF on day 30 after transplantation was determined with the use of error-corrected sequencing interrogating single-nucleotide variant mutations identified by enhanced exome sequencing of samples before transplantation. Patients are grouped according to the presence of positive (+) or negative (−) results for at least one mutation VAF of at least 0.5% (red lines) or all VAFs less than 0.5% (blue lines) and according to whether the patient received a reduced-intensity conditioning regimen (RIC, solid lines) or myeloablative conditioning (MAC, dashed lines). The rates of disease progression (Panel A) and disease progression or death (Panel B) are shown.

Fig. 9.1 Figure 3 of Duncavage and Others (2018)

subgroups (15% and 10%). It is misleading, though not manifestly, when it is applied to subjects who received either reduced-intensity or myeloablative conditioning regimen.

The ratio of the cumulative incidence rates of the mutation-positive and mutation-negative subjects equals 53.1%/13.0% = 4.08. The ratio of the cumulative incidence rates of the mutation-positive and mutation-negative subjects equals 75%/15% = 5.0 among the subgroup of subjecting who received reduced-intensity conditioning regimen and 15%/10% = 1.5 among the subgroup of subjects who receive the myeloablative conditioning regimen. They differed manifestly and suggest that the ratio of the adjusted cumulative incidence rates 53.1%/13.0% = 4.08 is an oversimplification and is misleading when it is applied to subgroups of subjects who received reduced-intensity conditioning regimen or myeloablative conditioning regimen.

The adjusted hazard ratio 3.86 is close to the ratio of adjusted incidence rates 4.08. It probably is also an oversimplification and misleading when it is applied to subgroups of subjects who received reduced-intensity conditioning regimen or myeloablative conditioning regimen.

To report informatively, it is more prolific to refer to Figure 3 and stress how the incidence of MDS progression differed between mutation-positive and mutation-negative subjects in sub-cohort of subjects who received a reduced-intensity conditioning (RIC) and the sub-cohort of subjects who received the myeloablative conditioning regimen (MAC).

Example 9.5.2
One feature of the study reported by Quinn and Others (1988) is that it performed univariate as well as multivariate analysis. The following is a narrative of the results of a multivariate analysis:

> Among women, parental drug use or status as a sexual partner of a bisexual man or a parenteral drug user was independently predictive of HIV seropositivity (Table 4). Of the sexual transmitted diseases, only a history of genital warts was independently associated with HIV seropositivity in women.

It is unclear what is meant by "independently predictive" and "independently associated." Does it mean that the association of HIV seropositivity with each variable was not affected by the other two variables?

Table 4 (Table 9.16) shows, for women, β-coefficients, P-values, and odds ratios of three variables: intravenous drug use, intravenous drug user as sex partner, and genital warts. These are the results of a multivariate regression analysis that used the three traits as its explanatory variables and presumed that the odds ratios of each variable are identical in subgroups of subjects specified by each other variable. That is, the associations of HIV seropositivity with the three variables are independent in the special sense that the association with each variable is not affected by the status of the other variable. As whether this presumption of the analysis is realistic is unknown, it is uncertain whether the result of the analysis is reliable.

It is more productive to show the odds ratios of each variable in subgroups of subjects specified by the other variables. The associations are indeed independent if the odds ratios of each variable in the subgroups specified by the variables are close. For instance, the association with genital warts would be "independent" of intravenous drug use and intravenous drug user as sex partner if the odds ratios of genital warts were close between the subgroups of subjects who did and did no use intravenous drug and between subgroups of subjects who did and did not have intravenous drug user as sex partner.

Example 9.5.3
The study reported by Goldman and Others (1988) (Example 9.4.1) evaluated in several ways the computer protocol for the diagnosis of myocardial infarction. Reliability measures were determined retrospectively by applying the protocol to the 1739 subjects from whose data the protocol was constructed and externally by applying the protocol to 4770 subjects whose data were not involved in the

Table 9.16 Table 4 of Quinn and Others (1988)

Table 4. Multivariate Logistic Regression Analysis of HIV Seropositivity.

Variable	β-Coefficient	P Value	Odds Ratio (95% Confidence Interval)
Men			
Race (white vs. nonwhite)	2.12	0.0420	8.3 (1.1–63.8)
Age (four groups)*	0.59	<0.0001	1.8 (1.5–2.3)
Homosexual or bisexual activity	2.66	<0.0001	14.2 (9.1–22.4)
Intravenous drug use	0.80	0.0038	2.2 (1.3–3.8)
History of syphilis	0.67	0.0057	2.0 (1.2–3.2)
Seropositivity for syphilis	1.20	<0.0001	3.3 (2.0–5.5)
Women			
Intravenous drug use	1.99	<0.0001	7.3 (2.9–18.2)
Intravenous drug user as sex partner	1.03	0.0206	2.8 (1.2–6.7)
Genital warts	1.42	0.0050	4.1 (1.5–11.1)

*Age groups were 15 to 19, 20 to 24, 25 to 29, and 30 years of age or more.

construction of the protocol. The external reliability measures were also compared with reliability measures of physicians' actual decisions to admit the 4770 patients to coronary care unit. The article stated:

> As compared with the physicians' actual decisions to admit patients to the coronary care unit, the computer protocol had a significantly higher specificity and overall accuracy, a marginally higher positive predictive value, and minimally higher sensitivity (Table 2).

It seems that, compared with physicians' decision, the computer protocol had markedly higher specificity and overall accuracy but only slightly higher positive predictive value and sensitivity. To read intelligently, it is critical to check the magnitude of the distinctions. Table 2 (Table 9.17) shows that all distinctions are small. The distinctions in specificities (74% vs. 71%), overall accuracies (76% vs. 73%), and positive predictive values (32% vs. 29%) are all 3 percentage points. The distinctions in specificities and overall accuracies were declared statistically significant, but the distinction in positive predictive values was not.

P-values of the distinctions in specificity and overall accuracy (71% vs. 74% and 73% vs. 76%) are small because they are the results of large numbers of observations (4194 and 4770); *P*-value of distinction in positive predictive value (29% vs. 32%) are not small because it is a result of smaller numbers of observations (1730 and 1590).

Table 9.17 Table 2 of Goldman and Others (1988)

Table 2. Comparison of Physicians' Judgment with Computer Predictions in Deciding Whether to Admit 4770 Patients to the Coronary Care Unit at Six Hospitals.

	Sensitivity*	Specificity†	Positive Predictive Value‡	Overall Accuracy
	number of infarctions/total number of patients (percent)			
Physicians	506/576 (87.8)	2970/4194 (71)	506/1730 (29)	3476/4770 (73)
Computer protocol	507/576 (88.0)	3111/4194 (74)	507/1590 (32)	3618/4770 (76)
P value	NS	<0.00001	0.10	<0.00001

*Percentage of patients with myocardial infarction who were admitted to the coronary care unit.

†Percentage of patients without myocardial infarction who were not admitted to the coronary care unit.

‡Percentage of patients with myocardial infarction among the total number of patients admitted to the coronary care unit.

To report informatively, it is more forthright to cite values of measures of reliability and note that all measures of the computer protocol were just slightly higher than those of physicians' decision.

Review Questions

1. How do the data analyzed to evaluate the association between two qualitative variables differ from the data analyzed to evaluate distinction between two unpaired qualitative data sets?
2. How useful are contingency tables for the purpose of depicting association between two qualitative variables?
3. How does the indication of ratio of odds of YES differ from the indication of ratio of percentages of YES?
4. Under what condition is an adjusted rate ratio, adjusted odds ratio, or adjusted hazard ratio a single convenient measure of distinction applicable to subgroups of subjects specified by its adjusting variables?
5. How may the influence of a factor on the association between two qualitative variables be portrayed informatively?
6. Is a small *P*-value an affirmation that an association is strong and clinically important?

Exercise

9.E.1. Review Fig. 3 of Duncavage and Others (Fig. 9.1).

(a) Determine the approximate values of cumulative incidence rates of MDS progression at 2 years among mutation-positive and mutation-negative subjects in the subgroup of subjects who received RIC and the subgroup of subjects who received MAC. Discuss what the rates suggest.

(b) Compute the ratio of the cumulative incidence rates between mutation-positive and mutation-negative subjects in the subgroup of subjects who received RIC and the subgroup of subjects who received MAC. Discuss what the ratios suggest.
(c) Suggest likely values of the crude cumulative incidence rates of MDS progression at 2 years among mutation-positive and mutation-negative subjects when conditioning regimen and other factors are not considered. Compute the ratio of the crude rates. Discuss usefulness of the crude rates and their ratio suggest.
(d) Suggest likely values of the adjusted cumulative incidence rates of MDS progression at 2 years among mutation-positive and mutation-negative subjects when conditioning regimen is the adjusting variable. Compute the ratio of the adjusted rates. Discuss the adjusted rates and their ratio are more useful than the crude rates and their ratio.

9.E.2. Bjerregaard and Others (2018) (Example 9.1.6) reported that the hazard ratios assessing distinction in risks of having type 2 diabetes diagnosed at 30–60 years of age in subjects whose educational levels were medium and high relative to the risk in subjects whose education levels were low are 0.86 and 0.70, respectively. Elaborate the suggestions of the hazard ratios and discuss how the association of having type 2 diabetes diagnosed at 30–60 years of age with a level of education may be depicted more informatively.

9.E.3. Table 3 of Young and Others (1993) (Table 9.2) shows the percentages and numbers of subjects whose apnea–hypopnea scores belonged to three categories by female and male subjects separately.

(a) Use the available information to compute crude percentages of habitual snorers and nonhabitual snorers whose apnea–hypopnea scores belonged to three categories when sex and other potentially related factors are ignored.
(b) Discuss whether the crude percentages and their ratio are oversimplifications.
(c) Suggest likely values of adjusted percentages of subjects whose apnea-hypopnea scores belonged to three categories when sex is the adjusting variable.
(d) Discuss whether the adjusted percentages and their ratio are oversimplifications.

9.E.4. The following statement was presented by Quinn and Others (1988) immediately following the statement cited in Example 9.1.3: *Similarly, HIV seroprevalence was significantly higher among men who acknowledged using parenteral drugs since 1978, as compared with those who did not.* Table 2 shows that percentages of HIV seropositivity were 15.2% among 224 male subjects who acknowledged intravenous drug use and 5.3% among 2358 who did not. Odds ratio equals 3.2, and P-value is <0.001. Table 3 shows that percentages of HIV seropositivity were 21.5% among 65 women who acknowledged intravenous drug use and 1.9% among 1214 who did not. Odds ratio equals 14.2, and P-value is <0.001.

(a) Use a table to display the percentages and numbers that constitute a comprehensive delineation of the association of HIV seropositivity with intravenous drug use and sex. Demonstrate how the odds ratios were computed.
(b) Use the percentages of HIV seropositive men and women to depict the association of HIV seropositivity with intravenous drug use and sex.
(c) Use the odds ratios to depict how HIV seropositivity was associated with intravenous drug use and sex.
(d) Discuss the relative merit of using ratios of percentages and ratios of odds to depict the association of HIV seropositivity with intravenous drug use and sex.
(e) Use a table to display the percentages and numbers that constitute a comprehensive delineation of the association of HIV seropositivity with intravenous drug use when sex and other factors are ignored.
(f) Discuss relative advantages when the ratio of the percentages and odds ratio is used to assess the association when effects of sex and other factors are not concerned.
(g) Suggest likely values of adjusted percentages of HIV seropositive subjects among subjects who did and did not acknowledge intravenous drug use and their ratio and odds ratio adjusted for sex. Elaborate their suggestions.

9.E.5. Review Table 2 of Goldman and Others (1988) (Table 9.17).

(a) Use a table to display the numbers used to compute measures of reliability of physicians' decision and demonstrate how the measures of reliability were computed.
(b) Elaborate the suggestions of the measures of reliability.

9.E.6. Table 2 of Fenske and Others (2018) (Example 9.4.2) shows that the measures of reliability of the water derivation–stimulated test in distinguishing primary polydipsia from central diabetes insipidus. Diagnostic accuracy = 44.0 (62/141), sensitivity = 98.3% (58/59), specificity = 5.0% (4/80), positive predictive value = 43.3% (58/134), and negative predictive value = 80.0% (4/5).

(a) Use a table to display the numbers used in the computations of the measures of reliability and demonstrate how the measures were computed.
(b) Elaborate the suggestions of the measures of reliability.

References

Bjerregaard, L. G., et al. (2018). Change in overweight from childhood to early adulthood and risk of type diabetes. *The New England Journal of Medicine, 378*(14), 1302–1312.

Callaghan, N., et al. (2004). Withdrawal of anticonvulsant drugs in patients free of seizure for two years. *The New England Journal of Medicine, 318*(15), 942–946.

Duncavage, E. J., et al. (2018). Mutation clearance after transplantation for myelodysplastic syndrome. *The New England Journal of Medicine, 378*(11), 1028–1041.

Fenske, W., et al. (2018). A copeptin-based approach in the diagnosis of diabetes insipidus. *The New England Journal of Medicine, 379*(5), 428–439.

Goldman, L., et al. (1988). A computer protocol to predict myocardial infarction in emergency department patients with chest pain. *The New England Journal of Medicine, 318*(13), 797–803.

Krolewski, A. S., et al. (1988). Epidemiology of diabetes and its complications. *The New England Journal of Medicine, 318*(24), 1619–1620.

Quinn, T. C., et al. (1988). Human immunodeficiency virus infection among patients attending clinics for sexually transmitted disease. *The New England Journal of Medicine, 318*(4), 197–203.

Young, T., et al. (1993). The occurrence of sleep-disorder breathing among middle-aged adults. *The New England Journal of Medicine, 328*(17), 1230–1235.

Part III
P-Value and 95% Confidence Interval

P-values and 95% confidence intervals are regularly presented to corroborate descriptions of revelations of data. Revelations of data are declared "significant" when *P*-values are below 0.05% and 95% confidence intervals exclude the null values of the statistics portraying data revelations. Descriptions of "significant" data revelations are frequently ambiguous and hyperbolic. To read intelligently, it is vital to know what *P*-values and 95% confidence intervals suggest.

This part probes suggestions of *P*-value and 95% confidence interval. The foundation of the methods for determinations of *P*-value and 95% confidence interval is the sampling distribution of the sample statistic portraying data revelation. Chapter 10 presents simple examples of sampling distribution. The suggestion of *P*-value is explored in Chap. 11. Use of 95% confidence intervals to assess reproducibility of data revelations is examined in Chap. 12.

Chapter 10
Sampling Distribution

Determination of P-values and 95% confidence intervals require the condition that the statistics portraying revelations of data are statistics of random samples. They are derived from sampling distributions of statistics of random samples. This chapter uses simple examples to demonstrate what constitutes a random sample and what constitutes the sampling distribution of the statistic of a random sample. Section 10.1 uses a simple example to exemplify random sample and universe. Examples of three fundamentally important sampling distributions are reviewed in Sects. 10.2, 10.3, and 10.4. The standard error of the mean of a random sample is sometimes cited in descriptions of data revelations. Its use is examined in Sect. 10.5.

10.1 Random Sample

Random sample is a required condition for statistical significance tests and methods of constructing construction of 95% confidence interval. This section uses simple examples to demonstrate what constitutes a random sample.

- *Sample and Universe*

A set of elements selected from a collection of elements is called a sample; the collection of elements is called a universe or a population. The elements may be observational units such as patients, students, or blood samples. A universe consisting of a countable number of elements is a finite universe. The exact number may be unknown. This book assumes that universes are finite for convenience.

Remark Universes are referred to as populations in many statistical texts. However, the subjects of clinical studies are often dubbed populations. They are samples when statistical significance is tested and confidence intervals are constructed. For this reason, the term "universe" is used in this book instead of population.

P. C. Chang, *Data Analysis of Medical Studies*,
https://doi.org/10.1007/978-3-031-49984-5_10

- *Universe Parameters and Sample Statistics*

In statistics, synoptic descriptions of observations such as the mean, standard deviation, medium, range, and percentage are referred to as sample statistics or simply statistics when the observations are considered elements of samples; they are referred to as universe parameters or simply parameters when they are synoptic descriptions of observations of universes. This book uses Latin letters to denote sample statistics and Greek letters to denote universe parameters. Some examples are shown in the following table.

Symbols for some sample statistics and universe parameters

Descriptive measures	Sample statistic	Universe parameters
Size	n	η
Mean	MEAN	μ
Variance	SD^2	σ^2
Standard deviation	SD	σ
Proportion	P	π

Example 10.1.1

Table 10.1 presents elements of unrealistically small finite universes fabricated for the purpose of this chapter. Its first row shows identifications of the subjects that are the observational units of the subject universe. The second row exhibits elements of the BMI universe consisting of body mass indices of the subjects, and the third row elements of the AHI universe consisting of apnea–hypopnea indices of the subjects. The 0s and 1s displayed in the fourth row are elements of the obesity universe; 0 indicates that the body mass index of a subject is below 30, and 1 indicates that the body mass index of a subject is greater than or equal to 30. The 0s and 1s displayed in the fifth row are elements of the apnea universe; 0 indicates that the apnea–hypopnea score of a subject is below 20 and 1 that the score of a subject is greater than or equals 20.

Means, variances, and standard deviations of the universes are also exhibited in Table 10.1. The variances and standard deviations were computed by the numbers of elements as their denominators.

The means, variances, and standard deviations of the universes were computed as follows:

BMI universe:

$$\mu_{(\mathrm{BMI})} = \frac{20 + 24 + 28 + 32 + 36 + 40}{6} = 30.0$$

Table 10.1 Elements and parameters of universes

Universe	Elements						Parameters			
Subject	A	B	C	D	E	F	$\eta = 6$			
BMI	20	24	28	32	36	40	$\eta_{BMI} = 6$	$\mu_{BMI} = 30$	$\sigma^2_{BMI} = 56.0$	$\sigma_{BMI} = 7.5$
AHI	10	15	20	22	23	30	$\eta_{AHI} = 6$	$\mu_{AHI} = 20$	$\sigma^2_{AHI} = 6.7$	$\sigma_{AHI} = 6.8$
Obesity	0	0	0	1	1	1	$\eta_{Obesity} = 6$	$\mu_{Obesity} = 0.5$	$\sigma^2_{Obesity} = 0.25$	$\sigma_{Obesity} = 0.05$
Apnea	0	0	1	1	1	1	$\eta_{Apnea} = 6$	$\mu_{Apnea} = 0.67$	$\sigma^2_{Apnea} = 0.22$	$\sigma_{Apnea} = 0.47$

$$\sigma^2{}_{(\mathrm{BMI})} = \frac{(20-30)2+(24-30)2+(28-30)2+(32-30)2+(36-30)2+(40-30)2}{6}$$
$$= 46.7.$$

$$\sigma_{(\mathrm{BMI})} = \sqrt{46.7} = 6.8.$$

AHI universe:

$$\mu_{(\mathrm{AHI})} = \frac{10+15+20+22+23+30}{6} = 20.0$$

$$\sigma^2{}_{(\mathrm{AHI})} = \frac{(10-20)2+(15-20)2+(20-20)2+(22-20)2+(23-20)2+(30-20)2}{6}$$
$$= 47.6.$$

$$\sigma_{(\mathrm{AHI})} = \sqrt{47.6} = 6.3.$$

Obesity universe:

$$\mu_{\mathrm{O}} = \frac{0+0+0+1+1+1}{6} = 0.5,$$

$$\sigma^2{}_{\mathrm{O}} = \frac{(0-0.5)2+(0-0.5)2+(0-0.5)2+(1-0.5)2+(1-0.5)2+(1-0.5)2}{6} = 0.25,$$

and

$$\sigma_{(\mathrm{O})} = \sqrt{0.25} = 0.5.$$

Apnea universe:

$$\mu_{\mathrm{A}} = \frac{0+0+1+1+1+1}{6} = 0.67,$$

$$\sigma^2{}_{\mathrm{O}} = \frac{(0-0.67)2+(0-0.67)2+(1-0.67)2+(1-0.67)2+(1-0.67)2+(1-0.67)2}{6}$$
$$= 0.22$$

and

$$\sigma_{\mathrm{A}} = \sqrt{0.22} = 0.47.$$

Remark In this book, the variance and standard deviation of a set of quantitative observations are computed by using the number of observations in the set minus one as their denominators when the set of observations is considered a sample and by the number of observations in the set as their denominators when the set of observations is considered a universe. The variance and standard deviation of a set of binary observations are computed by using the number of observations in the set as their denominators whether the set of observations is considered a sample or universe.

- *Random Sample*

Whether a sample is a random sample depends on how it was selected. Simple random sample is a fundamentally important type of random sample. This section uses simple examples to cultivate a grasp of random sample.

Definition: Simple Random Sampling Procedure

A simple random sampling procedure selects a sample from a universe in such a way that every possible sample of the same size has the same chance of being selected.

When a sample is selected from a universe by a simple random sampling procedure, every element of the universe has the same chance of being selected in the sample. A simple random sampling procedure may also be defined as:

A simple random sampling procedure selects a sample from a universe in such a way that every element of the universe has the same chance of being selected.

Definition: Simple Random Sample

A sample selected from a universe by a simple random sampling procedure is a simple random sample.

A simple random sampling procedure is also called a random sampling procedure, and a simple random sample is called a random sample.

- *Number of Possible Samples*

When a sample is selected from a universe by a simple random sampling procedure, samples consisting of the same elements selected in different orders are considered one possible sample. If elements of the universe are selected one by one, the selected elements are not returned to the universe and are no longer available for selection. The procedure is referred to as the without-replacement sampling procedure.

If a simple random sample of size n is selected from a universe of size η by a simple random sampling procedure, the number of possible samples is:

$$\text{Number of possible samples of size } n \text{ from a universe of size } \eta = \frac{\eta!}{n!(\eta - n)!} \tag{10.1.1}$$

Here, $\eta!$ denotes the product of η, $(\eta - 1)$, $(\eta - 2)$, ... and 3, 2, and 1 and $(\eta - n)!$ the product of $(\eta - n)$, $(\eta - n - 1)$, $(\eta - n - 2)$, ... 3, 2 and 1. By definition, $0! = 1$.

Example 10.1.2 $n = 2$

When a simple random sample of size $n = 2$ is selected from the subject universe of Table 10.1, the universe size is $\eta = 6$, and the sample size is $n = 2$. The number of possible simple random samples equals:

$$\frac{6!}{2! \times (6-2)!} = \frac{6 \times 5 \times 4 \times 3 \times 2 \times 1}{(2 \times 1)\ (4 \times 3 \times 2 \times 1)} = \frac{6 \times 5}{2} = 15.$$

They are listed in Table 10.2. Each of the 15 samples has the same chance of being selected. Suppose that the sample (C, D) was selected. The BMI values of the two subjects (28, 32) are a simple random sample of size $n = 2$ from the BMI universe, and the AHI values of the two subjects (20, 22) are a simple random sample of size $n = 2$ from the AHI universe. The obesity values of the two subjects (0, 1) are a simple random sample of size $n = 2$ from the obesity universe, and the apnea values of the two subjects (1, 1) are a simple random sample of size $n = 2$ from the apnea universe.

Example 10.1.3 $n = 4$

When a simple random sample of size $n = 4$ is selected from the subject universe of Table 10.1, the number of possible simple random samples is:

$$\frac{6!}{4! \times (6-4)!} = \frac{6 \times 5 \times 4!}{4! \times 2!} = \frac{6 \times 5}{2 \times 1} = 15.$$

They are listed in Table 10.3. Each of the 15 samples has the same chance of being selected. Suppose that the sample (A, C, D, F) was selected. The BMI values of the four subjects (20, 28, 32, 40) constitute a simple random sample of size $n = 4$ from the BMI universe. The AHI values of the four subjects (10, 20, 22, 30) constitute a simple random sample of size $n = 4$ from the AHI universe. The obesity values of the four subjects (0, 0, 1, 1) constitute a simple random sample of size $n = 4$ from the obesity universe. The apnea values of the four subjects (0, 1, 1, 1) constitute a simple random sample of size $n = 4$ from the apnea universe.

10.2 Sampling Distribution of the Mean of a Simple Random Sample

The sampling distribution of the mean of a random sample is fundamentally important. This section uses the sampling distribution of the mean of a simple random sample from the universes exhibited in Table 10.1 to exemplify the properties of the sampling distribution of the mean of a random sample.

Table 10.2 Possible samples of size $n = 2$ from the universes of Table 10.1

Subject	(A, B)	(A, C)	(A, D)	(A, E)	(A, F)	(B, C)	(B, D)	(B, E)	(B, F)	(C, D)	(C, E)	(C, F)	(D, E)	(D, F)	(E, F)
BMI	20, 24	20, 28	20, 32	20, 36	20, 40	24, 28	24, 32	24, 36	24, 40	28, 32	28, 36	28, 40	32, 36	32, 40	36, 40
AHI	10, 15	10, 20	10, 22	10, 23	10, 30	15, 20	15, 22	15, 23	15, 30	20, 22	20, 23	20, 30	22, 23	22, 30	23, 30
Obesity	0,0	0, 0	0, 1	0, 1	0,1	0, 0	0, 1	0, 1	0, 1	0, 1	0, 1	0, 1	1 1,	1, 1	1, 1
Apnea	0, 0	0, 1	0, 1	0, 1	0, 1	0, 1	0, 1	0,1	0, 1	1, 1	1, 1	1, 1	1,1	1, 1	1, 1

Table 10.3 Possible samples of size $n = 4$ from the universes of Table 10.1

Subject	(A, B, C, D)	(A, B, C, E)	(A, B, C, F)	(A, B, D, E)	(A, B, D, F)	(A, B, E, F)	(A, C, D, E)	(A, C, D, F)
BMI	20, 24, 28, 32	20, 24, 28, 36	20, 24, 28, 40	20, 24, 32, 36	20, 24, 32, 40	20, 24, 36, 40	20, 28, 32, 36	20, 28, 32, 40
AHI	10, 15, 20, 22	10, 15, 20, 23	10, 15, 20, 30	10, 15, 22, 23	10, 15, 22, 30	10, 15, 23, 30	10, 20, 22, 23	10, 20, 22, 30
Obesity	0, 0, 0, 1	0, 0, 0, 1	0, 0, 0, 1	0, 0, 0, 1	0, 1, 1, 1	0, 0, 1, 1	0, 0, 1, 1	0, 0, 1, 1
Apnea	0, 0, 1, 1	0, 0, 1, 1	0, 0, 1, 1	0, 0, 1, 1	0, 0, 1, 1	0, 0, 1, 1	0, 1, 1, 1	0, 1, 1, 1

Subject	(A, C, E, F)	(A, D, E, F)	(B, C, D, E)	(B, C, D, F)	(B, C, E, F)	(B, D, E, F)	(C, D, E, F)
BMI	20, 28, 36, 40	20, 32, 36, 40	24, 28, 32, 36	24, 28, 32, 40	24, 28, 36, 40	24, 32, 36, 40	28, 32, 36, 40
AHI	10, 20, 23, 30	10, 22, 23, 30	15, 20, 22, 23	15, 20, 22, 30	15, 20, 23, 30	15, 22, 23, 30	20, 22, 23, 30
Obesity	0, 1, 1, 1	0, 1, 1, 1	0, 0, 1, 1	0, 0, 1, 1	0, 0, 1, 1, 0, 1		
Apnea	0, 1, 1, 1	0, 1, 1, 1	0, 1, 1, 1	0, 1, 1, 1	0, 1, 1, 1	0, 0, 1, 1	1, 1, 1, 1

Definition: The Sampling Distribution of the Mean of a Simple Random Sample

The sampling distribution of the mean of a simple random sample from a universe is the distribution of the means of all possible samples of the given size from the universe.

The mean and standard deviation of the sampling distribution of the mean of a simple random sample from a universe is related to the mean and standard deviation of the universe. If the number of elements in a finite universe is η, the mean, variance, and standard deviation of the universe are μ, σ^2, and σ, respectively, and those of the sampling distribution of the mean of a random sample of size n from the universe are $\mu_{M(n)}$, $\sigma^2_{M(n)}$, and $\sigma_{M(n)}$, respectively; they are related as follows:

$$\mu_{M(n)} = \mu, \tag{10.2.1}$$

$$\sigma^2_{M(n)} = \frac{\sigma^2}{n}\left(\frac{\eta - n}{\eta - 1}\right), \text{ and} \tag{10.2.2}$$

$$\sigma_{M(n)} = \sqrt{\frac{\sigma^2}{n}\left(\frac{\eta - n}{\eta - 1}\right)} = \frac{\sigma}{\sqrt{n}}\sqrt{\left(\frac{\eta - n}{\eta - 1}\right)} \tag{10.2.3}$$

The fraction $\left(\frac{\eta - n}{\eta - 1}\right)$ is known as the finite universe correction factor. When the size of the sample is small relative to the size of the universe, it is close to 1.0. The standard deviation of the sampling distribution of the mean of a simple random sample of size n approximately equals:

$$\sigma_{\mathrm{M}(n)} = \frac{\sigma}{\sqrt{n}} \tag{10.2.4}$$

Equation 10.2.4 is used as the standard deviation of the sampling distribution of a random sample from a universe when the size of the universe is unknown.

Equations 10.2.1 and 10.2.3 submit the following two important properties of the mean of a random sample:

- *The mean of the sampling distribution of the mean of a random sample from a universe equals the mean of the universe.*
- *The standard deviation of the sampling distribution of the mean of a simple random sample is smaller when the size of the sample is larger.*

Example 10.2.1

Example 10.1.2 shows that there are 15 possible samples if a simple random sample of size $n = 2$ is selected from the BMI universe of Table 10.1. The samples and their means, variances, and standard deviations are shown in Table 10.4.

The distribution of the means of the 15 possible samples constitutes the sampling distribution of the mean of a simple random sample of size $n = 2$ from the BMI universe. Table 10.5 shows that the distribution is symmetric and varies from 22 to 38. The mean, variance, and standard deviation of the sampling distribution samples are:

$$\mu_{\mathrm{BMI}(n=2)} = \frac{22+24+2\times 26+2\times 28+3\times 30+2\times 32+2\times 34+36+40}{15} = 30,$$

$$\sigma^2{}_{\mathrm{BMI}(n=2)} = \frac{\begin{array}{c}(22-30)^2+(24-30)^2+2(26-30)^2+2(28-30)^2\\ +3(30-30)^2+2(32-30)+2(34-30)+(36-30)^2+(38-30)^2\end{array}}{15} = 18.7,$$

and

$$\sigma_{\mathrm{BMI}(n=2)} = \sqrt{18.7} = 4.3.$$

They are the same as those suggested by Eqs. 10.2.1, 10.2.2, and 10.2.3. Indeed,

$$\mu_{\mathrm{BMI}(n=2)} = 30 = \mu_{\mathrm{BMI}},$$

$$\sigma^2{}_{\mathrm{BMI}(n=2)} = 18.7 = \frac{\sigma^2}{n}\left(\frac{\eta-n}{\eta-1}\right) = \frac{46.7}{2}\left(\frac{6-2}{6-1}\right), \text{ and}$$

$$\sigma_{\mathrm{BMI}(n=2)} = 4.3 = \sqrt{\frac{\sigma^2}{n}\left(\frac{\eta-n}{\eta-1}\right)} = \sqrt{\frac{46.7}{2}\left(\frac{6-2}{6-1}\right)}.$$

Table 10.4 Means of possible samples of size $n = 2$ from the BMI universes

Subject	(A, B)	(A, C)	(A, D)	(A, E)	(A, F)	(B, C)	(B, D)	(B, E)	(B, F)	(C, D)	(C, E)	(C, F)	(D, E)	(D, F)	(E, F)
BMI	20, 24	20, 28	20, 32	20, 36	20, 40	24, 28	24, 32	24, 36	24, 40	28, 32	28, 36	28, 40	32, 36	32, 40	36, 40
Mean	22	24	26	28	30	26	28	30	32	30	32	34	34	36	38

Table 10.5 Distribution of the means of simple random samples of $n = 2$ from the BMI universe

Sample mean	22	24	26	28	30	32	34	36	38
Frequency	1	1	2	2	3	2	2	1	1
Relative frequency	7%	7%	13%	13%	20%	13%	13%	7%	7%

Table 10.6 Means, variances, and standard deviations of possible samples of size $n = 4$ from the BMI universes

Subject	(A, B, C, D)	(A, B, C, E)	(A, B, C, F)	(A, B, D, E)	(A, B, D, F)	(A.B. E, F)	(A, C, D, E)	(A, C, D, F)
BMI	20, 24, 28, 32	20, 24, 28, 36	20, 24, 28, 40	20, 24, 32, 36	20, 24, 32, 40	20, 24, 36, 40	20, 28, 32, 36	20, 28, 32, 40
Mean	26	27	28	28	29	30	29	30

Subject	(A, C, E, F)	(A, D, E, F)	(B, C, D, E)	(B, C, D, F)	(B, C, E, F)	(B, D, E, F)	(C, D, E, F)
BMI	20, 28, 36, 40	20, 32, 36, 40	24, 28, 32, 36	24, 28, 32, 40	24, 28, 36, 40	24, 32, 36, 40	28, 32, 36, 40
Mean	31	32	30	31	32	33	34

Table 10.7 Sampling distribution of the mean of a simple random sample of size $n = 4$ from the BMI universe

Sample mean	26	27	28	29	30	31	32	33	34
Frequency	1	1	2	2	3	2	2	1	1
Relative frequency	7%	7%	13%	13%	20%	13%	13%	7%	7%

Table 10.3 shows that there are 15 possible samples if a simple random sample of size $n = 4$ is selected from the BMI universe. The 15 possible samples and their means, variances, and standard deviations are displayed in Table 10.6. The distribution of the means of the 15 possible samples constitutes the sampling distribution of the mean of a simple random sample of size $n = 4$ from the BMI universe. It is displayed in Table 10.7, which shows that the distribution is symmetric and varies from 26 to 34.

The mean, variance, and standard deviation of the sampling distribution of a simple random sample of size $n = 4$ from the BMI universe equal:

$$\mu_{\mathrm{BMI}(n=4)} = \frac{26 + 27 + 2\times 28 + 2\times 29 + 3\times 30 + 2\times 31 + 2\times 32 + 33 + 34}{15} = 30,$$

$$\sigma^2_{\mathrm{BMI}(n=4)} = \frac{\begin{array}{c}(26-30)^2 + (27-30)^2 + 2(28-30)^2 + 2(29-30)^2 + 3(30-30)^2 \\ +2(31-30) + 2(32-30) + (33-30)^2 + (34-30)^2\end{array}}{15} = 4.7,$$

and

$$\sigma_{\mathrm{BMI}(n=4)} = \sqrt{4.7} = 2.2.$$

They are the same as those suggested by Eqs. 10.2.1, 10.2.2, and 10.2.3. Indeed,

$$\mu_{\mathrm{BMI}(n=4)} = 30 = \mu,$$

$$\sigma^2_{\mathrm{BMI}(n=4)} = 4.7 = \frac{\sigma^2}{n}\left(\frac{\eta - n}{\eta - 1}\right) = \frac{46.7}{4}\left(\frac{6-4}{6-1}\right), \text{ and}$$

$$\sigma_{\mathrm{BMI}(n=4)} = 2.2 = \sqrt{\frac{\sigma^2}{n}\left(\frac{\eta - n}{\eta - 1}\right)} = \sqrt{\frac{46.7}{4}\left(\frac{6-4}{6-1}\right)}.$$

Example 10.2.2

Table 10.2 shows that there are 15 possible samples if a simple random sample of size $n = 2$ is selected from the AHI Universe of Table 10.1. The samples and their means, variances, and standard deviations are displayed in Table 10.8. The distribution of the means of the 15 samples constitutes the sampling distribution of the mean of a simple random sample of size $n = 2$ from the AHI universe. It is depicted in Table 10.9.

The distribution of the means of the possible samples of size $n = 2$, the sampling distribution of the mean if a simple random sample of size $n = 2$ is selected from the AHI universe, varies from 13 to 29 and is asymmetric.

Table 10.9 yields that the mean, variance, and standard deviation of the sampling distribution of the mean of a simple random sample of size $n = 2$ from the AHI universe are:

$$\mu_{\mathrm{AHI}(n=2)} = \frac{13+14+15+16+17+18+19+20+21+22+2\times 23+24+25+26+29}{15} = 20,$$

$$\sigma^2_{\mathrm{AHI}(n=2)} = \frac{\begin{array}{c}(13-20)^2+(14-20)^2+\ldots+(21-20)^2+(22-20)^2+2(23-20)^2\\ +(24-20)^2+(25-20)^2+(26-20)^2+(29-20)^2\end{array}}{15} = 19.7,$$

and

$$\sigma_{\mathrm{AHI}(n=2)} = \sqrt{19.7} = 4.4$$

They are the same as those suggested by Eqs. 10.2.1, 10.2.2, and 10.2.3. Indeed,

$$\mu_{\mathrm{AHI}(n=2)} = 20 = \mu,$$

$$\sigma^2_{\mathrm{AHI}(n=2)} = 19.7 = \frac{\sigma^2}{n}\left(\frac{\eta - n}{\eta - 1}\right) = \frac{49.3}{2}\left(\frac{6-2}{6-1}\right), \text{ and}$$

Table 10.8 Means of possible samples of size $n = 2$ from the AHI universes

Subject	(A, B)	(A, C)	(A, D)	(A, E)	(A, F)	(B, C)	(B, D)	(B, E)	(B, F)	(C, D)	(C, E)	(C, F)	(D, E)	(D, F)	(E, F)
AHI	10, 15	10, 20	10, 22	10, 23	10, 30	15, 20	15, 22	15, 23	15, 30	20, 22	20, 23	20, 30	22, 23	22, 30	23, 30
Mean	12.5	15.0	16.0	16.5	20.0	17.5	18.5	19.0	22.5	21.0	21.5	25.0	22.5	26.0	26.5

Table 10.9 Sampling distribution of the mean of a simple random sample of size $n = 2$ from the AHI universe

Mean	13	14	15	16	17	18	19	20	21	22	23	24	25	26	27	28	29
Frequency	1	1	1	1	1	1	1	1	1	1	2	1	1	1	0	0	1
Rel. frequency	7%	7%	7%	7%	7%	7%	7%	7%	7%	7%	13%	7%	7%	7%	0%	0%	7%

Table 10.10 Means of possible samples of size $n = 4$ from the AHI universe

Subject	(A, B, C, D)	(A, B, C, E)	(A, B, C, F)	(A, B, D, E)	(A, B, D, F)	(A.B. E, F)	(A, C, D, E)	(A, C, D, F)
AHI	10, 15, 20, 22	10, 15, 20, 23	10, 15, 20, 30	10, 15, 22, 23	10, 15, 22, 30	10, 15, 23, 30	10, 20, 22, 23	10, 20, 22, 30
Mean	16.75	17.00	18.75	17.50	19.25	19.50	18.75	20.50

Subject	(A, C, E, F)	(A, D, E, F)	(B, C, D, E)	(B, C, D, F)	(B, C, E, F)	(B, D, E, F)	(C, D, E, F)
AHI	10, 20, 23, 30	10, 22, 23, 30	15, 20, 22, 23	15, 20, 22, 30	15, 20, 23, 30	15, 22, 23, 30	20, 22, 23, 0
Mean	20.75	21.25	20.00	21.75	22.00	22.50	23.75

$$\sigma_{\text{AHI}(n=2)} = 4.4 = \sqrt{\frac{\sigma^2}{n}\left(\frac{\eta - n}{\eta - 1}\right)} = \sqrt{\frac{49.3}{2}\left(\frac{6-2}{6-1}\right)}.$$

Table 10.3 shows that there are 15 possible samples when a simple random sample of size $n = 4$ is selected from the AHI universe. The samples and their means, variances, and standard deviations are exhibited in Table 10.10. The distribution of the means of the 15 samples is the sampling distribution of the mean of a simple random sample of size $n = 4$ from the AHI universe. It is depicted in Table 10.11.

The sampling distribution of the mean of a simple random sample of size $n = 4$ from the AHI universe varies from 15.5 to 23.5. The mean, variance, and standard deviation of the sampling distribution of the mean of a random sample of size $n = 4$ are denoted by $\mu_{\text{AHI }(n\,=\,4)}$, $\sigma^2_{\text{AHI }(n\,=\,4)}$, and $\sigma_{\text{AHI }(n\,=\,4)}$, respectively. They can be computed from the means of possible samples shown in Table 10.11 as follows:

$$\mu_{\text{AHI}(n=4)} = \frac{\begin{array}{c}15.5 + 17.0 + 18.0 + 2 \times 18.5 + 19.0 + 19.5 + 20.0 + 20.5\\ +21.0 + 21.5 + 22.0 + 22.5 + 23.0 + 23.5\end{array}}{15} = 20$$

$$\sigma^2_{\text{AHI}(n=4)} = \frac{\begin{array}{c}(15.5 - 20)^2 + (17 - 20)^2 + (18.0 - 20)^2 + 2(18.5 - 20)^2 + (19.0 - 20)^2 + \ldots\\ +(21.5 - 20)^2 + (23.0 - 20)^2 + (23.5 - 20)^2\end{array}}{15} = 4.9.$$

$$\sigma_{\text{AHI}(n=4)} = \sqrt{4.9} = 2.2$$

They are the same as those suggested by Eqs. 10.2.1, 10.2.2, and 10.2.3. Indeed,

Table 10.11 Sampling distribution of the mean of a simple random sample of size $n = 4$ from the AHI universe

Mean	15.5	17.0	18.0	18.5	19.0	19.5	20.0	20.5	21.0	21.5	22.0	22.5	23.0	23.5
Frequency	1	1	1	2	1	1	1	1	1	1	1	1	1	1
Rel. frequency	7%	7%	7%	13%	7%	7%	7%	7%	7%	7%	7%	7%	7%	7%

$$\mu_{\mathrm{AHI}(n=4)} = 20 = \mu,$$

$$\sigma^2_{\mathrm{AHI}(n=4)} = 4.9 = \frac{\sigma^2}{n}\left(\frac{\eta - n}{\eta - 1}\right) = \frac{49.3}{4}\left(\frac{6-4}{6-1}\right), \text{ and}$$

$$\sigma_{\mathrm{AHI}(n=4)} = 2.2 = \sqrt{\frac{\sigma^2}{n}\left(\frac{\eta - n}{\eta - 1}\right)} = \sqrt{\frac{49.3}{4}\left(\frac{6-4}{6-1}\right)}.$$

10.3 Sampling Distribution of the Proportion of YES in a Random Sample

Revelation of a set of dichotomous observations is informatively manifested by its proportion of YES. The sampling distribution of the proportion of YES in a simple random sample is another fundamentally important sampling distribution of the statistic of a random sample.

If the values 1 and 0 are assigned to each YES and NO observation of a set of dichotomous observations, the mean, variance, and standard deviation of the resulting set of binary observations consisting of 1s and 0s. 0s are related to the proportion of YES as follows:

Mean of Binary Observation = Proportion of 1's

Variance of Binary Observation = (Proportion of 1's)(1–Proportion of 1's),

and

$$\text{Standard Deviation of Binary Observations} = \sqrt{(\text{Proportion of } 1'\text{s})(1 - \text{Proportion of } 1'\text{s})}.$$

If π denotes the proportion of YES in a dichotomous universe and μ, σ^2, and σ denote the mean, variance, and standard deviation, respectively, of the resulting binary universe when the values 1 and 0 are assigned to the YES and NO observations of the universe, they are related as follows:

$$\mu = \pi \tag{10.3.1}$$

$$\sigma^2 = \pi\,(1-\pi) \tag{10.3.2}$$

$$\sigma = \sqrt{\pi\,(1-\pi)} \tag{10.3.3}$$

Note In this book, the variance and standard deviation of a binary data set are computed by using the number of observations in the data set as their divisors whether the data set is considered a sample or a universe.

Definition: The Sampling Distribution of the Proportion of YES in a Simple Random Sample

The distribution of the proportions of YES in all possible samples of a given size from a dichotomous universe constitutes the sampling distribution of the proportion of YES in a simple random sample of the given size from the universe.

The mean and standard deviation of the sampling distribution of the proportion of YES in a simple random sample from a dichotomous universe are related to the proportion of YES in the universe and the size of the sample. If η is the number of elements in the dichotomous universe, π is the proportion of YES in the universe, and $\mu_{P(n)}$, $\sigma^2_{P(n)}$, and $\sigma_{P(n)}$ are the mean, variance, and standard deviation of the sampling distribution of the proportion of YES in a random sample of size n from the universe, respectively, they are related as follows:

$$\mu_{P(n)} = \pi, \tag{10.3.1}$$

$$\sigma^2_{P(n)} = \frac{\pi\,(1-\pi)}{n}\left(\frac{\eta-n}{\eta-1}\right) \tag{10.3.2}$$

$$\sigma_{P(n)} = \sqrt{\frac{\pi\,(1-\pi)}{n}\left(\frac{\eta-n}{\eta-1}\right)} \tag{10.3.3}$$

The fraction $\frac{\eta-n}{\eta-1}$ is known as the finite universe correction factor. When the size of sample n is small relative to the size of the universe η, it is close to 1, and the standard deviation equals approximately:

$$\sigma_{P(n)} = \sqrt{\frac{\pi\,(1-\pi)}{n}} \tag{10.3.4}$$

Equation 10.3.4 is used to compute the standard deviation of the sampling distribution of the proportion of YES in a random sample selected from a finite universe when the size of the universe is unknown.

Equations 10.3.1 and 10.3.3 submit the following two important properties of the proportion of YES in a random sample:

- *The mean of the sampling distribution of the proportion of YES in a random sample from a universe equals the proportion of YES in the universe.*
- *The standard deviation of the sampling distribution of the proportion of YES in a random sample is smaller when the size of the sample is larger.*

Example 10.3.1

The obesity universe of Table 10.1 is the result of assigning the value 1 to each subject whose BMI value is 30 or larger and the value 0 to each subject whose BMI value is below 30. The proportion of 1 in the obesity universe is $\pi_O = 0.5$. The mean, variance, and standard deviation of the obesity universe are written as $\mu_{O,}$ σ_{2O}, and σ_O, respectively:

$$\mu_O = \frac{0+0+0+1+1+1}{6} = 0.5.$$

$$\sigma^2{}_O = \frac{(0-0.5)^2 + (0-0.5)^2 + (0-0.5)^2 + (1-0.5)^2 + (1-0.5)^2 + \ (1-0.5)^2}{6} = 0.25, \text{ and}$$

$$\sigma_O = \sqrt{0.25} = 0.5.$$

They are related to the proportion of YES in the dichotomous universe as follows:

$$\mu_O = \pi_O = 0.5,$$

$$\sigma^2{}_O = \pi_O(1\text{–}\pi_O) = \ = 0.5(1\text{–}0.5) = 0.25, \text{ and}$$

$$\sigma_O = \sqrt{0.5(1\text{–}0.5)} = \sqrt{0.25} = 0.5$$

- *Sample of Size 2*

Table 10.2 shows that there are 15 possible samples if a simple random sample of size $n = 2$ is selected from the obesity universe. Table 10.12 shows the 15 possible samples and their proportions of YES.

The distribution of the 15 proportions constitutes the sampling distribution of the proportion of YES in a simple random sample of size $n = 2$ from the obesity universe. It is depicted in Table 10.13

The mean, variance, and standard deviation of the sampling distribution, denoted by $\mu_{O(n\,=\,2)}$, $\sigma^2{}_{O(n\,=\,2)}$, and $\sigma_{O(n\,=\,2)}$, are equal to:

$$\mu_{O(n=2)} = \frac{3\times 0.0 + 9\times 0.5 + 3\times 1.0}{15} = 0.50,$$

$$\sigma^2{}_{O(n=2)} = \frac{3\times(0-0.5)^2 + 9\times(0.5-0.5)^2 + 3\times(1-0.5)^2}{15} = 0.10, \text{ and}$$

$$\sigma_{O(n=2)} = \sqrt{0.10} = 0.32.$$

They are the same as those suggested by Eqs. 10.3.1, 10.3.2, and 10.3.3. Indeed,

$$\mu_{O(n=2)} = 0.5 = \pi_O$$

$$\sigma^2{}_{O(n=2)} = 0.10 = \frac{0.5\ (1\text{–}0.5)}{2}\left(\frac{6-2}{6-1}\right)$$

$$\sigma_{O(n=2)} = 0.32 = \sqrt{\frac{0.5\ (1\text{–}0.5)}{2}\left(\frac{6-2}{6-1}\right)} = \sqrt{0.10}$$

Table 10.12 Possible samples of size $n = 2$ from the obesity universes of Table 10.1

Subject	(A, B)	(A, C)	(A, D)	(A, E)	(A, F)	(B, C)	(B, D)	(B, E)	(B, F)	(C, D)	(C, E)	(C, F)	(D, E)	(D, F)	(E, F)
Obesity	(0, 0)	(0, 0)	(0, 1)	(0, 1)	(0, 1)	(0, 0)	(0, 1)	(0, 1)	(0, 1)	(0, 1)	(0, 1)(	0, 1)	(1, 1)	(1, 1)	(1, 1)
Proportion	0	0	0.5	0.5	0.5	0	0.5	0.5	0.5	0.5	0.5	0.5	1.0	1.0	1.0

Table 10.13 Sampling distribution of the proportion of YES in a simple random sample of size $n = 2$ from the obesity universe

Proportion of 1 (Mean)	0.0	0.5	1.0
Frequency	3	9	3
Relative frequency	20%	60%	20%

Table 10.14 Possible samples of size $n = 4$ from the obesity universe of Table 10.1

Subject	(A, B, C, D)	(A, B, C, E)	(A, B, C, F)	(A, B, D, E)	(A, B, D, F)	(A.B. E, F)	(A, C, D, E)	(A, C, D, F)
Obesity	0, 0, 0, 1	0, 0, 0, 1	0, 0, 0, 1	0, 0, 1, 1	0, 0, 1, 1	0, 0, 1, 1	0, 0, 1, 1	0, 0, 1, 1
Proportion	0.25	0.25	0.25	0.5	0.5	0.5	0.5	0.5

Subject	(A, C, E, F)	(A, D, E, F)	(B, C, D, E)	(B, C, D, F)	(B, C, E, F)	(B, D, E, F)	(C, D, E, F)
Obesity	0, 0, 1, 1	0, 1, 1, 1	0, 0, 1, 1	0, 0, 1, 1	0, 0, 1, 1	0, 1, 1, 1	0, 1, 1, 1
Proportion	0.5	0.75	0.5	0.5	0.5	0.75	0.75

- *Sample of Size: 4*

Table 10.3 shows that there are 15 possible samples if a simple random sample of size $n = 4$ is selected from the obesity universe. The 15 possible samples and their proportions of 1 are shown in Table 10.14.

The distribution of the 15 proportions constitutes the sampling distribution of the proportion of YES in a simple random sample of size $n = 4$ from the obesity universe. It is depicted in Table 10.15. The mean, variance, and standard deviation of the sampling distribution, denoted by $\mu_{O\ (n\ =\ 4)}$, $\sigma^2_{O\ (n\ =\ 4)}$, and $\sigma_{O\ (n\ =\ 4)}$, are equal:

$$\mu_{O(n=4)} = \frac{3 \times 0.25 + 9 \times 0.50 + 3 \times 0.75}{15} = 0.50,$$

$$\sigma^2_{O(n=4)} = \frac{3 \times (0.25 - 0.5)^2 + 9 \times (0.5 - 0.5)^2 + 3 \times (0.75 - 0.5)^2}{15} = 0.025, \text{ and}$$

$$\sigma_{O(n=4)} = \sqrt{0.025} = 0.16.$$

They are the same as those suggested by Eqs. 10.3.1, 10.3.2, and 10.3.3. Indeed,

$$\mu_{O(n=4)} = 0.5 = \pi_O$$

$$\sigma^2_{O(n=4)} = 0.025 = \frac{0.5\ (1–0.5)}{4} \left(\frac{6-4}{6-1}\right)$$

$$\sigma_{O(n=2)} = 0.16 = \sqrt{\frac{0.5\ (1–0.5)}{2} \left(\frac{6-4}{6-1}\right)} = \sqrt{0.025}$$

Table 10.15 Sampling distribution of the mean of a simple random sample of size $n = 4$ from the obesity universe

Proportion (mean)	0.25	0.50	0.75
Frequency	3	9	3
Relative frequency	20%	60%	20%

Example 10.3.2

The Apnea universe of Table 10.1 is the result of assigning the value 1 to each element of the subject universe whose AHI score is 20 or larger and the value 0 to each subject whose AHI score is below 20. Its proportion of 1 is the proportion of YES in the apnea universe ($\pi_A = 0.67$).

When the mean, variance, and standard deviation of the apnea universe are written as $\mu_{A,}$ $\sigma^2{}_A$, and $\sigma_{A,}$ respectively, they equal:

$$\mu_A = \frac{0+0+1+1+1+1}{6} = 0.67,$$

$$\sigma^2{}_A = \frac{(0-0.67)^2+(0-0.67)^2+(1-0.67)^2+(1-0.67)^2+(1-0.67)^2+(1-0.67)^2}{6} = 0.22, \text{and}$$

$$\sigma_A = \sqrt{0.22} = 0.47.$$

They are related to the proportion of 1 in the universe as follows:

$$\mu_A = \pi_A = 0.67,$$

$$\sigma^2{}_A = \pi_A(1\text{–}\pi_A) = 0.67(1.0\text{–}0.67) = 0.22, \text{ and}$$

$$\sigma_A = \sqrt{0.67(1.0\text{–}0.67)} = \sqrt{0.22} = 0.47.$$

- *Sample of Size: 2*

Table 10.2 shows that there are 15 possible samples if a simple random sample of size $n = 2$ is selected from the apnea universe. The samples and their proportions of 1 (means) are shown in Table 10.16.

The distribution of the 15 proportions constitutes the sampling distribution of the proportions of YES in a random sample of size 2 from the universe. It is displayed in Table 10.17.

The mean, variance, and standard deviation of the sampling distribution are equal:

$$\mu_{A(n=2)} = \frac{0.0 + 8 \times 0.5 + 6 \times 1.0}{15} = 0.67,$$

Table 10.16 Possible samples of size $n = 2$ from the apnea universe

Subject	(A, B)	(A, C)	(A, D)	(A, E)	(A, F)	(B, C)	(B, D)	(B, E)	(B, F)	(C, D)	(C, E)	(C, F)	(D, E)	(D, F)	(E, F)
Obesity	0, 0	0, 1	0, 1	0, 1	0, 1	0, 1	0, 1	0, 1	0, 1	1, 1	1, 1	1, 1	1, 1	1, 1	1, 1
Proportion	0	0.5	0.5	0.5	0.5	0.5	0.5	0.5	0.5	1.0	1.0	1.0	1.0	1.0	1.0

Table 10.17 Sampling distribution of the proportion of YES in a simple random sample of size $n = 2$ from the apnea universe

Proportion (mean)	0.0	0.5	1.0
Frequency	1	8	6
Relative frequency	6.7%	53.3%	40.0%

Table 10.18 Possible samples of size $n = 4$ from the apnea universe of Table 10.1

Subject	(A, B, C, D)	(A, B, C, E)	(A, B, C, F)	(A, B, D, E)	(A, B, D, F)	(A.B. E, F)	(A, C, D, E)	(A, C, D, F)
Obesity	0, 0, 1, 1	0, 0, 1, 1	0, 0, 1, 1	0, 0, 1, 1	0, 0, 1, 1	0, 0, 1, 1	0, 1, 1, 1	0, 1, 1, 1
Proportion	0.5	0.5	0.5	0.5	0.5	0.5	0.75	0.75

Subject	(A, C, E, F)	(A, D, E, F)	(B, C, D, E)	(B, C, D, F)	(B, C, E, F)	(B, D, E, F)	(C, D, E, F)
Obesity	0, 1, 1, 1	0, 1, 1, 1	0, 1, 1, 1	0, 1, 1, 1	0, 1, 1, 1	0, 1, 1, 1	1, 1, 1, 1
Proportion	0.75	0.75	0.75	0.75	0.75	0.75	1.0

$$\sigma^2{}_{A(n=2)} = \frac{(0-0.67)^2 + 8\times(0.5-0.67)^2 + 6\times(1.0-0.67)^2}{15} = 0.09, \text{ and}$$

$$\sigma_{A(n=2)} = \sqrt{0.09} = 0.30.$$

They are the same as those suggested by Eqs. 10.3.1, 10.3.2, and 10.3.3. Indeed,

$$\mu_{A(n=2)} = 0.67 = \pi_O$$

$$\sigma^2{}_{A(n=2)} = 0.09 = \frac{0.67\ (1\text{–}0.67)}{2}\left(\frac{6-2}{6-1}\right) = \frac{0.2211}{2}\left(\frac{6-2}{6-1}\right)$$

$$\sigma_{O(n=2)} = 0.30 = \sqrt{\frac{0.67\ (1\text{–}0.67)}{2}\left(\frac{6-2}{6-1}\right)} = \sqrt{0.09}$$

- *Sample Size: 4*

If a simple random sample of size $n = 4$ is selected from the apnea universe, there are 15 possible samples. Table 10.18 shows the possible samples and their proportions of 1.

The mean, variance, and standard deviation of the sampling distribution are equal:

$$\mu_{A(n=4)} = \frac{6\times 0.50 + 8\times 0.75. + 1.00}{15} = 0.67,$$

$$\sigma^2{}_{\mathrm{A}(n=4)} = \frac{6 \times (0.50 - 0.67)^2 + 8 \times (0.75 - 0.67)^2 + (1.00 - 0.67)^2}{15} = 0.02, \text{ and}$$

$$\sigma_{\mathrm{A}(n=4)} = \sqrt{0.02} = 0.15.$$

They are the same as those suggested by Eqs. 10.3.1, 10.3.2, and 10.3.3. Indeed,

$$\mu_{\mathrm{A}(n=4)} = 0.67 = \pi_{\mathrm{O}}$$

$$\sigma^2{}_{\mathrm{A}(n=4)} = 0.02 = \frac{0.67\ (1\text{–}0.67)}{4}\left(\frac{6-4}{6-1}\right) = \frac{0.2211}{4}\left(\frac{6-4}{6-1}\right) = 0.0221$$

$$\sigma_{\mathrm{O}(n=4)} = 0.15 = \sqrt{\frac{0.67\ (1\text{–}0.67)}{4}\left(\frac{6-4}{6-1}\right)} = \sqrt{0.0221}$$

- *Two Important Properties of Proportions of Random Samples*

Examples 10.3.1 and 10.3.2 demonstrate that the proportion of YES of a set of dichotomous (YES or NO) observations is the mean of the resulting observations when the values 1 and 0 are assigned to YES and NO observations. The sampling distribution of the proportion of YES of a random sample from a universe of YES and NO observations has the same property as the sampling distribution of the mean of a random sample.

- *The mean of the sampling distribution of the proportion of YES of a random sample of size n from a universe equals the mean of the universe.*
- *The range of the sampling distribution of the proportion of YES of a random sample is narrower and the standard deviation of the sampling distribution is smaller when the size of the sample is larger.*

10.4 Sampling Distribution of the Mean of a Large Random Sample

The universes and samples of the above examples are unrealistically small. They are used as examples to demonstrate what constitutes possible samples and the sampling distribution of sample statistics.

The use of P-values of statistical significance tests and 95% confidence intervals assume that observations are elements of random samples. The sizes of the samples are generally larger than 10, and elements of the universes are unavailable. It is not feasible to examine the sampling distributions of a sample statistic by enumerating values of the statistic computed from all possible samples. If a revelation of a set of observations of a study is portrayed by a descriptive statistic of the observations and the set of observations may be considered a random sample, the results of the central limit theorem are particularly useful.

The central limit theorem is powerful and yields useful results pertaining to sampling distributions of many statistics under broad conditions. The case of sampling distribution of the mean of a random sample is reviewed here as an example.

- *Sampling Distribution of the Mean of a Large Random Sample*

The Central Limit Theorem asserts that the sampling distribution of the mean of a random sample from a universe with a finite standard deviation is characterized by a Gaussian distribution approximately when the size of the sample is large. The mean of the Gaussian distribution equals the mean of the universe, and the standard deviation of the Gaussian distribution equals the standard deviation of the universe divided by the square root of the size of the sample.

If the mean and standard deviation of a universe are μ and σ and the mean and standard deviation of the sampling distribution of the mean of a random sample of size n from the universe are $\mu_{M(n)}$ *and* $\sigma_{M(n)}$, the central limit theorem asserts:

$$\mu_M(n) = \mu \tag{10.4.1}$$

and

$$\sigma_{M(n)} = \frac{\sigma}{\sqrt{n}} \tag{10.4.2}$$

The condition that the standard deviation of the universe is finite is met in most applications. If the set of observations being analyzed is a sample from an existing universe, the standard deviation of the universe is finite. If the set of data being analyzed is a sample from a perceived target universe, it is rational to assume that the standard deviation of the universe is finite. The condition that the size of the random sample is large is not demanding. Generally, the sampling distribution of the mean of a random sample consisting of more than 20 observations is adequately characterized by a Gaussian distribution.

- *Sampling Distribution of the Proportion of YES in a Large Random Sample*

The proportion of YES in a random sample from a dichotomous universe is the mean of the resulting binary observations when the values 1 and 0 are assigned to YES and NO observations.

The central limit theorem asserts that the sampling distribution of the proportion of YES in a random sample is adequately characterized by a Gaussian distribution when the size of the sample is sufficiently large. The mean of the sampling distribution equals the universe proportion, and the standard deviation of the sampling distribution equals $\sqrt{\frac{(\text{Universe Proportion})(1-\text{Universe Proportion})}{\text{Sample Size}}}$.

If the mean and standard deviation of a universe are μ and σ and the mean and standard deviation of the sampling distribution of the mean of a random sample of size n from the universe are $\mu_P(n)$ and $\sigma_{P(n)}$, the Central Limit Theorem asserts:

> The sampling distribution of the proportion of YES in a random of size n is adequately characterized by a Gaussian distribution if n is sufficiently large. The mean and standard deviation of the sampling distribution equal

$$\mu_{P(n)} = \pi \tag{10.4.3}$$

and

$$\sigma_{P(n)} = \sqrt{\frac{\pi(1-\pi)}{n}}. \tag{10.4.4}$$

- *Empirical Support of the Central Limit Theorem*

Whether the distribution of a set of observations is adequately characterized by a Gaussian distribution may be assessed crudely by comparing the curve of the Gaussian distribution and a comprehensive description of the distribution of the observations. Another method is to compare the fractions of observations of the data set that are included in selected regions with the percentages of the total area under the curve of the Gaussian distribution. These two methods are used here to demonstrate that the central limit theorem is supported by the distributions of the proportions obtained in the two sampling experiments.

Remark Independent random samples

A rigorous definition of "independent random samples" is beyond the scope of this book. A loose criterion is that if the selection of any one sample is not in any way affected by the selection of any other sample, the samples may be considered "independent."

Example 10.4.1 Two sampling experiments

Two sampling experiments were conducted by a class of 25 students. Each student was asked to take four samples of size $n = 10$ and four samples of size $n = 20$ from a box containing 100 blue and 100 red marbles. A board with 10 holes of identical size was used to take samples of size $n = 10$, and a board with 20 holes was used to take samples of size $n = 20$. After each draw, the numbers of blue marbles were noted and recorded. The marbles were returned to the box and thoroughly mixed. The proportions of blue marbles in the samples were collected from all students. The distributions of the proportions are depicted in Tables 10.19 and 10.20.

The shapes and sizes of the marbles are identical. The 200 marbles constitute a dichotomous universe. Table 10.19 presents a description of the distribution of the proportions of YES in 100 independent random samples of size $n = 10$ from the

Table 10.19 Distribution of proportions of blue marble in 100 random samples of size $n = 10$

Sample proportion	0.1	0.2	0.3	0.4	0.5	0.6	0.7	0.8	0.9
Frequency	1	6	11	20	26	18	12	5	1
Relative frequency	1%	6%	11%	20%	26%	18%	12%	5%	1%

universe. Table 10.20 presents a description of the distribution of the proportions of YES in 100 independent random samples of size $n = 20$ from the universe.

When the mean, variance, and standard deviation of the proportions in the samples of size $n = 10$ are denoted by $M_{P\,(n\,=\,10)}$, $SD^2{}_{P\,(n\,=\,10)}$, and $SD_{\,(n\,=\,10)}$, respectively, they are:

$$M_{P(n=10)} = \frac{0.1+6\times0.2+11\times0.3+20\times0.4+26\times0.5+18\times0.6+12\times0.7+5\times0.8+0.9}{100}$$
$$= 0.497$$

$$SD^2{}_{P(n=10)} = \frac{\begin{array}{c}(0.1-0.5)^2+6(0.2-0.5)^2+11(0.3-0.5)^2+\ldots\\ +12(0.7-0.5)^2+5(0.8-0.5)^2+(0.9-0.5)^2\end{array}}{99}$$
$$=0.026,$$

and

$$SD_{P(n=10)} = \sqrt{0.026} = 0.162.$$

They are close to the values asserted by the central limit theorem. Indeed,

$$M_{P(n=10)} = 0.497 \cong \mu_{P(n=10)} = \pi = 0.5,$$

$$SD^2{}_{P(n=10)} = 0.026 \cong \sigma^2{}_{P(n=10)} = \frac{0.5(1.0-0.5)}{10} = 0.025, \text{ and}$$

$$SD_{P(n=10)} = 0.162 \cong \sigma_{P(n=10)} = \sqrt{\frac{\pi(1.0-\pi)}{10}} = \sqrt{\frac{0.5(1.0-0.5)}{10}} = \sqrt{0.025}$$
$$=0.158.$$

When the mean, variance, and standard deviation of the proportions in the samples of size $n = 20$ are denoted by $M_{P\,(n\,=\,20)}$ $SD^2{}_{P\,(n\,=\,20)}$, and $SD_{P\,(n\,=\,20)}$, respectively, they are:

$$M_{P(n=20)} = \frac{\begin{array}{c}0.20+2\times0.25+5\times0.30+8\times0.35+10\times0.40+11\times0.45+205\times0.50\\ +15\times0.55+10\times0.60+9\times0.65+5\times0.70+0.75\end{array}}{100}$$
$$=0.497,$$

and

Table 10.20 Distribution of proportions of blue marble in 100 random samples of size $n = 20$

Proportion	0.20	0.25	0.30	0.35	0.40	0.45	0.50	0.55	0.60	0.65	0.70	0.75	0.80
Frequency	1	2	4	6	10	15	26	14	11	5	3	2	1
Percentage	1%	2%	4%	6%	10%	15%	26%	14%	11%	5%	3%	2%	1%

$$SD^2_{P(n=20)} = \frac{2(0.25-0.50)^2 + 4(0.30-0.50)^2 + \ldots + 3(0.70-0.50)^2 + 2\,(0.75-0.50)^2 + (0.80\text{–}0.50)^2}{99}$$
$$= 0.0125,$$

and

$$SD_{P(n=20)} = \sqrt{0.0126} = 0.112.$$

These agree with the values suggested by the central limit theorem. Indeed,

$$M_{P(n=20)} = 0.499 \cong \mu_{P(n=20)} = \pi = 0.5,$$

$$SD^2_{P(n=20)} = 0.0126 \cong \sigma^2_{P(n=20)} = \frac{0.5(1.0-0.5)}{20} = 0.0125, \text{ and}$$

$$SD_{P(n=20)} = 0.112 \cong \sigma_{P(n=20)} = \sqrt{\frac{\pi(1.0-\pi)}{20}} = \sqrt{\frac{0.5(1.0-0.5)}{20}} = \sqrt{0.0125}$$
$$= 0.112.$$

Figure 10.1 uses histograms to depict the distributions of the proportions of YES in the two sets of independent random samples and the curves of the Gaussian distributions suggested by the central limit theorem. When the sizes of the samples are $n = 10$ and $n = 20$, the histograms depicting the distribution of the proportions of YES in independent random samples resemble the curves of the Gaussian distributions asserted by the central limit theorem.

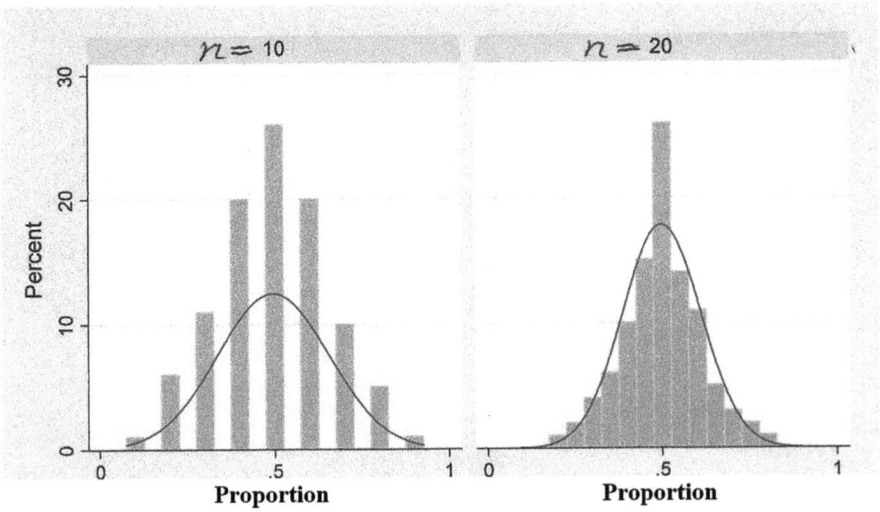

Fig. 10.1 Distributions of proportions of blue marble in 100 random samples

Table 10.21 Percentages of proportions in samples of size $n = 10$ and area under the curve of G [0.50, 0.16]

Region	% of proportions	Area under the curve of G[0.50, 0.16]
0.4–0.6	64%	$\mu_{P(n=10)} \pm 0.625 \times 0.16 = \mu_{P(n=10)} \pm 0.625 \times \sigma_{P(n=10)} \cong 47\%$
0.3–0.7	87%	$\mu_{P(n=10)} \pm 1.275 \times 0.16 = \mu_{P(n=10)} \pm 1.275 \times \sigma_{P(n=10)} \cong 80\%$
0.2–0.8	98%	$\mu_{P(n=10)} \pm 1.875 \times 0.16 = \mu_{P(n=10)} \pm 1.875 \times \sigma_{P(n=10)} \cong 94\%$

Table 10.22 Percentages of proportions in samples of size $n = 20$ and area under the curve of G [0.50, 0.11]

Region	% of proportions	Area under the curve of G[0.50, 0.11]
0.4–0.6	76%	$\mu_{P(n=20)} \pm 0.965 \times 0.11 = \mu_{P(n=20)} \pm 0.965 \times \sigma_{P(n=20)} = 68\%$
0.3–0.7	94%	$\mu_{P(n=20)} \pm 1.818 \times 0.11 = \mu_{P(n=20)} \pm 1.818 \times \sigma_{P(n=10)} \cong 94\%$
0.2–0.8	100%	$\mu_{P(n=20)} \pm 2.727 \times 0.11 = \mu_{P(n=20)} \pm 2.727 \times \sigma_{P(n=10)} \cong 99\%$

Tables 10.21 and 10.22 compare percentages of proportions of YES in regions with areas under the curve of the Gaussian distribution suggested by the central limit theorem.

Percentages of sample proportions in the regions [0.3 to 0.7] and [0.2 to 0.8] are close to the percentages of areas in the regions under the curves of the Gaussian distributions suggested by the central limit theorem when the sizes of the samples are $n = 10$ as well as when $n = 20$. The percentages of sample proportions in the region [0.4 to 0.6] are nevertheless larger than the percentages of areas in the region under the curves of the Gaussian distributions. The discrepancy is smaller when $n = 20$ (76% vs. 68%) than when $n = 10$ (64% vs. 47%).

- *Effect of Sample Size*

The number of subjects is a critical consideration of clinical studies. It is generally believed that the results of a study would be more reproducible if the number of subjects is larger. This would be true if the subjects of a study constitute a random sample. The sampling distribution of a descriptive statistic of a random sample varies in a narrower range and has a smaller standard deviation when the size of the samples is larger. This is demonstrated by Examples 10.2.1 and 10.2.2 as well as 10.3.1 and 10.3.2. It is also demonstrated by the two sampling experiments of Example 10.4.1.

Example 10.4.2

The two experiments described in Example 10.4.1 showed that the mean of the distribution of proportions of blue marbles in 100 independent random samples from a universe of marbles is close to the proportion of blue marbles in the universe when the sizes of the samples are $n = 10$ and $n = 20$, the standard deviation of the distribution is smaller and the percentage of proportion of blue marbles between 0.40 and 0.60 is larger when the size of the samples is $n = 20$. These are shown in Table 10.23.

Table 10.23 Proportions of blue marbles in 100 independent random samples

Size of sample	Mean of proportions	Standard deviation of proportions	Percentage of proportions in [$\pi - 0.1$ to $\pi + 0.1$]
$n = 10$	$M_{P(n = 10)} = 0.495$	$SD_{P(n = 10)} = 0.162$	64%
$n = 20$	$M_{P(n = 20)} = 0.499$	$SD_{P(n = 20)} = 0.112$	76%

10.5 Standard Error

The standard error of the mean of a set of observations is sometimes presented along with the mean of the observations. It is an estimate of the standard deviation of the sampling distribution of the mean of the observations if the observations constitute a random sample.

- *Standard Error of the Mean of a Random Sample*

The mean and standard deviation of the universe are usually unknown. The mean and standard deviation of a random sample are optimal estimates of the mean and standard deviation of the universe. The mean of a random sample is also an optimal estimate of the mean of the sampling distribution of the mean of the random sample; the standard deviation of a random sample divided by the square root of the size of the sample is an optimal estimate of the standard deviation of the sampling distribution of the mean of the random sample. It is known as the standard error of the mean. If n denotes the size of a random sample and SD denotes the standard deviation of the sample, the standard error of the mean of the random sample, denoted by SEM, equals:

$$\mathrm{SEM} = \frac{SD}{\sqrt{n}} \tag{10.5.1}$$

When the standard error of the mean of a random sample is smaller, it suggests that the standard deviation of the sampling distribution of the mean is smaller and there is a higher percentage of means of possible samples close to the universe mean.

When a revelation of a set of n observations of a study is portrayed by the mean of the observations, if it is rational to perceive the set of observations as a random sample, it is rational to use the sampling distribution of the mean of the random sample to mimic the distribution of the means of the observations if the study was replicated a score of times. A smaller standard error of the mean of observations suggests that the standard deviation of the distribution of the means of replicates of the study would be smaller. The revelation is more reproducible.

Example 10.5.1

Beck and Others (2014) presented the results of randomized clinical trials to evaluate the effect of dupilumab in adults with moderate-to-severe atopic dermatitis. Dupilumab was evaluated as monotherapy in a 4-week trial and a 12-week trial. It was also evaluated in combination with topical glucocorticoids in a 4-week trial.

Descriptions of the demographic and clinical characteristics of the subjects are presented in Table 1 of the article. For instance, the ages and affected body surface area of 51 subjects in the dupilumab group of the 4-week monotherapy trial were depicted by 42.6 ± 1.9 and 51.4 ± 3.5, respectively. A footnote of the table states: "Plus-minus values are means ± SEs." Thus, the values before the ± sign are means, and those after the sign are standard errors of the means.

The purpose of the table is to describe the subjects of the study. The means unveil the locations of the centers of the distributions of the ages and the affected body surface areas of the 51 subjects. The standard errors of the means are improvised assessments of the standard deviations of the means of replicates of the studies if they were replicated a score of times. They are not measures of the degrees of difference among of the ages and the affected body surface areas of the 51 subjects. It is unknown whether there were very young or very old subjects and whether the affected body surface areas of some subjects were little or vary large.

To garner some useful tips about variation of the ages and affected body surface areas, Eq. 10.5.1 was used to determine the standard deviations of age and affected body surface area.

The standard deviations of ages and affected body surface areas of the 51 subjects in the dupilumab group were written as $SD_{P(Age)}$ and $SD_{P(Area)}$. Equation 10.5.1 yields $SD_{D(Age)} = 1.9 \times \sqrt{51} = 13.6$ and $SD_{P(Area)} = 3.5 \times \sqrt{51} = 25.0$. The standard deviations are not small relative to the means. They suggest that the ages and affected body surface areas of the subjects varied widely.

The means and standard deviations were used to determine the 95% observation-regions speculated by the Gaussian model. Figure 10.2 shows the speculated observation-regions schematically. It suggest that there were probably subjects as young as 15 years of age and subjects as old as 70 years of age, and that there were probably subjects whose affected body surface areas were as little as 2% and subjects whose affected body surface areas were as large as 90%.

Example 10.5.2

Bwakura-Dangarembizi (2014) presented the results of a study evaluating the effects of stopping versus continuing daily open-label cotrimoxazole in children and adolescents. Participants were older than 3 years of age, had been receiving antiretroviral therapy for more than 96 weeks, were using insecticide-treated bed nets, and had not had *Pneumocystis jirovecti* pneumonia. One result was related as follows:

```
        Age                        Affected Body Surface Area
 [----------▲----------]      [-----------------------▲-----------------------]
 15.5     42.6     69.7      1.4                    51.4                 101.4
 42.6∓2×13.6years                             51.4∓2×25.0
```

Fig. 10.2 Gaussian model speculated 95% observation-regions of 51 subjects in the dupilumab group

> At 12 weeks after randomization, the hemoglobin level had increased from baseline in the prophylaxis-continued group but not in the prophylaxis-stopped group (mean [±SE] change, 0.16±0.05 vs. -0.07±0.06 g per deciliter; adjusted P = 0.03); . . . .

The values 0.16 ± 0.05 and -0.07 ± 0.06 denote the means of changes in hemoglobin levels in the two treatment groups and their standard errors.

The changes are observations of subjects who were randomly assigned to the treatment groups; it is rational to consider the two sets of changes random samples. The standard errors are estimates of the standard deviations of the sampling distributions of the means. They are improvised estimates of the standard deviations of the distributions of the means if the study was replicated a score of times and measures of the reproducibility of the means. They seem to be small and submit that the means of changes are relatively reproducible.

The standard errors of the means of changes are not measure of the degrees of changes among the subjects of the two treatment groups. They do not unveil whether the changes included both increases and decreases and whether there were some large increases and large decreases.

Equation 10.5.1 suggests that the standard deviation the changes of the 376 subjects in the prophylaxis-continued group equals $0.05 \times \sqrt{376} = 0.05 \times 19.4 = 0.97$ and that he standard deviation of the changes of the 382 subjects of prophylaxis-stopped group equals $0.06 \times \sqrt{382} = 0.0.6 \times 19.5 = 1.17$. They are large relative to the means and suggest that there were increases as well as decreases in both groups.

To ascertain whether there both increases and decreases, the standard deviations were used to determine 95% observation-regions speculated by the Gaussian model. The speculated observation-regions (are displayed schematically in Fig. 10.3. They suggest that the distributions of the two sets of changes varied widely and overlapped extensively. The changes in the two treatment groups included both increases and decreases. Most changes in the two treatment groups are comparable. The assertion that the hemoglobin levels increased in the prophylaxis-continued group increased but not in the prophylaxis-stopped group is misleading. It is more productive to depict the distributions of the two set of changes comprehensively and articulate the manifestations of the distributions. Percentages of relevant changes are informative synoptic descriptions of the two sets of changes and their distinction.

The assertion that the hemoglobin level had increased from baseline in the prophylaxis-continued group but not in the prophylaxis-stopped group is misleading. The changes in both groups include increases as well as decreases.

It is more productive to describe the distributions of the changes in the subjects of the two treatment groups and articulate the suggestions of the distributions.

```
Prophylaxis-continued group:        [----------------0-▲------------------]
    0.16∓2×0.97                   -1.78          0.16                  2.10
Prophylaxis-stopped group:        [------------------▲0 -----------------------]
   -0.07∓2 ×1.18                -2.43         -0.07                    2.29
```

Fig. 10.3 Gaussian model speculated 95% observation-regions for changes in hemoglobin level

Percentages of notable increases would be constructive synoptic descriptions of the two sets of changes and their distinction.

Review Questions

1. How are the universe and sample defined in statistics?
2. When are descriptive statistics such as the mean, median, and standard deviation universe parameters and sample statistics?
3. Under what condition is a sample a simple random sample?
4. What are the elements of the sampling distribution of the mean of a simple random sample?
5. What are the elements of the sampling distribution of the proportion of YES in a simple random sample?
6. How do the mean and standard deviation of the sampling distribution of the mean of a simple random sample relate to the mean and standard deviation of the universe?
7. How do the mean and standard deviation of the sampling distribution of the proportion of YES in a simple random sample relate to the proportion of YES in the universe?
8. How is the probability that the means of a random sample close to the universe mean affected by the size of the sample?
9. How is the probability that the proportion of YES in a random sample close to the universe proportion affected by the size of the sample?
10. How are the sampling distribution of the mean of a random sample and the distribution of the means of replicates of a study related?
11. Is the mean of a random sample representative? Why?
12. When can groups of subjects of a study be considered random samples?
13. How do indications of the standard deviation of a set of observations and the standard error of the mean of the observation differ?

References

Beck, L. A., et al. (2014). Dupilumab treatment in adults with moderate-to-severe atopic dermatitis. *The New England Journal of Medicine, 371*(2), 130–139.

Bwakura-Dangarembizi, M., et al. (2014). A randomized trial of prolonged co-trimoxazole in HIV-infected children in Africa. *The New England Journal of Medicine, 370*(1), 41–53.

Chapter 11
Statistical Null Hypothesis Testing

Statistical significance plays an important role in analysis of data of medical studies. Revelations of data are declared "significant" when *P*-values of statistical significance tests are below 0.05. Descriptions of "significant" data revelations are frequently ambiguous and hyperbolic. Statistics portraying revelations are not explicitly identified, and indications of revelations are not elucidated.

In examples of Part II (Chaps. 4, 5, 6, 7, 8 and 9) small *P-values* are used as suggestions that revelations of data would be unlikely if chance were the explanation. Declaring data revelations statistically significant when *P*-values are smaller than 0.05 is considered a declaration that the concern of incidental data revelation may be dismissed and the revelations may be inferred to appropriate individuals. The ground of this use of *P*-value and statistical significance is examined in this chapter.

Statistical significance tests are special applications of statistical hypothesis tests when the tested hypotheses assert data revelations incidental. Data revelations are portrayed by statistics. When statistical hypothesis tests are used to test the statistical significance of data revelations, it is assumed that the statistics portraying the data revelations are statistics of random samples. The tested hypotheses assert that the corresponding universe parameters, the values of the statistics computed from all observations of the universes, equal their null values (0 if a difference and 1.0 if a ratio). They are the null hypotheses of the tests and insinuate data revelations incidental. They are tested against the alternative hypotheses that they are false. The *P*-values of the tests are used as improvised appraisals of the likelihoods that the statistics portraying the data revelations deviate from their null values as much as or more than the statistic portraying the data revelations if the null hypotheses were true. *P*-values smaller than 0.05 are propositions that data revelations would be particularly unlikely if the null hypotheses were true. The null hypotheses are rejected because data revelations would be particularly unlikely if they were true data revelations are declared statistically significant. Declaration of statistical significance is a mesmerizing paraphrasing of the declaration that the null hypotheses are rejected. As the null hypotheses imply data revelations incidental,

P. C. Chang, *Data Analysis of Medical Studies*,
https://doi.org/10.1007/978-3-031-49984-5_11

declaration of statistical significance is a mesmerizing phrase of the declaration that the concern of incidental data revelations is dismissed.

An important property of *P*-value is that it relates to not only the magnitudes of the statistics portraying data revelations but also number of observations. The P-value of the same statistic portraying a data revelation is smaller if the statistic is a result of a larger number of observations.

There are many statistical significance tests. This chapter uses classic tests to demonstrate that it is rational to use *P*-values as improvised appraisals of likelihoods of data revelations being chance coincidences. They all have the following components:

1. *Required condition*: All statistical tests are derived from specific models. Their use requires the condition that observations are elements of a random sample from one universe or random samples from universes. The statistics portraying data revelations are estimates of universe parameters, the value of the statistic computed from data of the universe or universes. This assumption is met approximately when data are results of randomized clinical trials. It is disputable when the subjects of studies are available individuals.
2. *Null hypothesis*: A hypothesis that asserts the data revelation incidental is tested. It is the null hypothesis of the test and implies that chance is the explanation of the differences of the statistics portraying the data revelation among random samples and the differences among replicates of the study if the study were replicated a score of times.
3. *Test statistic*: The value of a function of the statistic portraying data revelation is computed. It is the test statistic of the test and is written as t_0 for convenience.
4. *Null distribution*: The sampling distribution of the test statistic under the condition that the null hypothesis is true—the distribution of the test statistics of all possible samples of the given size or all possible combinations of independent random samples of the given sizes under the condition that the null hypothesis is true is the null distribution of the test. It is used as a model of the distribution of the statistics of replicates of the study if the study were replicated a score of times and chance is the explanation.
5. *P-value*: An estimate of the probability that the test statistic deviates from its null value (0) as much as or more than t_0 if the null hypothesis were true was determined from the null distribution. It is the *P*-value of the test and an improvised appraisal of the likelihood of the statistic portraying the data revelation diverging from its null value (0 if a difference and 1.0 if a ratio) as much as or more than the one portraying the data revelation if chance were the explanation of the differences among possible samples. It is an improvised appraisal of the likelihood of the statistic deviating from its null value (0 if a difference and 1.0 if a ratio) as much as or more than the one portraying the data revelation if chance were the explanation of the differences among replicates of the study.
6. *Decision*: Reject the null hypothesis and declare the data revelation statistically significant if the *P*-value is sufficiently small, and do not reject the null hypothesis and do not declare the data revelation statistically significant if the *P*-value is not sufficiently small. $P \leq 0.05$ is a customary criterion of being sufficiently small.

In other words:

- *A small P-value insinuates that the statistic portraying a data revelation would be unlikely if chance were the explanation.*
- *Declaring a revelation of the data of a study statistically significant is a declaration that the data revelation is particularly unlikely if the study is replicated a score of times. It is not a declaration of clinical importance but a declaration that the concern of chance coincidence may be dismissed.*

Example 11.1

Hays and Others (2003) (Example 4.2.1) reported that there were small but statistically significant positive effects of estrogen plus progestin on several measures of health-related quality of life. The effects were measured by distinctions the means of post-treatment changes between the two treatment groups. Distinction in means of changes in scores on physical functioning (0.8 points) was cited as an example. The distinction in means of changes (0.8 points) is exceedingly small relative to the range of possible scores (0 to 100) and the ranges of the changes in the two treatment groups (−50 to 50 approximately). As a measure of treatment effect, it has little or no clinical importance. $P < 0.001$ suggests only that it would be particularly unlikely that the distinction in means of changes deviating from 0 as much as 0.8 points or more if chance were the only explanation. Being declared statistically significant only means that it is all right to dismiss the concern that the distinction in means of changes (0.8 points) is a chance coincidence. It is not an affirmation that the changes in the estrogen plus progestin group were larger improvements compared with those in the placebo group.

Figure 2A of the article (Fig. 2.14) shows that the distributions of the changes in physical function in the two treatment groups are totally overlapped and nearly identical. Although the distinction between the means of changes (0.8 points) could be declared statistically significant, it is minute relative to the ranges of the changes in the two treatment groups (−50 to +50 approximately) and does not suggest a clinically relevant treatment effect. One reason for the small P-value (< 0.001) is the large numbers of changes (7503 and 7160).

$P < 0.001$ was a result of using a linear model to test statistical significance. Several other tests could be used. They all have the same components. The large sample Gaussian test is used as an example here.

1. *Required condition*: The condition that the two groups of subjects are random samples of sizes 7503 and 7160 independently selected from universes is required. As the subjects were randomly assigned to the treatment groups, it is rational to consider this condition met. The distinction in means of changes (0.8 points) is a distinction in means between independent random samples.
2. *Null hypothesis*: The hypothesis that the means of the changes of the two universes equal was tested against the alternative that the means of the two universes do not equal. This is the null hypothesis of the test and insinuates that chance variation is the explanation of the differences among independent random samples of sizes 7503 and 7160 from the universes. Chance is the explanation of

the differences between the means of changes among replicates of the study if the study were replicated a score of times; the distinction between the means of changes (0.8 points) is incidental. The null hypothesis was tested against the alternative hypothesis that it is false.

3. *Test statistic*: The ratio of the distinction between the means of the two sets of changes (0.8 points) divided by the standard error of the distinction was used as the test statistic. Table 2 of the article sows that the standard error of the distinction between he means of changes equals 0.2. The value of the test statistic is $t_O = 0.8/0.2 = 4.0$
4. *Null distribution*: The sampling distribution of the test statistic under the condition that the null hypothesis is true—the distribution of the test statistics of all possible combinations of independent random samples of sizes 7503 and 7160 under the condition that the null hypothesis is true—is the null distribution of the test. It is characterized by the Gaussian distribution with mean 0 and standard deviation 1.0 and suggests that the Gaussian distribution with mean 0.8 and standard deviation 0.2 is an operative model of the distribution of the distinctions in means of changes between the two treatment groups if the study were repeated a score of times.
5. *P-value*: An estimate of the probability that the test statistics of independent random samples of sizes 7503 and 7160 from the universes diverge from the null value (0) as much as or more than 4.0 if the null hypothesis were true was determined from the null distribution. It is smaller than 0.001 and an improvised appraisal of the likelihood that the distinction in the means of changes between the two treatment groups would diverge from the null value (0) as much as or more than 0.8 points if chance were the explanation.
6. *Decision*: The null hypothesis was rejected because if it were true it would be particularly unlikely that the distinction between the means of the changes of the two treatment groups deviates from 0 as much as or more than 0.8. The concern that the small distinction in means of changes (0.8 points) is incidental was dismissed. Nevertheless, the distinction in the means of changes (0.8) is minute and trivial. It is more important to note that the distributions of the changes in the two treatment groups overlap completely and are similar. They suggest that the effects of the two treatments are comparable.

Example 11.2

Hsu and Others (2004) (Example 5.1.4) reported: "*Exercise time and capacity also increased significantly in both groups.*" The assertion was warranted by means and standard deviations of before-ablation and during-follow-up measurements and $P < 0.001$. The *P*-value is a result of testing the statistical significance of the distinction between the means of the before-ablation and the during-follow-up measurements. The assertion of significant increases is a stylish paraphrase of the declaration that the distinctions between the means of before-ablation and the during-follow-up measurements (11 vs. 14) may be declared statistically significant and the concern that it is incidental may be dismissed. It is not a certification that the changes of all subjects were noteworthy increases.

Example 5.1.4 used means and standard deviations of the before-ablation and the during-follow-up exercise times to determine speculated 95% observation-regions for the changes in exercise time. Schematic displays of the regions (Fig. 5.5) suggest that the distributions of the before-ablation and the during-follow-up changes in exercise time of subjects in the two groups overlap extensively. Probably there were both increases and declines. It is critical to note that the reported significant increase in exercise time alluded to the changes in means only. It would be a mistake if it were interpreted as a suggestion that exercise times of all subjects were noteworthy increases.

The before-ablation and the during-follow-up exercise times of a subject constitute a pair. The difference between the pair of exercise times of a subject constitutes a measure of the change in the subject. There were 58 subjects with congestive heart failure. The distinction in the before-ablation and the during-follow-up means equals the mean of the 58 changes. $P<0.001$ is a result of using the Student's test for paired data to test the statistical significance of the distinction between the means of before-ablation and during-follow-up exercise times (11 and 14 min). It comprised the following components:

1. *Required condition*: The condition that the group of 58 subjects with heart failure constitute a random sample from a universe of patients with congestive heart failure is required. It implies that, if the study were replicated a score of times, chance is the explanation of the differences among replicates of the study. Whether this condition was met is questionable, because the subjects were not randomly selected from a universe but consecutively available patients. Use of the t-test also requires the condition that the distribution of the changes in exercise time of the universe of subjects with heart failure is characterized by a Gaussian distribution. It is unknown whether this condition was met.
2. *Null hypothesis*: The hypothesis that the mean of the changes of the subjects of the universe equals its null value 0 was tested against the alternative that it is false. It is the null hypothesis of the test and intimates that chance variation among random samples is the explanation of the differences among all possible samples of size 58 from the universe and that chance is the explanation of the differences among replicates of the study if the study were replicated a score of times. The mean of the changes (3 min) is incidental.
3. *Test statistic*: The test statistic is a ratio of the mean of the changes (3 min) and the standard error of the mean. It was written as t_0 for convenience.
4. *Null distribution*: The sampling distribution of the test statistic if the null hypothesis is true—the distribution of the test statistics of all possible samples of size 58 under the condition that the null hypothesis is true is the null distribution of the test. It is the t-distribution with 57 degrees of freedom and is used as a model of the distribution of the test statistics of replicates of the study.
5. *P-value*: An estimate of the probability that the t-statistic deviates from 0 as much as t_0 or more if the null hypothesis were true was determined from the null distribution of the test. It is the *P*-value and an improvised appraisal of the likelihood of the mean of the changes diverging from the null value 0 as much

as or more than 3 min if chance variation is the explanation of the differences among replicates of the study. It is smaller than 0.001 and suggests that the distinction between the means of the before ablation and the during follow-up exercise times (11 vs. 14 minutes) would be particularly unlikely if chance were the explanation.

6. *Decision*: The null hypothesis was rejected because $P < 0.001$ met the customary criterion of ≤ 0.05 and suggest that the increase in the mean of exercise times (11 to 14 min) deviating from 0 as much as or more than 3 minutes or more would be particularly unlikely if the null hypothesis were true. The increase in mean was declared statistically significant, and the concern that it is incidental was dismissed. $P < 0.001$ is not a certification that all changes of exercise time are noteworthy increases. There were probably increases as well as decreases.

Example 11.3

The article by van Driel and Others (2018) (Example 6.4.2.4) uses the hazard ratio of 0.66 to assess the distinction in risks of the event of disease recurrence or death between the 122 subjects in the surgery plus HIPEC group and the 123 subjects in the surgery-only group. $P = 0.003$ and 95% confidence interval: [0.50 to 0.87] were presented. The hazard ratio 0.66 suggests that the risk of the event of disease recurrence or death of the surgery plus HIPEC group is 6.6-tenth of the risk of the surgery-only group. $P = 0.003$ and the 95% confidence interval suggest that the hazard ratio: 0.66 may be declared statistically significant and the concern that it is incidental may be dismissed. However, the 95% confidence interval is wide and suggests that the reproducibility of the hazard ratio is inadequate. It is astute to limit the hazard ratio to the subjects of the study. $P = 0.003$ is a result testing the statistical significance of the hazard ratio. The test comprised the following components:

1. *Required condition*: The condition that the 122 subjects of the surgery plus HIPEC group and the 123 subjects of the surgery group are elements of independent random samples from universes is required. It was reasonably met because the two treatment groups are the results of random assignment.
2. *Null hypothesis*: The hypothesis that the universe hazard ratio equals its null value 1.0 was tested against the alternative hypothesis that it is false. It is the null hypothesis of the test and intimates that chance variation among combinations of independent random samples of sizes 123 and 122 is the explanation of the difference among the hazard ratios of replicates of the study if the study were replicated a score of times. The null hypothesis submits that the hazard ratio of 0.66 is incidental.
3. *Test statistic*: The proportional hazard regression analysis was performed. A function of the hazard ratio was used as a test statistic. It was written as t_O for convenience.
4. *Null distribution*: The sampling distribution of the test statistic—the distribution of the test statistics of all possible combinations of independent random samples of size 122 and size 123—if the null hypothesis is true is the null distribution of

the test. It was used as a model of the distribution of the hazard ratios of replicates of the study if the study were replicated a score of times.

5. *P-value*: An estimate of the probability that the test statistic deviating from its null value as much as t_0 or more if the null hypothesis was true was determined from the null distribution. It is the *P*-value and an improvised appraisal of the probability likelihood of the hazard ratios of replicates of the study deviating from the null value 1.0 as much as or more than 0.66 if chance were the explanation.
6. *Decision*: The null hypothesis was rejected because $P = 0.003$ is below 0.05 and suggests that the hazard ratio deviating from 1.0 as much as 0.66 or more would be particularly unlikely if chance were the explanation. The hazard ratio of 0.66 was declared statistically significant. Declaration of statistical significance is a declaration of dismissal of the concern that the hazard ratio of 0.66 is incidental. It is not a declaration of clinical importance. The 95% confidence interval of the hazard ratio: [0.50 to 0.87] is wide and suggests inadequate reproducibility; it is astute to limit the hazard ratio: 0.66 to the subjects of the study and consider it a preliminary signal.

Example 11.4

Lockley and Others (2004) (Example 8.3.4) used $r = -0.57$ and $P < 0.001$ to corroborate the assertion that weekly durations of sleep and work were significantly inversely correlated. $P < 0.001$ is a result of testing the statistical significance of the correction coefficient $r = -0.57$. The correlation coefficient and its *P*-value are the results of the 40 pairs of weekly duration of sleep and durations of work of the 20 interns during two schedules. Figure 3C of the article (Fig. 8.10) shows that with only one exception, the mean weekly durations of work of the 20 interns during the intervention schedule are shorter than their mean weekly durations of work during the traditional schedule. The mean weekly durations of sleep of several interns during the intervention schedule are longer than their mean weekly durations of sleep during the traditional schedule. The mean weekly durations of sleep and the mean weekly durations of work of the 20 infants during the intervention schedule did not demonstrate a discernable relationship, and the mean weekly durations of sleep and the mean weekly durations of work of the 20 infants during the traditional schedule did not demonstrate a discernable relationship either. The correlation coefficient (−0.57), to a considerable extent, is a result of the distinction between the two schedules. Although the correlation coefficient was declared statistically significant, the assertion that weekly durations of sleep and work of the 20 interns were significantly inversely correlated is misleading.

The statistical significance test comprised the following components:

1. *Required conditions*: The condition that the set of 40 pairs of mean duration of sleep and mean duration of work constitute a random sample from a universe was required. This condition is not met. The 40 pairs of mean duration of sleep and mean duration of work are observations of the same 20 interns during two schedules, and the 20 interns were not selected by a random selection procedure.
2. *Null hypothesis*: The hypothesis that the correlation coefficient of the universe equals its null value 0 was tested against the alternative that it is false. It is the null

hypothesis of the test and intimates that chance variation among possible samples of size 40 is the explanation of the differences among correlation coefficients of replicates of the study if the study were replicated a score of times. The null hypothesis implies that the correlation coefficient −0.57 is incidental.

3. *Test statistic*: The value of a test statistic that is a function of the correlation coefficient –0.57 was computed and written as $t_{0.}$
4. *Null distribution*: The sampling distribution of the test statistic under the condition that the null hypothesis is true—the distribution of the test statistics of all possible samples of size 40 under the condition that the null hypothesis is true—is the null distribution of the test. It was used as a model of the distribution of the correlation coefficients of replicates of the study if the study was replicated a score of times.
5. *P-value*: An estimate of the probability that the test statistic diverges from 0 as much as t_0 or more if the null hypothesis were true was determined from the null distribution. It is the *P*-value and an improvised appraisal of the likelihood of the correlation coefficients of replicates of the study diverging from the null value 0 as much as or more than $r = -0.57$ if chance were the explanation.
6. *Result*: The null hypothesis was rejected because $P < 0.001$ met the customary criterion ≤ 0.05 and suggests that the correlation coefficient deviating from 0 as much as −0.57 would be particularly unlikely if chance were the explanation. The correlation coefficient of –0.57 was declared statistically significant, and the concern that it is incidental was dismissed. It is astute to note that the mean durations of sleep and mean durations of work of the 20 interns did not demonstrate a discernable relationship during the each schedule. The assertion that the weekly durations of sleep and work of the 20 interns were significantly inversely correlated is misleading.

Example 11.5

The article by the Stabilization of Atherosclerotic Plague by Initiation of Darapladib (STABILITY) Investigators (2014) (Example 6.7.5) used the *P*-value of the hazard ratio assessing the relative risk of myocardial infarction between the darapladib and the placebo group (P = 0.11) as an example to corroborate the assertion that there were no significant effects of darapladib on any of the components of the primary end point. P = 0.11 suggests that the probability of the hazard ratio deviating from 1.0 as much as 0.89 or more is not particularly low (lower than 0.05) and that the hazard ratio was not declared statistically significant. P = 0.11 is not a measure of the distinction in the risks of myocardial infarction between the two treatment groups and not a suggestion that the risks between the two groups are close. It suggests that the probability of the hazard ratio deviating from 1.0 as much as 0.89 or more would not be lower than 0.05 if chance were the explanation. The hazard ration was not declared statistically significant and the concern that it is incidental was not dismissed. Not declaring the hazard ratio: 0.89 statistically significant is not an affirmation that the risks of myocardial infraction of the two groups are comparable. That the risks of myocardial infarction is close between the two treatment groups is suggested by the hazard ratio: 0.8, which is relatively close to 1.0 and suggests that the risk of myocardial infarction of the darapladib group is relatively close to and about 8.9-tenth of the risk of the placebo group.

It is important to note that the *P*-value would be smaller and the hazard ratio: 0.9 would be declared statistically significant if the hazard ratio were a result of sufficiently larger number of subjects. Determination of P = 0.11 comprised of the following components:

1. *Required condition*: The condition that the two groups of subjects are random samples OF SIZES 7924 AND 7904 independently selected from universes was required. As subjects were randomly assigned to the treatment groups, it is rational to consider the condition is met and use the hazard ratio 0.89 an estimate of the universe hazard ratio.
2. *Null hypothesis*: The hypothesis that the universe hazard ratio equals the null value of 1.0 was tested against the alternative hypothesis that it is false. It is the null hypothesis of the test and intimates that chance variation is the explanation of the differences among the hazard ratios of the possible combinations of independent random samples of sizes 7924 and 7904 from the universes. In other words, the null hypothesis submits that chance variation is the explanation of differences among the hazard ratios of replicates of the study if the study is replicated a score of times. The null hypothesis implies that the hazard ratio 0.89 is incidental.
3. *Test statistic*: Cox proportional hazards regression analysis was performed, and a function of the hazard ratio was determined and used as the test statistic. It was written as t_O for convenience.
4. *Null distribution*: The null distribution of the test statistic—the distribution of the test statistics of all possible combinations of independent random samples of sizes 7924 and 7904 under the condition that the null hypothesis is true—was recognized. It was used as a model of the distribution of the hazard ratios of replicates of the study if the study was replicated a score of times.
5. *P-value*: An estimate of the probability that the hazard ratios of independent random samples of sizes 7924 AND 7904 would deviate from the null value (1.0) as much as or more than 0.89 was determined from the null distribution of the test. It is the *P*-value and an improvised appraisal of the likelihood of the hazard ratios of replicates of the study would deviate from the null value (1.0) as much as or more than 0.89 if chance variation among replicates of the study were the only explanation.
6. *Decision*: The null hypothesis was not rejected, and the hazard ratio of 0.89 was not declared statistically significant because $P = 0.11$ did not meet the customary criterion ≤0.05. However, the 95% confidence interval of the hazard ratio: 0.77 to 1.03 is moderately wide and suggests that the hazard ratio is moderately reproducible. It the study were replicated a score of times, the hazard ratios of many replicates of the study would confirm that the risks of myocardial infarction of the darapladib group is slightly lower than the risk of the placebo groups.

References

Hays, J., et al. (2003). Effects of estrogen plus progestin on health-related quality of life. *The New England Journal of Medicine, 348*(19), 1839–1854.

Hsu, L. F., et al. (2004). Catheter ablation for atrial fibrillation. *The New England Journal of Medicine, 351*(23), 2373–2383.

Lockley, S. W., et al. (2004). Effect of reducing interns' weekly work hours on sleep and attentional failure. *The New England Journal of Medicine, 351*(18), 1829–1837.

The STABILITY Investigators. (2014). Darapladib for preventing ischemic events in stable coronary heart disease. *The New England Journal of Medicine, 370*(18), 1702–1711.

van Driel, W. J., et al. (2018). Hyperthermic intraperitoneal chemotherapy in ovarian cancer. *The New England Journal of Medicine, 378*(3), 230–240.

Chapter 12
95% Confidence Interval

Examples of Part II (Chaps. 4, 5, 6, 7, 8 and 9) demonstrate that descriptions of revelations of data are frequently ambiguous and hyperbolic. The statistics portraying data revelations are not explicitly identified; revelations of data are not plainly described. The principle cause of such descriptions of data revelations is miss use of statistical significance. One way to circumvent such descriptions of data relations is to use 95% confidence intervals to assess reproducibility instead of use *P*-values to decide whether statistical significance is declared. One merit of using 95% confidence intervals to assess reproducibility is that the statistics portraying data revelation are explicitly identified. Another merit is that assessing reproducibility requires deliberate judgements. Also, the mesmerizing modifier "significant" is not involved.

Confidence intervals and *P*-values of statistical significance tests are based on the same theoretical ground and are closely related. They agree generally. Indeed, 95% confidence intervals exclude the null values of the statistics portraying data revelations when the *P*-values of statistical significance tests are smaller than 0.05, and the null values of the statistics portraying data revelations are included when *P*-values are not smaller than 0.05.

Unlike using *P*-values to decide whether revelations of data may be declared statistically significant, using 95% confidence intervals to assess reproducibility does not have a customary criterion for adequate reproducibility. Suggestions of the statistics portraying data revelations are reviewed, and the clinical importance of revelations is scrutinized when the reproducibility of the statistics portraying revelations of data is appraised.

Examples of Part II used an improvised scheme to rate reproducibility suggested by 95% confidence intervals when it is not obvious whether the intervals are narrow or wide. The scheme is used in this book because of the lack of better schemes. The rationale of the scheme is expounded in this chapter. Like testing statistical significance, a basic condition of the scheme is that it is rational to consider data elements of random samples. A limitation of the scheme is that it may not work well if the statistics portraying revelations are close to zero.

P. C. Chang, *Data Analysis of Medical Studies*,
https://doi.org/10.1007/978-3-031-49984-5_12

- *95% Confidence Interval*

Interval estimation is fundamentally important in statistics. When a revelation of the data of a study is portrayed by a statistic, and it is rational to consider observations elements of random sample, the statistic is an estimate of its corresponding universe parameters, the value of the statistic determined from the observations in the universe or universes. The 95% confidence interval of the statistic is an estimate of the universe parameter. It was determined from the sampling distribution of the statistic—the distribution of the statistics of all possible samples of the given size from the universe or all possible combinations of the given sizes from the universes. The percentage: 95%, the confidence level of the interval is the percentage of intervals that would include the universe parameter if 95% confidence intervals were determined from all possible samples of the given size or all possible combinations of random samples of the given sizes. It is not the probability that the interval would include the universe parameter; the interval is not a probability interval.

- *95% Confidence Interval and Reproducibility of Data Revelation*

One way to assess the reproducibility of a revelation of the data of a study is to replicate the study a score of times. The revelation would be considered adequately reproducible if it would be confirmed by most replicates. When a data revelation of is portrayed by a descriptive statistic, the reproducibility of the revelation is depicted by the distribution of the statistics of replicated studies. If it is rational to consider observations elements of random sample or samples, the sampling distribution of the statistic is a credible model of the distribution of the statistics of replicated studies. It is a viable description of the reproducibility of the revelation.

The 95% confidence interval of a data revelation is determined from an estimate of the sampling distribution of the statistic portraying the revelation. It is the region that would include the statistics of 95% of the possible samples of the given size or possible combinations of independent random samples of the given sizes. It is a contrived estimate of the region of the sampling distribution of the statistics of replicated studies that would include 95% of the statistics if the study were replicated a score of times. A narrow interval insinuates that the statistics of 95% of replicated studies would be close to the given statistic and are confirmations of the revelation; a wide interval insinuates that the statistics of replicated studies would vary widely and the revelation would be disputed by many replicated studies.

- *Three Crude Grades of Reproducibility*

Frequently, it is not obvious whether a 95% confidence interval is narrow or wide and a suggestion of adequate or inadequate reproducibility. In this case, using the interval to assess reproducibility is a challenging task and requires deliberate judgements. This book uses the following improvised scheme to rate reproducibility of data revelations when it is not obvious whether a 95% confidence interval suggests adequate reproducibility:

1. *Adequate reproducibility*: The 95% confidence interval of a data revelation a is considered a suggestion of adequately reproducibility if its boundaries

are between 90% and 110% of the statistic portraying the revelation. The revelation may be used to make inference.

2. *Moderate reproducibility*: The 95% confidence interval of a data revelation is considered suggestion of moderately reproducibility if one of its boundaries is between 75% to 89% or between 110% and 125% of the statistic portraying the revelation. It is astute to be cautious when the revelation is used to make inference.
3. *Inadequate reproducibility*: The 95% confidence interval of a data revelation is considered a suggestion of inadequate reproducibility if one of its boundaries is less than 75% or more than 125% of the statistic portraying the revelation. It is astute to limit the revelation to the subjects of the study and use it as a preliminary signal.

Note
The three crude grades of reproducibility may not work well if the statistic portraying data revelation is close to 0. When the statistic portraying a revelation of data is close to 0, boundaries of its 95% confidence interval may be close to 0 and suggest that most replicated studies would yield statistics close to 0 and confirmations of the revelation. But they may be lower than 75% or higher than 125% of the statistics portraying the revelation and suggest inadequate reproducibility.

Remark 95% credible intervals of Bayesian statistics may also be used to assess reproducibility of data revelations. The above improvised scheme may be used when it is difficult to assess whether a 95% credible interval suggest adequate reproducibility.

Using 95% confidence intervals to assess reproducibility is demonstrated in the following examples.

Example 12.1
Hays and Others (2003) (Example 4.2.1) used distinction in means of changes in scores of physical functioning (0.8 point) between treatment groups and $P < 0.001$ as an example to substantiate the perplexing assertion that there were small but statistically significant positive effects of estrogen plus progestin relative to placebo. The small but statistically significant effects alluded to the statistical significance of the minute distinctions in the means of changes in scores of physical functioning between the two treatment groups (0.8 point).

Figure 2A (Fig. 4.1) shows that the distributions of the changes in score of physical functioning of the two groups are nearly completely overlapped and are virtually identical. Although the small distinction in the means of changes between the treatment groups may be declared statistically significant, the distributions of the changes of the two treatment groups suggest that the changes of the subjects of the two treatment groups are comparable. Using the statistically significant distinction in the means of changes between the two treatment groups to assert a small but statistically significant effect of estrogen plus progestin relative to placebo is hyperbolic. It is productive to note the complete overlapping of the distributions of the two sets of changes.

If a 95% confidence interval were presented, it would suggest that the miniscule distinction in means of changes would be confirmed by most replicates of the study.

Table 2 of the article shows that the standard error of the distinction in means of changes equals 0.2. It yields *[0.8* ∓2×*0.2]* = *[0.4 to 1.02]*, a 95% confidence interval of the distinction in means of changes (0.8 point). Its boundaries are small relative to the range of the distributions of changes in the two treatment groups (−50 to 50 points approximately) and suggest the that the miniscule distinction in means of changes in physical function between the two treatment groups (0.8 points) would be confirmed by most replicates of the study if the study were replicated a score of times.

Using the 95% confidence interval [0.4 to 1.02] to assess reproducibility was based on the following considerations:

1. The 7503 women in the estrogen plus progestin group and 7160 women in the placebo group are the results of random allocation. It is rational to consider them independent random samples from target universes and the distinction in means of changes (0.8 point) a distinction between means of two independent random samples.
2. The number of subjects in the two treatment groups (7503 and 7160) are large; the Central Limit Theorem suggests that the sampling distribution of the distinction in the means of changes between the two groups of subjects—the distribution of distinctions in means of all possible combinations of independent random samples of sizes 7503 and 7160—is characterized by the Gaussian distribution with mean 0.8 and standard deviation 0.2. It was used a model of the distribution of the distinctions in means of changes of replicated studies if the study were replicated a score of times.
3. The 95% confidence interval *[0.8* ∓2×*0.2]* = *[0.4 to 1.02]* is a region that include approximately 95% of the observation of the Gaussian distribution with mean 0.8 and standard deviation 0.2. It is an improvised estimate of the region that would include 95% of the distinctions in means of changes of replicated studies.
4. The boundaries of the interval are small relative to the ranges of the distributions of changes (−50 to 50 approximately). The revelation of the study that the distinction in the means of changes between the estrogen plus progestin group and the placebo group is small would be confirmed by most replicates of the study if the study were replicated a score of times. The reproducibility of the distinction in means of changes between the two treatment groups (0.8 point) is adequate. It may be used to make inference.

Example 12.2

Gaudino and Others (2018) (Example 6.1.4) asserted that the incidence of the composite outcome of death, myocardial infarction, or repeat revascularization was significantly lower in the radial artery group than in the saphenous vein group. Incidence rates (25 vs. 39 events per 1000 patient-years), hazard ratio (0.67), 95% confidence interval of the hazard ratio: [0.49 to 0.90], and $P = 0.01$

were cited to corroborate the assertion. The 95% confidence interval excludes 1.0, and $P = 0.01$ is smaller than 0.05; they suggest that the hazard ratio may be declared statistically significant.

Example 6.1.4 demonstrated that the 95% confidence interval: [0.49 to 0.90] is more useful than just confirming the suggestion of $P = 0.01$ that the hazard ratio 0.67 may be declared statistically significant. It is rather wide and suggests that, although the hazard ratio may be declared statistically significant, its reproducibility is inadequate. It is astute to limit the hazard ratio to the subjects of the study and use it as a preliminary signal only.

Using the 95% confidence interval [0.49 to 0.90] to assess reproducibility involved the following considerations:

1. The 534 subjects in the radial artery group and the 502 in the saphenous vein groups are the results of random allocation. It is rational to consider them elements of independent random samples. The hazard ratio is an assessment of the distinction in risks between two independent random samples and an estimate of the universe hazard ratio.
2. It is rational to use the sampling distribution of the hazard ratio—the distribution of hazard ratios of all possible combinations of independent random samples of sizes 534 and 502—a model of the distribution of hazard ratios of replicates of the study if the study were replicated a score of times.
3. The 95% confidence interval [0.49 to 0.90] is an operative estimate of the region that would include approximately 95% of the hazard ratios of replicates of the study.
4. The boundaries of the 95% confidence interval are 73% and 134% of the reported hazard ratio (0.67). The reproducibility of the hazard ratio of 0.67 is deemed inadequate. Although it was declared "significant," it is astute to limit it to the subjects of the study and consider it a preliminary signal.

Example 12.3

Adams and Others (2018) (Example 8.4.1) reported that a correlation was observed between the degree of reduction in transthyretin levels from baseline and the changes in the mNIS+7 at 18 months. The observed correlation is depicted by Figure 3 (Fig. 8.12) which uses different symbols to depict pairs of mean post dose transthyretin level and change in mNIS+7 from baseline of 137 subjects in the partisan group and those of the 51 subjects in the placebo group. Pearson's r, 0.59 (95% CI , 0.49 to 0.68) are shown.

Pearson's r, 0.59, is the value of correlation coefficient computed from the 188 pairs of mean post dose transthyretin levels and changes in mNIS+7 from baseline. The 95% confidence interval excludes the null value 0. It suggests that the correlation coefficient may be declared statistically significant and the concern that its incidental may be dismissed. Example 8.4.1 suggested that the 95% confidence interval: [0.49 to 0.90] is moderately wide and a suggestion that the correlation coefficient is moderately reproducible. It is prudent to be cautious if it is inferred to individuals beyond the 188 subjects of the study.

One advantage of using the 95% confidence interval to assess reproducibility is that it enticed an examination of the indication of the correlation coefficient 0.59. It was noticed that the correlation coefficient 0.59 was determined from the 188 pairs of change in mNIS+7 from baseline and reduction in transthyretin levels of two groups of subjects. Figure 3 of the article (Fig. 8.11) suggests that the mean post dose transthyretin levels relative to baseline and the changes in mNIS+7 from baseline of the subjects in each group are not related. The correlation coefficient is, to a large extent, a result of the distinction between the two groups of subjects. The correlation coefficient is misleading; the changes in mNIS+7 from baseline and reductions in transthyretin levels of the subject are not related when the two groups of subjects are evaluated separately.

The reproducibility of the correlation coefficient was assessed by the following process:

1. It was assumed that the 188 pairs of observations constitute a random sample from a universe. This assumption is dubious. The 188 subjects included two groups of subjects randomly assigned to receive intravenous patisiran or placebo. They are elements of samples from two universes.
2. The sampling distribution of the correlation coefficient—the distribution of correlation coefficients of all possible random samples of size 188 from the universe—was used a model of the distribution of correlation coefficients of replicates of the study if the study were replicated a score of times.
3. The 95% confidence interval [0.49 to 0.68] was used as an estimate of the region of the distribution of the correlation coefficients of replicated studies that would include the correlation coefficients of 95% of the replicates. It suggests that about 95% of the correlation coefficients of replicates of the study would vary between 0.49 and 0.68.
4. The boundaries of the interval [0.49 to 0.68] are 83% and 115% of 0.59. The correlation coefficient (0.59) was deemed moderately reproducible.

Example 12.4

The article by the STABILITY Investigators (2014) (Example 11.5) used the hazard ratio of myocardial infarction (0.89) as one example to corroborate the assertion that there were no significant effects of darapladib on any of the components of the primary end point or on all-cause mortality. Both 95% confidence interval: [0.77to 0.60] and $P = 0.11$ -are shown in parenthesis. They suggest that the hazard ratio may not be declared statistically significant.

The 95% confidence interval [0.77 to 1.03] is more useful than simply agreeing with $P = 0.11$ that the hazard ratio may not be declared statistically significant. Its boundaries are 87% and 116% of the hazard ratio 0.89. They suggest that if the study were replicated a score of times, about 95% of the hazard ratios of the replicates would vary between 87% and 116% of the hazard ratio: 0.89. The hazard ratio 0.89 is deemed moderately reproducible. That the risk of myocardial infarction is slightly lower in the darapladib group than the risk in the placebo group would be confirmed by many replicates of the study if the study were replicated a score of times.

Using the 95% confidence to assess reproducibility involved the following considerations:

1. It is rational to consider the 7924 subjects in the darapladib group and the 7904 in the placebo group elements of independent random sample because they are the results of random allocation. The hazard ratio is a measure of the distinction between two independent random samples from the target universes and an estimate of the universe hazard ratio.
2. It is rational to use the sampling distribution of the hazard ratio—the distribution of hazard ratios of all possible combinations of independent random samples of sizes 7924 and 7902—as a model of the distribution of the hazard ratios of replicated studies if the study were replicated a score of times.
3. The 95% confidence interval [0.85 to 1.03] is an estimate of the region that would include 95% of the hazard ratios of possible independent random samples of sizes 7924 and 7904 from the universes. In other words, the 95% confidence interval [0.85 to 1.03] is an improvised estimate of the region that would include 95% of the hazard ratios of replicates of the study if the study were replicated a score of times.
4. The boundaries of the 95% confidence interval [0.77 to 1.03] are 87% and 116% of the hazard ratio: 0.89. It suggests that about 95% of the hazard ratios of replicated studies would vary between 89% and 116% of 0.89. The reproducibility of the hazard ratio of 0.89 is moderate.

References

Adams, D., et al. (2018). Patisiran, an RNAi therapeutic, for hereditary transthyretin amyloidosis. *The New England Journal of Medicine, 379*(1), 11–21.

Gaudino, M., et al. (2018). Radial-artery or saphenous-vein grafts in coronary-artery pass surgery. *The New England Journal of Medicine, 378*(22), 2069–2077.

Hays, J., et al. (2003). Effects of estrogen plus progestin on health-related quality of life. *The New England Journal of Medicine, 348*(19), 1839–1854.

The STABILITY Investigators. (2014). Darapladib for preventing ischemic events in stable coronary heart disease. *The New England Journal of Medicine, 370*(18), 1702–1711.

Index

P. C. Chang, *Data Analysis of Medical Studies*,
https://doi.org/10.1007/978-3-031-49984-5

MIX
Papier aus verantwortungsvollen Quellen
Paper from responsible sources
FSC® C105338
FSC
www.fsc.org

If you have any concerns about our products,
you can contact us on
ProductSafety@springernature.com

In case Publisher is established outside the EU,
the EU authorized representative is:
Springer Nature Customer Service Center GmbH
Europaplatz 3, 69115 Heidelberg, Germany

Printed by Libri Plureos GmbH
in Hamburg, Germany